W9-CZN-383

Clinical

Rheumatology

Clinical
Rheumatology

A Problem-Oriented Approach
to Diagnosis and Management

ROLAND W. MOSKOWITZ, M.D.

Professor of Medicine
Case Western Reserve University
School of Medicine
Director, Division of Rheumatic Diseases
University Hospitals
Cleveland, Ohio

Second Edition

LEA & FEBIGER · Philadelphia · 1982

Lea & Febiger
600 Washington Square
Philadelphia, Pa. 19106
U.S.A.

Library of Congress Cataloging in Publication Data

Moskowitz, Roland W.
  Clinical rheumatology.

  Bibliography: p.
  Includes index.
  1. Rheumatism. I. Title. [DNLM: 1. Arthritis—Diagnosis. 2. Arthritis—Therapy. 3. Rheumatism—Diagnosis. 4. Rheumatism—Therapy. WE 344 M911c]
  RC927.M64   1982   616.7′23   82-242
  ISBN 0-8121-0847-7   AACR2

Printed in the United States of America

Print Number 3 2 1

To my wife, Peta,

for her encouragement and the hours spent alone; to our children Joshua and Kara, whose smiles and enthusiasm brighten every day; and to my parents, who made this book possible.

FOREWORD TO THE FIRST EDITION

A distinct honor was extended to me by Dr. Moskowitz when he asked me to write a foreword for *Clinical Rheumatology*. This volume is a comprehensive and problem-oriented presentation of rheumatology, presenting clearly and completely what the clinician needs to know about all rheumatologic problems, not just the more common forms of arthritis. Starting with the symptoms and findings noted in each patient, through differential diagnosis and treatment, the approach is practical. The arrangement of chapters has been carefully planned with a few basic chapters describing the necessary clinical skills and how to develop them. This is followed by the most important section of the book: Clinical Presentations. These 18 chapters have been masterfully organized to deal with each type of clinical problems, discussing differential diagnostic points and objectives of therapy. The third section deals with specific management of various problems encountered in rheumatology, and special types of treatment such as physical and occupational therapy, local injection therapy, and proper use of steroids.

By writing the entire book himself, the author has avoided many of the difficulties encountered in editing a collection of contributor papers that present differing opinions. It was a tremendous task, but he has done it well. I congratulate Dr. Moskowitz on an excellent job.

JOSEPH LEE HOLLANDER, M.D., M.A.C.P.

PREFACE TO THE FIRST EDITION

Rheumatology, one of the youngest medical subspecialties, has seen a burgeoning growth over the past several decades. Clinical and basic investigations have been expanded and increased numbers of capable people attracted to the field of study. Pessimism has given way to optimism that much can be done to control many of the rheumatic disorders. Application of the basic scientific disciplines, particularly immunology and biochemistry, provides hope that prevention and cure are not unreasonable goals for the near future.

Intensified interest and study in the rheumatic disorders was necessary and warranted. A recent task force survey by the Arthritis Foundation demonstrated that in the United States alone, at least 20,230,000 people were suffering from arthritis and arthritis-like conditions. Among the commonest causes of disability, these diseases result in untold human suffering in addition to massive economic losses. Rheumatic diseases represent a major component of the patient population seen by practicing physicians. Provision of optimal care requires development of full training programs in rheumatology in all medical schools, and expanded programs of postgraduate education. It is toward this latter effort that this book is primarily devoted. Hopefully, it will provide a resource whereby additional education can be provided on a background of everyday practice and experience.

Several excellent textbooks on rheumatology are already available. They have been particularly helpful to physicians who have a primary interest in the rheumatic diseases, or as reference texts. This textbook represents an effort to provide the practicing physician with a new, additional dimension of information. The clinical discussions are based on a problem-oriented approach, paralleling the disease manifestations as they appear initially to the physician. It is designed to be a working text, to be kept close at hand for use on a day-to-day basis as a helpful guide in the management of problems as they appear.

Many of the chapters are based on material used by me in daily teaching discussions in clinics, at the bedside, or in small conferences, which has been expanded for completeness. Although this text was written primarily for the general practitioner and the internist, who provide the bulwark of care to arthritis patients, hopefully medical students, house officers, rheumatologists, orthopedists, pediatricians and other physicians who come into contact with patients with rheumatologic complaints will find it valuable.

My deep appreciation is extended to Drs. Beno Michel, Samuel J. Horwitz, Paul J. Vignos, Jr., Phillip I. Lerner, Victor M. Goldberg and Harvey M. Rodman for their review and comments on the sections related to laboratory diagnosis, dermatologic disorders, muscle disease, infectious arthritis, and steroid management in stress situations. Miss Betsy J. Fallon, R.P.T., M.A., Mrs. Charlotte Ryan, O.T.R., and Mrs. Maxine Landers, O.T.R., collaborated on the preparation of the chapter on physical and occupational therapy. I am indebted to Drs. Allen Mackenzie, Charles W. Denko, Beno Michel, Victor M. Goldberg, Mahmood Pazirandeh, Fred Bishko, Robert Gatter and the national office of the Arthritis Foundation* for making material available for illustrations. Their contributions are recognized in the legends where these illustrations are used. Dr. Sergio A. Murillo, Fellow in Rheumatology, and Miss Fallon were most helpful in the preparation of some of the illustrations relative to diagnosis. Mrs. Mary Lee Berman assisted in many administrative tasks of manuscript preparation.

Photography was performed by Mr. Donald Schad and his associates, Mr. Ken-Ichi Kondo and Mr. Joseph Molter, of the Department of Medical Photography, Case Western Reserve University School of Medicine. Typing of the manuscript through its inception and numerous revisions was done by Mrs. Carole Walters and Mrs. Sondra Patrizi. I am grateful to the publishers, Lea & Febiger, for advice and guidance throughout preparation of the text for publication.

To my former mentors, Dr. John Lansbury, formerly Professor of Medicine at Temple University, and Dr. Charles H. Slocumb and his colleagues at the Mayo Clinic, I owe a deep debt of gratitude for my basic training in rheumatology. The examples of excellence they provided have served as a continuing guide throughout my own career of study. To Dr. Joseph L. Hollander, whose textbook of rheumatology stands as an outstanding contribution to the study of the rheumatic diseases, I am grateful for the foreword to this text. The assistance of Dr. Michael G. Sheahan, Senior Fellow in Rheumatology, in proofreading the manuscript is gratefully acknowledged.

Manuscript preparation was supported in part through the Division of Research in Medical Education, Case Western Reserve University, Grant #LM 00673, National Library of Medicine.

Cleveland, Ohio　　　　　　　　　　　　ROLAND W. MOSKOWITZ

PREFACE

Rheumatology continues its almost exponential growth as a medical subspecialty. Advances in clinical and basic research have been exciting, and more rheumatologists are being trained than ever before. Unfortunately, the prevalence of patients suffering from arthritis has kept pace, with the latest survey by the United States Public Health Service listing approximately 31,000,000 people afflicted with this disorder. Advances in the biology, biochemistry, and immunology of the connective tissue diseases have been striking. Research by rheumatologists has played a leading role in definitions of disease relationships to histocompatibility antigens. Since the first edition of this book, a number of new connective tissue diseases have been described, new diagnostic tools discovered and major advances in therapeutic approaches described. The appearance of numerous new textbooks in the musculoskeletal disease field is testimony to this increased growth.

The response to this textbook has been most rewarding. It is utilized as a standard textbook by medical students in a number of schools and has found wide application by house officers in internal medicine and family medicine, rheumatology fellows, arthritis educators, and practicing physicians. The selection of this book as one of five recommended by the American College of Physicians as a core text in rheumatology for internists was particularly rewarding.

The second edition represents extensive revision and expansion. New clinical cases have been added where appropriate, and figures added or revised to better demonstrate text material. Chapter bibliographies have been extensively updated and the sections on therapy augmented.

The chapter on laboratory studies includes material on newly described antinuclear antibody studies such as anti-nRNP, anti-Sm, anti-SS-A, anti-SS-B, anti-Scl-70, and anti-RANA. Descriptive material on the complement system, immune complexes, cryoglobulins, histocompatibility antigens, and T and B cell interplays has been expanded or added. Sections on the use of new radiologic techniques, radioisotope diagnostic methods and arthroscopy are designed to acquaint the reader with exciting new diagnostic tools. New information on synovial fluid analysis updates information relative to use of short-chain fatty acids, and anti-teichoic acid anti-bodies for diagnosis of infectious arthritis. Descriptive material for the diagnosis of calcium apatite deposition disease is fully reviewed. New or expanded sections in subsequent chapters relate to such disorders as plica syndrome, osteonecrosis, arthritis associated with pancreatic and lipoprotein disorders, hereditary disorders of muscle due to abnormalities in glycogen and lipid metabolism, myopathies related to hyperparathyroidism, acromegaly and osteomalacia and the newly described inclusion myositis. Arthritis related to skin disease includes new observations on the use of capillary nail-fold changes in diagnosis, eosinophilic fasciitis, Lyme arth-ritis, subacute bacterial endocarditis, cryoglobulinemia, Sweet's syndrome and acne conglobata/fulminans. Yersinia arthritis, a relatively newly de-fined reactive arthropathy, has been added to the section on gastrointes-tinal-related disorders. The importance of excluding atrial myxoma and retroperitoneal fibrosis in patients with otherwise nondescript clinical dis-orders is stressed. Localized musculoskeletal syndromes include sections on shin splints, compartment syndromes, and localized entities related to sports injuries. In response to requests that the section on therapy be expanded, the chapter on disease management has been thoroughly updated to include not only well-accepted new drugs and modes of management, but also in-vestigational modalities likely to be soon available. Treatment of septic arthritis has been updated to keep pace with newly introduced antibiotics. The assistance of Dr. Jerrold Ellner, Associate Professor and Chief of the Division of Infectious Diseases, Department of Medicine at University Hospitals/Case Western Reserve University, is gratefully acknowledged. Indications for joint surgery and pre- and postoperative management are provided in greater detail. The use of transcutaneous nerve stimulation as a therapeutic modality in the physical therapy armamentarium, and the possibly expanded role for intra-articular use of radioisotope therapy further round out additions to this text. A chapter on eye disease as it so commonly relates to arthritic disorders represents a totally new area of text presentation. Dr. Jonathan H. Lass, Assistant Professor of Surgery, Division of Ophthalmology, kindly reviewed this new chapter contribution.

The initial objective of this textbook, to present clinical descriptions based on a problem-oriented approach, has been maintained. Hopefully this text will prove to be of even further value in this newly expanded and revised edition.

Appreciation is gratefully acknowledged to Ms. Bonnie Langevin for her dedicated help in the organization and typing of revised materials, and to Ms. Connie McSweeney for her professional editing. Drs. Alan M. Cohen, Scott R. Burg and Jeffrey Loman kindly assisted in preparation of new illustrations.

Cleveland, Ohio   ROLAND W. MOSKOWITZ

CONTENTS

INTRODUCTION

Medical textbooks are usually organized by topics based on specific disease entities. Most patients, however, do not come to the physician with a disease already diagnosed and given a name; rather, they more commonly have a complex of symptoms and physical abnormalities. This textbook is organized in a problem-oriented fashion on the basis of presenting signs and symptoms, in the way that medical problems are likely to appear to the physician.

The text is divided into three major divisions. The chapters in *Part I* review clinical examination, laboratory studies, and diagnostic techniques in specific relationship to rheumatic disorders. Special attention is given to synovial fluid analysis, an important study in the diagnosis of these disease states.

The chapters in *Part II* are devoted to common clinical presentations of rheumatic disorders. The chapters in this section have a common format, as follows:

A. Introduction. A brief general discussion of the problem at hand is presented.

B. Differential diagnosis. A listing of those entities most likely to provide the answer to the patient's problem is given. No attempt is made to list the diseases within this group according to frequency of occurrence. A clinical description of diseases to be considered in diagnosis follows. This information is designed to provide important clues to diagnosis and direction to further clinical and laboratory investigation necessary for accurate diagnosis. Some repetition of these clinical outlines occurs in the various chapters; this repetition is deliberate. It allows variation in emphasis on salient features of the disease states, depending upon the nature of the problem under discussion. In addition, it lessens the need for the reader to move back and forth between chapters for clinical information. Hopefully, this aspect of the book, in which each chapter provides a relatively

1

complete discussion of the problem under investigation, will prove especially valuable to the physician using the text on a day-to-day basis.

Additional possible diagnoses, to be considered after the more common causes have been excluded, are noted for completion but are generally discussed in lesser detail. These latter entities are less likely to represent the diagnosis at hand, either because the diseases themselves or their symptomatic presentation as the type of problem under discussion are uncommon.

C. Diagnostic studies to be considered in the evaluation. A comprehensive discussion of diagnostic studies with a detailed discussion of their application for most appropriate and effective use is given.

D. Therapy. Discussion of therapy is directed toward two phases of management. In the first phase, therapeutic procedures directed toward *symptomatic* relief *prior* to specific diagnosis are outlined. Great care has been exercised to avoid those measures which, though providing symptomatic help, would interfere with further clinical and laboratory diagnostic measures. The use of the recommended agents and procedures for temporary relief of pain and disability allows time for further clinical observation and diagnostic study, as well as time to carry out appropriate literature research into the patient's problem if required.

The second phase of therapy relates to *specific* measures of management to be utilized *after the diagnosis* has been made. In some instances, these specific therapeutic programs are outlined in detail in the chapter itself. Additional details regarding specific management of the more common rheumatic diseases are given in more complete form in the chapters on therapy in Part III.

Following the material in each chapter of Part II, representative cases typifying some of the problems under discussion are presented. These cases, based on patients seen in practice, demonstrate the clinical and laboratory aspects of diagnosis and management both before and after diagnosis has been made.

The chapters in *Part III* describe specific detailed management of some of the more common rheumatic diseases after the diagnosis has been made. In addition, special chapters are devoted to physical therapy, occupational therapy and supportive appliances, and to local injection therapy, extremely important adjuncts to rheumatic disease care. The final chapter describes the management of corticosteroid therapy in patients in stress situations, with particular reference to its use in surgery and obstetrics.

References to available textbooks and key articles in medical journals are provided for more detailed study after each chapter.

This textbook is designed to provide practical information that will allow judicious and appropriate study and management of the more commonly seen rheumatic disease problems. The more difficult or uncommon problems may require more extensive reading or, when indicated, referral to specialists in the rheumatic diseases.

This text represents a distillate of prevailing diagnostic and therapeutic philosophies as viewed and practiced by a single author. There is always a danger that such an approach will be dogmatic regarding both methods of evaluation and therapy. Realizing this danger, an attempt has been made to avoid this insofar as possible. It is hoped that most authorities in the field will agree in general with the concepts of management and treatment outlined. Of course, individual variations and preferences are to be expected. Material of controversial nature is specifically described as such when discussed.

PART I

CLINICAL EXAMINATION, LABORATORY STUDIES AND DIAGNOSTIC TECHNIQUES

CHAPTER 1

HISTORY AND PHYSICAL EXAMINATION

HISTORY OF PRESENT ILLNESS

Effective history-taking in patients with rheumatic disorders requires paying attention both to the usual general inquiries and to specific symptoms. Close attention must be paid to the location, nature and course of the joint involvement. Important determinations include the duration of joint symptoms, the location of the joints first involved, the pattern of progression to other joints, and the acute, subacute or chronic nature of the symptoms observed. Frequency and periodicity of attacks are other important considerations. The examiner should inquire about anatomic areas other than the musculoskeletal system, because joint manifestations are similar, if not identical, in many of these disorders. Diagnosis often depends on the demonstration of important ancillary findings. The age, sex and race of the patient may influence the consideration of certain diseases. Fever, weakness, fatigue and weight loss indicate systemic disease. Fibrositis or stiffness is a characteristic manifestation of many of the rheumatic diseases; when generalized, it suggests a systemic disorder. The patient complains of gelling of the muscles and joints, which occurs most prominently upon awakening in the morning. Stiffness is also present following inactivity, with improvement following increased physical activity. It is more pronounced preceding stormy weather, when the barometric pressure falls and humidity is high. Commonly, cool, damp weather accentuates the stiffness and heat relieves it. Raynaud's phenomenon with its typical color changes is likely to herald the presence of a serious systemic disorder; cold is the most common precipitating factor. A suspected diagnosis of systemic lupus erythematosus is strengthened by the presence of sun sensitivity, pleurisy, drug allergy, or hair loss. Photophobic reactions or a long history of nausea and dizziness on sun exposure do not have the import of sun sensitivity reactions characterized by rash, fever, or arthritis. Skin rash is an important clue to the diagnosis of such entities as psoriatic arthritis, systemic lupus erythematosus, scleroderma and dermatomyositis, to name only a few. Gastrointestinal symptoms of chronic diarrhea and bleeding, when associated with joint symptoms, suggest a diagnosis of ulcerative colitis or regional enteritis. Frequent aphthous ulcers, commonly called canker sores by the patient, are seen in Behçet's and Reiter's syndromes. Renal stones may be the first manifestation of gout. Ophthalmologic findings including conjunctivitis, episcleritis, and iritis are common in a number of systemic rheumatic disorders. Urethritis suggests the presence of gonococcal arthritis or Reiter's syndrome.

A complete rheumatologic history should include current and past details regarding dose, effectiveness and toxicity of antiarthritic agents used in the management of the patient's symptoms. In particular, specific information regarding the use of analgesics, aspirin and other nonsteroidal anti-inflammatory drugs, oral, intramuscular and intra-articular corticosteroids, antimalarials, gold, D-penicillamine, and immunosuppressive agents should be obtained. Medications that the patient may be taking for unrelated illnesses should be noted for several reasons: Firstly, contraindicated drug combinations can be avoided. Secondly, certain drugs such as oral contraceptive agents, hydralazine, anticonvulsant medications and procainamide may be precipitating or causative factors in the patient's connective tissue disease symptoms.

SYSTEMS REVIEW

A complete review of systems is required. However, certain points of information command particular interest in this group of patients. Headaches and tenderness in the temporal area suggest a diagnosis of temporal (cranial) arteritis. The importance of eye symptoms characteristic of conjunctivitis, episcleritis or iritis was previously noted. Persistent dryness of the eyes and mouth should lead to a consideration of Sjögren's syndrome. Dysphagia as a result of esophageal dysfunction is a common manifestation of several connective tissue disorders, such as dermatomyositis and scleroderma. Symptoms of peptic ulcer disease are important to note because many of the medications commonly considered in the treatment of arthritis may be contraindicated. Symptoms of colitis are a clue to the diagnosis of enteropathic arthritis, such as the arthritis associated with ulcerative colitis. Dysuria and urinary frequency may indicate urethritis, a prominent manifestation of gonococcal infection and Reiter's syndrome. Cutaneous lesions on the genitalia are seen in Reiter's and Behçet's syndromes. Sensory symptoms such as burning and paresthesia of the extremities are common manifestations of neurologic complications associated with arthritic disorders. Specific muscle weakness should direct attention to the presence of either a primary myopathy or neurogenic atrophy secondary to involvement of the nervous system.

PAST MEDICAL HISTORY

In addition to the usual review of the patient's medical history, a history of acute rheumatic fever, other forms of arthritis, or trauma is often helpful in delineating the patient's problem. Detailed information regarding past surgery or fractures should be elicited. Knowledge of prior roentgenograms and their availability is useful because they can be obtained for review if necessary. Drug allergies should be noted.

FAMILY HISTORY

A number of articular disorders such as gout, ankylosing spondylitis and osteoarthritis of the distal interphalangeal joints (Heberden's nodes) have an hereditary background. Their presence in other family members is supportive in diagnosis.

SOCIOECONOMIC HISTORY

Questions regarding the ability of the patient to perform the usual activities of daily living such as bathing, dressing, toileting, transfer, and feeding provide information about the impact of the disease in limiting daily function. In addition, these parameters of function can be used as a guide to the progress of the disease. The patient's emotional response to the disease and the presence of complicating premorbid psychiatric disturbances should be ascertained. The effect of the disease on the family and on financial stability should be noted. Knowledge of the patient's occupation may have etiologic importance. In addition, limitations resulting from the patient's arthritis may require consideration of job alteration or total job retraining.

PHYSICAL EXAMINATION

One of the most serious errors a physician can commit in the diagnosis of rheumatic disorders is to look only at the principal site of complaint or at a limited number of joints. An evaluation of all components of the locomotor system is necessary to assess disease affecting any one joint. A complete examination of other systems is also required, since many of the rheumatic disorders have associated general findings. The patient should be fully undressed except for a short gown. Joint assessment includes observations related to erythema, increased warmth, swelling, tenderness on direct palpation, pain on movement, joint range of motion, instability and deformity. *Erythema* of the skin commonly occurs over acutely inflamed joints but is frequently absent in the presence of chronic inflammation. *Increased skin warmth* is a sensitive indicator of inflammation, but

Figure 1-1. Bulge sign. (A) Fluid is compressed to one side of the knee. (B) Pressure on the opposite aspect of the knee produces a small fluid wave or bulge.

changes may be subtle. Care must be taken to exclude externally applied heat or cold as a cause of temperature differences. Comparing the same joint on the opposite side of the body is helpful when changes are minimal. *Swelling* reflects a number of joint abnormalities, including synovial inflammation, increased amounts of synovial fluid or proliferation of cartilage and bone. Inflamed synovium has a boggy edematous feel. Increased mobility of articular structures, such as the patella, suggests the presence of fluid. The patella can often be ballotted when fluid is present. Using one hand to compress the suprapatellar pouch in order to concentrate the fluid in the main compartment of the knee, the patella is then forcefully directed downward to demonstrate the sensation of bone riding on fluid. Small amounts of fluid in the knee can be detected by the "bulge sign." Fluid is compressed with the hands to one side of the knee (Fig. 1-1,A). This side is then gently tapped or compressed, following which a small fluid wave or bulge can be detected on the opposite aspect of the knee (Fig. 1-1,B). Small amounts of fluid, generally 15 ml or less, can be detected by this simple maneuver. The maneuver is not applicable in the presence of large fluid collections, since fluid displacement is resisted. Bony enlargements are palpated as hard, irregular swellings. They occur most commonly in osteoarthritis and reflect the presence of proliferating spurs of cartilage and bone.

Tenderness, an important sign of joint disease, is tested by direct pressure. Mild tenderness may require a significant amount of pressure to elicit an abnormal response. Comparing the findings with joints on the opposite side of the body is important in determining the significance of the response when changes are subtle. Tenderness can be graded in a gross fashion according to the degree of pressure required to elicit pain. More accurate grading can be performed by the use of an instrument called a dolorimeter, which numerically determines the amount of pressure required to bring on pain. The degree of tenderness parallels the severity of the inflammation. Localization of findings is extremely important, because disease of para-articular structures such as tendons or bursae may be misinterpreted as evidence of primary articular disease. Certain joints may not be tender to palpation but will be painful on *active or passive motion*. Crepitus (crepitation) may be felt or heard as a crackling, grating sensation associated with joint motion. Fine crepitus is seen in the presence of surface granulation tissue or early cartilage erosion; prominent, coarse crepitus indicates more severe cartilage and bone irregularity. Snapping, clicking, or cracking sounds related to slipping of ligaments or tendons over articular surfaces, not uncommon in normal joints, are to be differentiated.

Measurement of joint *range of motion* is important not only in defining the presence of joint disease, but also in providing an important parameter of disease progression or response to therapy. Familiarity with normal range of motion is essential to evaluate the significance of measurements in the presence of joint disease. Comparison with similar opposite joints is helpful in differentiating abnormal from normal findings. The preferred system for joint measurement is based on the neutral zero method, whereby the normal anatomic position of the joint is defined as zero. For example, the flat position of the wrist would be defined as zero degrees. From this position, motion is recorded as the number of degrees of flexion or extension. When extension is an unnatural movement for a given joint, the term hyperextension is used and appropriately recorded. Accurate measurement of range of motion requires the use of a goniometer, a hinged device with a scale showing the angle formed between two linear arms.

The presence of *instability* is usually demonstrated most readily by various stress maneuvers. These abnormalities in stability may reflect intra-articular changes, such as loss of cartilage and bone substance, or loss of integrity of supporting joint structures, such as capsule and ligaments. Instability may be obvious on joint use, but it is most readily demonstrated by fixing one component of the joint and testing for increased motion in various planes. Fixed joint *deformity* is usually obvious on inspection.

Completion of the musculoskeletal examination requires evaluation of the muscles for both atrophy and weakness. In patients in whom pathologic changes are located primarily in joints, atrophy and weakness are usually localized to those muscles associated with the affected joints. Erroneous misinterpretations of muscle atrophy may be made when joint swelling is present and the associated muscles look smaller in size by comparison. Generalized atrophy and weakness reflect primary muscle disorders. Tenderness due to muscle disease per se is uncommon except in patients with inflammatory muscle disease. More often, such tenderness on pressure reflects local or systemic fibrositis involving associated fascial tissue.

As noted earlier, proper examination of the patient with arthritis requires evaluation not only of the musculoskeletal system, but of other systems as well. The following is a description of a suggested routine for examination of patients with musculoskeletal complaints. The procedure can be varied to suit the individual examiner, but I have found it useful as an effective routine.

The examination is begun as the patient enters the room. Abnormalities in gait and the ability to perform certain activities such as undressing, sitting and rising from a chair, and getting up on the examining table are observed. Direct study begins with an examination of the hands. The nails are examined for evidence of anemia, paronychial rash, psoriasis and subungual infarcts. The presence or absence of clubbing is noted. Tapering of the distal phalanges is characteristic of scleroderma. Observation of the palms may reveal rash, palmar erythema, subcutaneous nodules, and thickenings due to tenosynovitis or Dupuytren's contracture. Muscle atrophy should be noted. Ruptured tendons may be revealed by loss of active motion. The extent to which the patient can make a complete fist bilaterally is recorded. Grip strength can be evaluated by having the patient attempt to squeeze the examiner's second and third fingers. At the same time, crepitus due to tenosynovitis may be observed. More accurate assessment of grip strength can be carried out by having the patient squeeze a sphygmomanometer cuff which has been folded twice and partially inflated to 20 mm Hg. Mercury column elevation is noted, and the average of three readings for each hand recorded. Each joint should be specifically evaluated for erythema, heat, swelling, tenderness, instability and deformity. Carpal and wrist joints are similarly examined. The primary motions at the wrist are flexion and extension, but radial and ulnar movement should also be evaluated. Wrist swelling may not be apparent on simple examination in the anatomic wrist position. Flexion of the wrist will frequently result in a dorsal protrusion of inflamed synovium and fluid, allowing demonstration of early joint disease. Elbow motion should normally allow movement from full extension (0°) to 150° flexion. In some normal individuals, however, 5° lack of full extension, or 5° of hyperextension may be noted. Swelling is most readily palpated in the regions between the medial and lateral epicondyles and the olecranon process (Fig. 1-2). Tenderness over the epicondyles themselves reflects epicondylitis with inflammation of tendon attachments, as occurs in patients with tennis elbow. When examining the elbow joint, special note should be taken of the presence of rheumatoid nodules, gouty tophi or other subcutaneous swellings. Rheumatoid nodules may be truly subcutaneous and mobile, but they are frequently fixed to periosteum. Nonspecific bony irregularities may cause diagnostic confusion, but they usually can be readily differentiated, especially if they are present bilaterally. Rheumatoid nodules most often occur on the extensor surface of the ulna in a subolecranon distribution (Fig. 1-3). Localization here is usually related to pressure exerted on arm rests while sitting. Later, nodules may occur over the olecranon area itself. In contrast, gouty tophi usually occur first in the olecranon area; later, tophi develop distally in the subolecranon areas as well. Nodules of other origin,

Figure 1-2. Rheumatoid arthritis, right elbow. Swelling is readily palpated between the lateral epicondyle and the olecranon process.

Figure 1-3. Subcutaneous nodules, rheumatoid arthritis. Lesions appear in both the subolecranon and the olecranon areas. (Courtesy, the Arthritis Foundation)

Figure 1-4.   Olecranon bursal swelling in a patient with rheumatoid arthritis.

Figure 1-5.   Shoulder abduction. The examiner fixes the left scapula of the
patient with downward pressure.
Abduction at the glenohumeral
joint was limited to 70°.

such as xanthomata, amyloid deposits, granuloma annulare, epidermoid cysts and subcutaneous nodules of rheumatic fever may be present. Olecranon bursitis may be observed as a swelling at the posterior aspect of the elbow, over the tip of the olecranon process (Fig. 1-4).

Swelling of the shoulder joint is often difficult to detect. It is seen most readily at the anterior aspect of the joint. Tenderness may be due to intrinsic joint disease, bursitis or tendinitis. Shoulder motions are a combination of glenohumeral and scapulothoracic motions. Glenohumeral motion is tested after first fixing the scapula by downward pressure. Motions to be evaluated include abduction, adduction, flexion, extension, and internal and external rotation. Abduction is tested by moving the shoulder away from the body with the elbow in 90° flexion (Fig. 1-5). Movement to 90° abduction is normal. Rotation upward measures external rotation (normal, 80° to 90°); rotation downward measures internal rotation (normal, 80° to 90°). Pure adduction is obstructed by the thorax but can be measured by bringing the arm across the front of the chest. Swinging the arm forward and backward measures flexion and extension respectively. Following the examination for glenohumeral motion, total functional shoulder motions of flexion, extension, abduction and hyperabduction are tested without scapular fixation. Pain patterns associated with active and passive shoulder motion may provide a clue to disease origin. Intra-articular disease is associated with pain both on active and passive motion. In patients with extra-articular disease, as in supraspinatus tendinitis, active

Figure 1-6. Screening maneuver for testing deltoid muscle weakness.

Figure 1-7. Multiple tophi in a patient with gout. Deposits were opaque to transillumination. (Courtesy, Dr. A. Mackenzie)

motion is painful but minimal or no pain is seen with passive abduction. Palpation of the acromioclavicular and sternoclavicular joints is performed for evidence of tenderness and swelling. Disease of the acromioclavicular joint is often misinterpreted as disease of shoulder origin, due to its proximity to the latter joint. Atrophy and strength of the deltoid muscles are determined as a screening maneuver for the presence of myopathy (Fig. 1-6).

Following these studies, the attention of the examiner is directed to the head. The ears are evaluated for the presence of gouty tophi (Fig. 1-7) and scalp for rash or hair loss. Early small tophi may be difficult to differentiate from localized thickenings of ear cartilage. Differentiation is aided by use of transillumination, during which tophi are opaque. Tophi must be differentiated from calcification of the pinna of the ear, seen in a number of diverse disease states including Addison's disease, ochronosis, acromegaly, relapsing polychondritis, and hyperthyroidism. Eyes, ears, nose and throat are examined as part of the routine general exam. Temporomandibular joint swelling is uncommon. Limitation of motion can be readily assessed by noting the distance between the upper and lower incisors with the mouth open maximally. This vertical movement is variable, but serial measurement in a given patient is a valuable indicator of changes in joint range of motion associated with disease activity. The joint is most readily palpated with the mouth open. Synovitis, tenderness, and warmth can be noted, and dislocations felt as the joint is put through range of motion. Palpable clicking, often felt and of concern to the patient, is usually a normal finding. The neck is palpated for evidence of thyroid enlargement and lymphadenopathy. Cervical spine motion is tested for flexion (normal = 45°), extension (normal = 45°), rotation right or left (normal = 60°) and lateral bending with ear towards the shoulder (normal = 45°). The posterior cervical and upper trapezius muscles are palpated for the presence of tenderness, spasm or nodules. Cardiorespiratory examination and blood pressure readings follow. The patient is then asked to lie down and an abdominal examination and evaluation of the lower extremities can be carried out.

Hip motions to be tested include flexion, extension, abduction, adduction, and internal and external rotation. Hip flexion is measured by moving the flexed knee toward the abdomen. Fixed flexion deformities of the hip may be masked if the patient tilts the pelvis to the affected side. Accurate testing can be accomplished by holding the opposite hip in full flexion while attempting full extension of the hip being examined. Lack of full extension is a measure of the fixed deformity (Fig. 1-8). Extension is

Figure 1-8.   Flexion deformity of left hip in a patient with rheumatoid arthritis. The right hip is held in full flexion to avoid compensatory pelvic tilt.

Figure 1-9.   Fabere-Patrick maneuver. (A) Normal. The right knee can be brought almost to the horizontal position. (B) Rheumatoid arthritis. Hip disease prevents rotation of the right knee toward the horizontal position.

tested by drawing the leg backward as the patient lies on the opposite side. To test abduction, the leg is moved laterally. Adduction is evaluated by moving the leg medially in front of the opposite leg. Rotation may be measured with the leg extended or with the knee flexed to 90°. The limb is rolled outward to test for external rotation and inward for internal rotation. Abnormalities in hip motion can be rapidly screened by asking the patient to place the heel on the opposite knee while rotating the hip outward, in an attempt to bring the ipsilateral knee horizontal to the examining table (Fabere-Patrick maneuver). Normal hip rotation should allow the knee to be brought almost completely horizontal (Fig. 1-9). Tests of hip motion may be somewhat invalidated by disease of the knee, since pain in the latter joint may prevent full hip movement. Interpretation of the findings requires caution. Similarly, inflammation of the greater trochanteric bursa may limit hip motion due to pain, despite the absence of

Figure 1-10.   Ballottement of the patella. The suprapatellar pouch is first compressed with the left hand, following which sharp pressure is exerted on the patella directly towards the femur.

intrinsic hip disease. Tenderness on pressure applied over the bursa at the trochanteric area is characteristic.

Measurements of leg length are important. The distance between the anterior-superior iliac spine and the medial malleolus reflects true leg length. Apparent leg length is measured from the umbilicus to the medial malleolus. Differences in true leg length occur in disease in or near the hip joint; differences in apparent leg length alone may reflect pelvic tilt or scoliosis. The strength of the iliopsoas muscle is determined to complete the screening for proximal muscle weakness. This is evaluated by applying downward pressure on the anterior aspect of the thigh as the patient holds the knee and hip at 90° angles.

The knee lends itself readily to full examination. Clinical findings may be generalized but efforts should be made to define symptoms according to the medial femorotibial, lateral femorotibial, and patellofemoral compartments into which the knee is anatomically divided. Obvious deformities such as genu varus (bowleg) or genu valgus (knock knee) are readily noted. The knee should be inspected for erythema and palpated for increased warmth, tenderness and swelling. Early swelling is often most obvious in the suprapatellar extension of the joint beneath the quadriceps tendon. As noted earlier, joint swelling may be due to synovial inflammation, increased amounts of joint fluid, or bony proliferation. Small amounts of fluid may be detected by the "bulge sign" maneuver (see Fig. 1-1, page 10). Ballottement of the patella whereby the patella can be readily displaced in an anteroposterior position against the femur can be carried out in the presence of large fluid collections (Fig. 1-10).

Palpation at the posterior aspect of the knee is important to detect the presence of popliteal cysts (Fig. 1-11). Circumferential measurement of the thigh at a specific distance above the knee and at the knee joint itself is valuable in patient follow-up. Patellofemoral disease is suggested by pain and crepitus produced when the patella is moved forward over the femur. Abnormal patellar motion is detected by attempts at medial and lateral displacement. Instability of the collateral ligaments is tested by forcing medial and lateral motion with the knee slightly flexed; abnormal findings are accentuated with the patient in a standing position. Cruciate ligament instability is tested by moving the tibia forward and backward on the femur, which is held fixed (Fig. 1-12). Excessive forward motion reflects disease of the anterior cruciate ligament; excessive backward motion, disease of the posterior cruciate ligament. A positive McMurray maneuver suggests a meniscal lesion. To perform this test (Fig. 1-13), one hand is placed over the anterior aspect of the fully flexed knee, placing the index finger and thumb on opposite sides of the joint for palpation purposes. The ankle is then grasped with the other hand, and the knee moved back and forth from full flexion to extension, while rotating the leg medially and laterally. A positive test is characterized by a palpable or audible click or

Figure 1-11. Popliteal cyst, right knee. Swelling behind the knee extends into the calf.

Figure 1-12. Firm anterior pull on the tibia tests instability of the anterior cruciate ligament.

Figure 1-13. McMurray maneuver. A palpable or audible click or pop, often associated with pain and local tenderness at the site of the damaged meniscus as the knee is moved back and forth while rotating the leg represents a positive test.

pop, often associated with pain and local tenderness at the site of the damaged meniscus. Snapping of the popliteus tendon, a generally benign event, should be differentiated. Quadriceps atrophy, common in the presence of knee arthritis, should be noted.

Swelling of the ankle may be difficult to detect. It is most commonly seen at the anterior aspect of the joint only. Swelling of tendons due to tenosynovitis in this area is not uncommon. The Achilles tendon should be examined for the presence of tenderness; it is a common site for rheumatoid nodule formation. Flexion and extension motions at the ankle are tested. Subtalar disease is indicated by pain and limitation of inversion and eversion. Tarsal disease may lead to swelling and tenderness. The latter can be readily tested by firm compression of the entire tarsal area in the palm of the examiner. The tarsal joints are usually considered en masse since they do not lend themselves to separate examination. Heel tenderness should be noted. The metatarsophalangeal joints are each examined separately by palpation and pressure. The interphalangeal joints should be similarly observed for swelling and tenderness, and the toenails examined.

The musculoskeletal examination is completed by evaluation of the dorsolumbar spine and sacroiliac joints. The latter are tested for tenderness by direct pressure. Pain on sacroiliac motion may be elicited by having the patient lie on the back in a supine position near the edge of the examining table. Each leg is then separately moved off to the side and below the surface of the table. This maneuver distorts the pelvis and causes pain in the affected joint. Straight leg raising is an important maneuver to test for nerve root irritability in patients with suspected back disorders. The spine itself is examined with the patient in a standing position. Postural abnormalities including kyphosis (forward curvature), lordosis (backward curvature), or scoliosis (lateral curvature) are noted. Localized angulations may be seen. Tenderness over the spine is tested by direct percussion, using either the side of the fist or a percussion hammer. Flexion, extension, rotation and lateral motions are tested. In testing for flexion motions, it is important to fix the hips by grasping the patient from behind over the hip area. Otherwise, flexion limitations may be obscured by bending forward at the hip joints (Fig. 1-14, A and B). In normal persons forward flexion should allow the fingertips to be approximated to the feet,

Figure 1-14. Examination of lumbar spine motion. Fixation of hips by the examiner (A) eliminates hip flexion. Compare motion with hips free (B).

and often to the floor. Measurement of the distance from floor to fingertips is a useful indicator of disease-incurred limitations in function. Spine flexion can also be assessed by the Schober test, in which the distance between the 7th cervical and 1st sacral vertebrae is compared in erect versus flexed positions. An increase in length of 10 cm is normal. Persons without spine disease should be capable of 25° spinal extension and 30° lateral flexion. Chest expansion measured at the nipple line is an index of costovertebral joint motion. In normal patients, the difference between inspiration and expiration varies, measuring 5 to 10 cm depending on the age and size of the patient being tested.

In addition to the screening procedures for proximal muscle strength outlined previously, all muscles should be evaluated for weakness and atrophy. Neurologic examination includes evaluation of deep tendon reflexes, pathologic reflexes such as the Babinski sign, and evaluation of pain, touch, vibration, and position senses. The state of the vascular system is evaluated by palpation of radial, ulnar, temporal, carotid, femoral, popliteal, and pedal pulses. Bruits heard on auscultation indicate abnormal flow and are consistent with vessel narrowing. Temporal artery examination is of particular interest, because tenderness and nodularity support a suspected diagnosis of temporal (cranial) arteritis. Rectal and pelvic examination completes the over-all evaluation.

Forms utilized by me for the initial history and physical examination appear in the Appendix. I have found these helpful as a guide for interviewing the patient and recording physical findings.

CHAPTER **2**

LABORATORY STUDIES AND DIAGNOSTIC TECHNIQUES: INDICATIONS AND INTERPRETATIONS

GENERAL STUDIES

A number of routine general laboratory tests are helpful and indicated in the diagnosis of patients with rheumatic disorders. Baseline studies should include white blood cell and differential cell counts, hematocrit, erythrocyte sedimentation rate, and urinalysis. Leukopenia suggests a diagnosis of systemic lupus erythematosus. The presence of a severe anemia militates against a benign localized disorder, and the patient should be scrupulously studied for serious systemic disease. Similarly, an elevated erythrocyte sedimentation rate is strong evidence for the presence of a more generalized disorder. Abnormal findings on urinalysis favor a diagnosis of systemic lupus erythematosus, vasculitis, or scleroderma rather than rheumatoid arthritis.

When suggested by clinical findings, other studies to be considered are serum protein electrophoresis, calcium, phosphorus, alkaline phosphatase, creatinine, antistreptolysin O (ASO) titer, thyroxine, cholesterol, triglycerides, lipoprotein electrophoresis, serum glutamic oxaloacetic transaminase, and hepatitis-associated antigen (HB$_s$Ag). Serum protein immunoelectrophoresis, serum complement and immune complex determinations are of particular value in the diagnostic assessment of a number of systemic connective tissue disorders. Chest roentgenograms should be obtained if systemic disease is suspected. Roentgenograms of involved joints are indicated.

Certain diagnostic studies are particularly important in the study of rheumatic disorders. These are discussed in greater detail.

URIC ACID STUDIES

Serum Uric Acid

Routine determination of the serum uric acid is valuable in patients with articular symptoms to determine whether symptoms are due to gout. In addition, many medications affect the serum uric acid level. Determining the true baseline serum uric acid level is cumbersome and often difficult at a later time after such medications have been begun.

Serum uric acid determinations are usually made by the colorimetric method. A more accurate study is obtained using the enzymatic spectrophotometric method in which uric acid levels are determined both before and after uricase digestion. The latter method eliminates the effect of non-urate substances, which produce a spuriously high reading. Normal values vary, depending on the technique used. Automated techniques provide more reproducible results. It is important for the physician to know the normal values obtained by the laboratory in which the test is conducted as they vary from laboratory to laboratory. Normal levels also differ in males

Table 2-1. Drugs and Disease States Associated with Secondary Elevation of Serum Uric Acid

Drugs

    Diuretics (e.g., chlorothiazide, hydrochlorothiazide, chlorthalidone, furosemide, triamterene, ethacrynic acid)
    Low dose salicylate therapy
    Pyrazinamide
    Ethambutol[1]
    Levodopa[2]
    Nicotinic acid[3]

Disease states

    Obesity[4]
    Myeloproliferative and lymphoproliferative disorders (lymphomas, multiple myeloma, polycythemia vera)
    Malignant tumors[5]
    Lead intoxication (saturnine gout)[6]
    Psoriasis
    Glycogen storage disease (type 1)[7]
    Bartter's syndrome[8]
    Hyperlactacidemia (acute ethanol ingestion, toxemia of pregnancy, exercise)
    Increased blood levels of beta hydroxybutyrate and acetcacetate (diabetic ketoacidosis, starvation)
    Chronic renal failure
    Essential and renal hypertension[9]
    Postadrenalectomy for hypertension[10]
    Hyperparathyroidism[11]
    Hypoparathyroidism[12]
    Myxedema[13]
    Paget's disease[14]
    Cystinuria[15]
    Down's syndrome[16]

Table 2-2.   Drugs and Disease States that Lower Serum Uric Acid

Drugs

    Probenecid

    Sulfinpyrazone

    Allopurinol

    High dose salicylate therapy

    Coumarin derivatives

    Phenylbutazone

    Adrenal corticosteroids

    Radiocontrast agents[17]

    Glyceryl guaiacholate[18]

    High dose ascorbic acid[19]

    Estrogens[20]

Disease States

    Purine enzyme deficiency states[21]

    Wilson's disease[22]

    Fanconi's syndrome

    Xanthine oxidase deficiency

    Neoplasms (carcinoma,[23] Hodgkin's disease[24])

    Laennec's cirrhosis[25]

    Jaundice[26]

and females. Using colorimetric methods, the normal value for males is 4 to 6 mg/100 ml; for postmenopausal females, 3.5 to 5.5 mg/100 ml; and for premenopausal females, 3 to 5 mg/100 ml. Values tend to be higher with automated colorimetric techniques, and standardization of normal levels at 7 to 8 mg/100 ml is not uncommon. There is a mild to moderate variation in serum uric acid levels throughout the day and at various times of the year. Although these variations are not marked, it is worth rechecking several uric acid determinations obtained at a similar time each day if the initial study is only slightly abnormal.

Hyperuricemia may indicate primary gout or may represent an elevation secondary to various medications or disease states (Table 2-1).[1-16] A low or normal serum uric acid, on the other hand, may indicate (1) a normal state, (2) patients with an early stage of gout in which the serum uric acid is normal between attacks, or (3) patients in whom the uric acid has been lowered by certain drugs or disease processes (Table 2-2).[17-26]

Urinary Uric Acid

Information regarding the quantitative daily excretion of uric acid has diagnostic and therapeutic importance. In patients whose clinical symptoms suggest gout but whose serum uric acid is high normal or only slightly elevated, an increase in urinary uric acid excretion supports the diagnosis. In patients with a confirmed diagnosis of gout, the quantitative urinary uric acid determination is helpful in deciding the most appropriate drug to use in an interval therapy program. In those patients with a definitely elevated urinary uric acid, allopurinol is usually the drug of choice, since this agent lowers both serum and urinary uric acid and diminishes the hazard of kidney stone formation. In contrast, uricosuric agents such as probenecid and sulfinpyrazone increase urinary uric acid output and may increase the tendency to develop stones. Since most gouty patients excrete normal amounts of uric acid, a normal excretion level does not exclude the diagnosis. On a purine-free diet, the mean daily excretion should not exceed 600 mg. In patients on an average normal daily diet, the daily uric acid excretion should not exceed 900 mg.

Determination of urinary excretion of uric acid requires collection of a 24-hour urine specimen. It has been suggested that uric acid overexcretion can be more simply determined by evaluation of spot mid-morning serum and urine samples.[27] Values in which the product of urinary uric acid and serum creatinine concentrations, divided by urinary creatinine (all concentrations in mg/100 ml) exceeded 0.7 mg/100 ml of glomerular filtrate were considered abnormally high, consistent with uric acid overexcretion. More recent studies, however, have not confirmed the utility of this technique in assessing uric acid overexcretion.[28]

RHEUMATOID FACTORS

Abnormal proteins are found in the sera of many patients with rheumatoid arthritis. These circulating proteins, heterogeneous in type, have been classified as antibodies on the basis of their physical, chemical and behavioral characteristics. They have been named rheumatoid factors because they were first described in rheumatoid arthritis. Most rheumatoid factors are the IgM (19S macroglobulin) type. Less commonly, rheumatoid factors are the IgG or IgA variety. In the test tube, rheumatoid factor reacts with IgG (7S) gamma globulin. This reaction is the basis of most tests for rheumatoid factor. The technique most commonly used to identify the presence of rheumatoid factor uses agglutination of latex particles to demonstrate that the rheumatoid factor–IgG interaction has occurred. Specifically, latex particles are coated with IgG, which has been denatured to increase the sensitivity of the reaction. Sera to be tested are heated to eliminate prozone reactions, and then added to the suspension of globulin-coated latex particles. If rheumatoid factor is present, it will react with IgG and cause agglutination of the latex particles. The results can be observed macroscopically. The test for rheumatoid factor is considered positive if agglutination occurs in a serum dilution of 1:40 or higher. Rheumatoid factor is seen in approximately 40 to 50% of patients with rheumatoid arthritis during the early stages of the disease. In later stages, a positive rheumatoid factor test is seen in 80 to 90% of cases. Once present, the factor usually persists.

Although the presence of rheumatoid factor supports a diagnosis of

Table 2-3. Conditions Other than Rheumatoid Arthritis Associated with Rheumatoid Factor

Normal persons (2 to 4% of the population)
Relatives of rheumatoid arthritis patients
Aging (10 to 20% positive over age 65 years)[30]
Systemic lupus erythematosus
Scleroderma
Dermatomyositis
Sarcoidosis[31]
Leprosy
Dysproteinemias and paraproteinemias
Liver disease (infectious hepatitis, cirrhosis)
Syphilis
Idiopathic pulmonary fibrosis
Pneumoconiosis
Acute pulmonary tuberculosis[32]
Acute viral infections
Parasitic diseases
Following prophylactic vaccinations[33]
Subacute bacterial endocarditis[34]
Diabetes mellitus patients on insulin therapy[35]
Psychiatric disorders (schizophrenia, endogenous depression)[36]
Following multiple blood transfusions[37]
Parenteral narcotic addiction[38]
Renal transplantation[39,40]

rheumatoid arthritis, rheumatoid factor may be associated with many other disease states (Table 2-3).[29-40] In these other conditions, titers are usually low, but not always.

ANTINUCLEAR ANTIBODIES AND LE CELL STUDIES

Antinuclear antibodies are abnormal circulating proteins that react with nuclei and with individual constituents of nuclei such as nucleoprotein, DNA and histone. Antinuclear antibodies are usually IgG (7S) in character, but IgM (19S) antibodies also occur. They are a heterogeneous group of antibodies with varying specificities for various nuclear constituents and for different sites on a particular nuclear constituent. To detect the presence of antinuclear antibody, the fluorescent antibody technique has been utilized. The test is performed as a two-stage procedure. The test serum is first applied to tissue sections containing nucleated cells. If antinuclear antibody is present, it will bind with the nuclei. Following this, fluorescein-labeled antiserum to human gamma globulin is applied to the cells. This anti-human gamma globulin will react with the antinuclear antibody and result in fluorescence of the nuclei. Patterns of localization of fluorescent stain may be helpful in diagnosis. Homogeneous patterns (Fig. 2-1) are least specific. A peripheral rim pattern (Fig. 2-2) suggests the

Figure 2-1. Antinuclear antibody, homogeneous stain. (Courtesy, the Arthritis Foundation)

Figure 2-2. Antinuclear antibody, peripheral rim pattern. (Courtesy, the Arthritis Foundation)

Table 2-4.   Conditions Other than Systemic Lupus Erythematosus (SLE) Associated with Antinuclear Antibodies

---

Other connective tissue diseases (rheumatoid arthritis, scleroderma, dermatomyositis, mixed connective tissue disease)

Sjögren's syndrome

Relatives of patients with SLE

Aging (antinuclear antibodies seen in up to 25% of normal females over 60 years; anti-DNA and LE cell studies normal)[54]

Chronic liver disease, infectious hepatitis

Idiopathic pulmonary fibrosis[55]

Pneumoconiosis[56]

Neoplasia[57]

Leprosy[58]

Drug-related SLE (certain drugs may induce formation of antinuclear antibodies and a clinical syndrome similar to spontaneously occurring SLE):

  Hydralazine[59]
  Procainamide[60]
  Isoniazid[61]
  Anticonvulsant drugs (e.g., diphenylhydantoin, mephenytoin, trimethadione)[62]
  Antibiotics (penicillin, sulfonamides, tetracycline)
  Propylthiouracil[63]
  Methimazole[64]
  Methyl dopa[65]
  Oral contraceptive pills[66]
  Phenothiazines[67]
  D-penicillamine[68]
  Quinidine[69]
  Clofibrate[70]
  Oxyphenisatin[71]
  Griseofulvin
  Nalidixic acid[72]

---

presence of systemic lupus erythematosus. Staining of nucleoli or a speckled pattern suggests a diagnosis of scleroderma or Sjögren's syndrome. A speckled pattern also occurs in systemic lupus erythematosus and mixed connective tissue disease. Qualitative reactions overlap, however, and diagnoses made on this basis should be done with caution.

Antinuclear antibodies are present in almost all patients with acute active systemic lupus erythematosus. In patients with subacute or chronic disease, the antibodies may be absent or present only in low titer. Although these antibodies are seen most frequently and to highest titer in systemic lupus erythematosus, they are associated with a number of other disease states[54-72] (Table 2-4).

Using various immunologic techniques such as immunofluorescence, complement fixation, immunodiffusion, and hemagglutination, immunologic specificities of different antinuclear antibodies have been identified. Antibody to native (double-stranded) DNA is seen primarily in lupus. It occurs less frequently and to a lower titer in other connective tissue diseases. This antibody produces a nuclear rim pattern of staining by immunofluorescence (Fig. 2-2). Antibodies to denatured (single-stranded) DNA are nonspecific and are found in a variety of rheumatic and nonrheumatic diseases. In addition to the commonly employed methods utilizing radioisotope labeling for anti-DNA determinations, an immunofluorescent method for detection of antibodies to double-stranded DNA which employs the kinetoplast of the flagellate Crithidia luciliae as substrate has been introduced.[41,42] Active LE disease, particularly if associated with nephritis, is likely to be associated with high titers of anti-DNA antibody.

Antibodies to deoxyribonucleoprotein are the serum factor which gives rise to the LE cell and can be found in patients with a positive LE cell test. Antibodies to histones have been shown to occur with high frequency in patients with drug-induced SLE and may be useful in differentiating patients with drug-induced from spontaneously occurring disease.[43]

Antibodies to nonhistone (acidic) nuclear proteins appear to have sufficient specificity to promise usefulness in differential diagnosis. When present, they all give a speckled pattern of nuclear staining. Anti-Sm antibody is highly specific for SLE,[44,45] and may be a marker for a subset of SLE patients with milder renal and central nervous system disease.[45] Antibody to nuclear-ribonucleoprotein, anti-nRNP, is characteristically present in high titer in mixed connective tissue disease.[46] It is, however, seen in systemic lupus erythematosus, scleroderma, Sjögren's syndrome and other rheumatic diseases, generally in lower titer. The term anti-ENA antibody, defining antibody to extractable nuclear antigen, originally denoted the presence of antibodies to Sm and RNP antigen.

Antibodies to other nonhistone nuclear proteins have been described. Antibodies to SS-A and SS-B antigens have been reported in the sera of patients with Sjögren's syndrome.[47-49] Anti-SS-A occurs in a broad spectrum of connective tissue disease. Anti-SS-B is more specific and is seen in a majority of patients with primary Sjögren's syndrome or with Sjögren's syndrome plus SLE. Antibody to rheumatoid arthritis nuclear antigen (anti-RANA, rheumatoid arthritis precipitin),[50] antibody to scleroderma-70 antigen (anti-Scl-70),[51] and antibody to polymyositis antigen[52] (anti-PM-1) appear to have some specificity for rheumatoid arthritis, scleroderma, and polymyositis, respectively. Antibody to Scl-70 antigen, although present in only approximately 20% of patients with scleroderma has not been observed in studies of large numbers of patients with systemic lupus erythematosus or rheumatoid arthritis. Accordingly, this antibody may represent a marker for scleroderma disease. This marker does not, however, differentiate between patients with diffuse scleroderma and those with CREST variant.[51] On the other hand, a high frequency of antibody to chromosomal centromere (anti-centromere antibody) has been reported in patients with

Figure 2-3. LE cell (arrow) surrounded by polymorphonuclear leukocytes in form of rosette.

Figure 2-4. Extracellular altered nuclear material (arrow), with beginning rosette formation.

CREST syndrome (57%), compared to only an 8% frequency in diffuse scleroderma.[51]

The sensitive and quantitative tests available for determination of antinuclear antibody and anti-DNA have largely replaced the LE cell test which is based on an interaction between antinuclear antibody, nuclear material, and phagocytic white cells.[53] A characteristic LE cell consists of a polymorphonuclear leukocyte which contains an inclusion hematoxylin body (Fig. 2-3). Rosettes of polymorphonuclear leukocytes may surround the LE cell, in response to chemotactic activity of the altered nuclear material in the hematoxylin body (Fig. 2-3). At times, altered nuclear material will remain free (Fig. 2-4). When present, it has the same diagnostic significance as fully-formed LE cells. LE cells must be differentiated from tart cells which result from ingestion of nuclear material by leukocytes as a normal phagocytic process.[53] In the latter cells, the chromatin structure of the enclosed nuclear material retains its fine fibrillar pattern.

SKIN BIOPSY

Routine histopathologic study of material obtained on skin biopsy is helpful in the diagnosis of a number of rheumatic disorders, such as systemic lupus erythematosus, scleroderma (Fig. 2-5), vasculitis, sarcoid arthritis and psoriatic arthropathy. Specimens for study can be obtained readily by use of a punch biopsy needle under local anesthesia. Further aid in differential diagnosis can be obtained by immunofluorescent staining techniques to identify immunoglobulins and complement in the area of the basement membrane at the epidermal-dermal junction (the lupus band test).[73,74] The immunoglobulin deposits may be either antinuclear antibody or antibasement membrane antibody. Immunofluorescent study requires the use of skin that has been frozen rather than fixed, or that has been preserved in a special solution.[75] The skin sample is placed on a glass slide, over which is placed a solution containing fluorescein-labeled anti-whole human gamma globulin antibody. Positive tests reveal a band of immunofluorescence at the epidermal-dermal junction (Fig. 2-6). Immunoglobulin deposits can be more specifically identified by use of fluorescein-labeled antibodies to IgG, IgM, IgA and complement. A positive reaction is seen in 90 to 95% of biopsies taken from the site of clinical rash in patients with systemic lupus erythematosus. A positive test occurs in 75 to 80% of SLE patients in biopsies from normal sun-exposed skin and in up to 50% of patients in biopsies derived from normal non-sun-exposed skin.[76] A positive band reaction in normal non-sun-exposed skin may correlate with LE renal involvement. In patients with chronic discoid lupus, a positive reaction occurs similarly in 85% of patients when areas of clinical involvement are studied. Normal skin, however, yields negative findings. Basement membrane immunofluorescence occurs in only a few other diseases, including bullous pemphigoid and lepromatous leprosy.

Figure 2-5. Skin biopsy, scleroderma. Characteristic changes include thinning of the epidermis, loss of rete pegs, atrophy of dermal appendages, and a marked increase in dermal collagen. (Hematoxylin and eosin) (Courtesy, Dr. A. Mackenzie)

Figure 2-6. Skin, systemic lupus erythematosus. A band of immunofluorescence appears at the epidermal-dermal junction. (Courtesy, the Arthritis Foundation)

Other patterns of immunofluorescent skin staining in connective tissue diseases have been identified.[77,78] Positive staining of epidermal nuclei is associated with the presence of serum antibody to nuclear-ribonucleoprotein (anti-n-RNP) and has similar diagnostic significance. It is seen in a number of connective tissue diseases. A third staining pattern, characterized by immunofluorescent staining of the nucleoli of epidermal cells, appears specific for patients with scleroderma.[78]

COMPLEMENT

The complement system consists of a series of interacting proteins which are related to both immune and inflammatory responses. The system was originally described as being activated by antigen-antibody complexes at the C1 site (the classical pathway of activation) (Fig. 2-7). More recent studies have demonstrated that later components are activated directly (alternate pathway activation) (Fig. 2-7). The classical complement pathway appears to play a central role in tissue injury mediated by antibodies and immune complexes. The sequence of complement activation generates several small polypeptides, C3a, C5a, and C567, that have chemotactic activity. C3a and C5a also stimulate histamine release. The final reaction of the complement system produces a complex which is capable of lysing

Figure 2-7. Schematic representation of classical and alternate complement pathways. (Bar across number indicates activation of component.) The lack of normal numerical sequence in the classical system reflects the fact that specific components were numbered in the sequence of discovery.

cell membranes. The role of the alternate complement pathway in producing immune-mediated injury is unclear. Activation at the C3 level may be initiated by C3b component derived from the classical pathway, or by a number of other substances including zymosan and other complex polysaccharides, endotoxin, and noncomplement-fixing antibodies such as IgA and IgE.

Complement levels are measured either by testing the total hemolytic activity of serum incubated with a standard preparation of sensitized sheep erythrocytes (CH^{50} whole hemolytic complement activity), or by radioimmunodiffusion to assay individual complement components, principally C1q, C3 and C4. The CH^{50} study is the most sensitive indicator of functional integrity of the complement system, but the study requires technical expertise and the use of fresh or frozen serum to maintain the integrity of component labile proteins. Radioimmunodiffusion studies, on the other hand, do not require fresh serum. CH^{50} activity reflects the interaction of all nine components of the classical system. Activation of the classical pathway is associated with reduction of complement components C1q, C4, C2 and C3. Activation of the alternate pathway, on the other hand, is associated with reduction of C3 and later components, with normal C1q, C4 and C2.

Changes in serum complement level are seen in certain connective tissue diseases and their study is helpful both in diagnosis and the evaluation of disease activity. Low serum complement levels are characteristic of active systemic lupus erythematosus, particularly when lupus glomerulonephritis is present. Low serum complement levels occur sometimes in patients with rheumatoid arthritis when the titer of serum rheumatoid factor is high.[79] Synovial fluid complement has some value in differential diagnosis. Low synovial fluid complement levels occur in systemic lupus erythematosus and seropositive rheumatoid arthritis. Synovial fluid complement is characteristically elevated in many patients with Reiter's syndrome. Hereditary deficiencies of specific complement components have been described and should be considered when there is an unexplained lack of parallel between disease activity and complement levels.

IMMUNE COMPLEXES AND CRYOGLOBULINS

Immune complexes are thought to induce tissue damage in a variety of human diseases. Complexes may form in the circulation and then become localized in tissues or may be formed locally, initiating an inflammatory response by activation of complement and other mediators. The importance of immune complexes in disease pathogenesis has led to a number of assays related to their detection. The labeled C1q binding technique and Raji cell radioimmunoassay are frequently utilized. In the C1q-binding study, isolated C1q globulin labeled with I^{125} binds to immune complexes in the serum of the patient. The I^{125} C1q-bound complex is precipitated and the radioactivity in the precipitate counted. The level of immune complexes in the serum directly relates to the amount of I^{125} C1q globulin in the precipitate. In the Raji cell radioimmunoassay complement-containing immune complexes interact with complement receptors on the membrane of Raji cells, a B lymphocyte line maintained in tissue culture. I^{125}-labeled rabbit anti-human IgG is added, which binds to the immune complexes on the cell surface. Radioactivity is counted to assess the level of immune complexes in the test serum.

The various assays for circulating immune complexes have limitations and thus disparate results are often noted. To obviate these difficulties, research laboratories may run multiple techniques for study of the same set of serum samples.

Cryoglobulins are proteins which have the property of precipitating when cooled and redissolving when warmed. Small amounts of serum cryoglobulins are normal. Increased cryoglobulins may be a secondary manifestation of connective tissue disorders, hematologic diseases or infection. Not infrequently, no underlying associated disease is found and a diagnosis of essential or idiopathic cryoglobulinemia is made.

Monoclonal cryoglobulins are most commonly associated with lymphomas, multiple myeloma and Waldenstrom's macrogobulinemia. Cryoglobulins associated with various connective tissue diseases are more likely to contain a mixture of immune complexes. In testing for cryoglobulins, blood should be drawn into a warmed syringe and allowed to clot at 37°C so as not to precipitate the cryoglobulin into the fibrin clot. The clear serum should be stored for at least 48 hours at 4°C. The presence of cryoglobulin precipitate can be noted and critically defined by further immunologic studies.

TESTS OF CELL-MEDIATED IMMUNITY

Cell-mediated immunity is closely related to a functioning T-cell lymphocyte system. Normally, more than 75% of the lymphocytes in peripheral blood are T-lymphocytes. These cells can be assayed by mixing purified peripheral blood lymphocytes with sheep erythrocytes. Lymphocytes that have bound three or more erythrocytes are considered to be T cells. B-lymphocytes, identified primarily with humoral immunity, can be identified and counted by detecting membrane-bound immunoglobulin synthesized by B-cells but not by other cells.

In vitro assessment of cell-mediated immunity can be performed by observing T-cell response to various appropriate stimuli. Commonly used reactions include determinations of the rate of lymphocyte transformation to lymphoblasts in the presence of nonspecific mitogens such as phytohemagglutinin (PHA), or concanavalin A (ConA), or to antigens such as

PPD to which the cells have had a prior encounter. The rate of lymphocyte transformation is estimated from the amount of tritiated thymidine incorporated into newly synthesized DNA. Inhibition of leukocyte migration can also be studied as a measure of cellular immunity (migration inhibition factor, MIF). Migration of leukocytes placed in capillary tubes is inhibited in proportion to the degree of sensitivity of the cell to the test antigen.

Studies of B and T cells and their interactions remain primarily of value in investigations of disease pathogenesis and pathophysiology. Assays for changes in B-cell and T-cell number, and evaluation of the function of helper and suppressor subsets of T-cells have provided insights into primary and secondary immunodeficiency diseases.

Histocompatibility (HLA) Antigens

An important observation which substantiated the suspected interrelationship of the various spondylitic disorders was the demonstration of a strong association between these diseases and the human leukocyte antigen (HLA) system, particularly HLA-B27. These antigens are controlled by genes located in at least four major loci situated close together on chromosome 6 in the human. Until recently, serologic methods have been available to identify only antigens of the A, B, and C series. D locus antigens have been characterized by use of the mixed lymphocyte culture (MLC) reaction. More recently, serologic techniques to identify human B-lymphocyte allo-antigens have been devised. These allo-antigens are strongly associated with the HLA-D system. To reflect this relationship, the nomenclature HLA-DRw (1, 2 . . . etc.) has been assigned to the known B-lymphocyte allo-antigens. Strong associations have been noted between various HLA antigens and connective tissue disease (see Table 2-5).

Table 2-5.   Associations of HLA Antigens and Rheumatic Disease

Antigen	Disease Associations
B-27	Ankylosing spondylitis
	Reiter's syndrome; Yersinia arthritis
	Spondylitis associated with juvenile rheumatoid arthritis, psoriasis, or inflammatory bowel disease
B-5	Behçet's syndrome
B-8	Sjögren's syndrome; systemic lupus erythematosus
*DRw4, Bw35, Dw3, DRw5, DRw8[80,81]	Juvenile rheumatoid arthritis
DRw2, DRw3	Systemic lupus erythematosus
Dw3	Sjögren's syndrome

*Associations vary depending upon clinical presentation as pauci-articular, polyarticular or systemic disease forms

Several pathogenic mechanisms may explain the interrelationship of these antigens and disease. Certain HLA antigens may share antigenic determinants with infectious agents, leading to an immunologic tolerance by the host; HLA antigens may have antigenic determinants which are similar to certain viruses or bacteria, leading to antibody cross reaction; HLA antigens may provide receptor sites for infectious agents on cell membrane surfaces; the HLA antigen may act only as a marker which is closely linked to abnormal immune response genes; and, finally, susceptibility may be related to a genetically-related deficiency of a complement system component.

It should be stressed that none of the associations of disease and HLA antigens is absolute. Accordingly, although they help to define the degree of susceptibility of a patient to a given disease, positive findings do not confirm nor do negative findings exclude a given clinical diagnosis.

SEROLOGIC TEST FOR SYPHILIS

Serologic studies for syphilis have some diagnostic value, because a false positive serologic test for syphilis (STS) is seen in as many as 10 to 15% of patients with various forms of connective tissue disease.[82] A false positive test is most often associated with systemic lupus erythematosus, but it also occurs in the presence of rheumatoid arthritis, scleroderma and sarcoidosis. The routine serologic test for syphilis (STS) is performed first. If positive, the fluorescent treponema antibody absorbed test (FTA-ABS) should be carried out. A negative FTA-ABS study excludes the presence of luetic infection in almost all cases. A positive study characterized by a *uniform treponemal fluorescence* indicates syphilis in all but rare instances. Positive fluorescence may be seen in patients with rheumatoid arthritis and systemic lupus erythematosus but the treponemal fluorescence in these connective tissue disorders usually has a *nonuniform beaded pattern.*[83] Uniform treponemal fluorescence in patients with connective tissue disease has been described, but is extremely rare. The treponema pallidum immobilization test (TPI) is utilized when the interpretation is still in doubt. This latter test, though more costly and difficult to perform, is highly specific for treponemal disease.

In some patients, a positive STS is noted by chance as part of the routine physical examination of otherwise healthy persons. If follow-up studies reveal a false positive test, the patient should be carefully evaluated for clinical evidence of one of the connective tissue diseases. Further studies helpful in clarifying the issue include a white blood cell count and differential cell count, hematocrit, urinalysis, erythrocyte sedimentation rate, serum studies for rheumatoid factor and antinuclear antibodies, and serum protein electrophoresis. If all findings are negative, the clinical examination and laboratory studies should be repeated at periodic intervals.

The underlying systemic disease, if present, may take years to become apparent.

DIAGNOSTIC STUDIES FOR MUSCLE DISEASE

Serum Muscle Enzymes

Measurement of serum muscle enzymes is important in the diagnosis of muscle disorders.[84,85] Elevated values commonly occur in the primary myopathies, but are unusual in neurogenic atrophy. In the latter, elevations are usually mild when present. The three serum muscle enzymes most commonly employed for study are serum glutamic oxaloacetic transaminase (SGOT), aldolase and creatine phosphokinase (CPK). Although all three enzymes may be elevated simultaneously in patients with primary myopathy, elevation of only one or two enzymes is not uncommon. Thus, diagnostic accuracy is enhanced if all three enzymes are routinely studied.

The CPK is the most sensitive and SGOT the least sensitive determination. CPK is the most specific for muscle disease, but all may be elevated by a number of causes.[86-92] The SGOT is increased in patients with myocardial disease or hepatic cell breakdown. Serum aldolase may be elevated if hepatic cell damage is present. In addition, a rise in serum aldolase occurs in the presence of a hemolytic anemia or if a hemolyzed blood specimen is sent to the laboratory, due to enzyme release from erythrocytes. CPK elevations occur in the presence of myocardial disease and following frequent intramuscular injections,[86] and it may be significantly elevated following prolonged strenuous exercise.[87] Elevated blood levels have been noted in association with strokes and subarachnoid hemorrhage[88] and in patients with acute psychosis.[89] Other nonmyopathic causes of a rise in serum CPK include pulmonary infarction and acute pneumonia. Patients with hypoparathyroidism may have elevated CPK levels,[90] even in the absence of overt muscle symptoms. Unexplained elevation of CPK has been described in patients with ankylosing spondylitis.[91] Finally, elevated levels of CPK may be associated with large muscle mass in heavy-framed normal individuals.[92] Measurement of CPK isoenzymes produced by different tissues (BB = brain, MB = cardiac, MM = skeletal muscle) will allow more accurate utilization of this study as a diagnostic procedure. Determination of enzymes more specific for liver injury, such as 5'-nucleotidase or γ-glutamyl transpeptidase, is helpful in differentiating the source of elevated levels of serum SGOT or aldolase.

Elevation of these enzymes occurs as a result of either the release of enzyme from degenerating muscle fibers or the escape of enzymes from muscle with increased membrane permeability. Although elevated levels support a diagnosis of myopathy, normal levels may occur in the presence of active muscle disease.

Creatine-Creatinine Ratio

Creatine is formed primarily in the liver and is converted into creatinine by muscle. In the presence of muscle disease, creatine conversion decreases and its urinary excretion subsequently increases. In studies of the creatine-creatinine ratio, the 24-hour urinary creatinine excretion is first determined. Urinary creatine is then converted to creatinine and the analysis repeated. The resulting value represents total urinary creatine plus creatinine. The original creatinine value is subtracted from the total to provide an absolute measure of creatine excreted. The creatine value divided by total creatine plus creatinine yields percent creatinuria:

$$\% \text{ Creatinuria} = \frac{\text{creatine (mg/24 hrs)}}{[\text{creatine} + \text{creatinine}] \ (\text{mg/24 hrs})} \times 100$$

The values for percent creatinuria in both males and females should not exceed 6%. Excretion is somewhat higher in pregnant females. Children have a physiologic creatinuria, with values up to 40% at age three years, 20% at age eight years, and normal adult values at age 15. Patients on androgen therapy may demonstrate an elevated excretion of urinary creatine due to stimulation of creatine formation in the liver. Two 24-hour urine determinations of creatine-creatinine ratio should be obtained routinely in order to confirm results and also because slight variations in the amount of creatinine excreted occur from day-to-day. The two daily values should not vary by more than 10% if accurate urine collections have been obtained. Creatine-creatinine ratios are increased not only in primary myopathies but also in disuse and neurogenic atrophy. Elevations generally appear earlier in the primary myopathies. The study is valuable not only as a diagnostic tool, but also in disease follow-up during therapy.

Electromyogram and Nerve Conduction Velocities

The electromyogram is utilized to study the electrical activity of skeletal muscle. Abnormalities appear both in primary myopathic disorders and in neurogenic atrophy. In patients with primary myopathy, the size of the individual motor unit potentials associated with voluntary contraction is decreased, and a relative increase occurs in the number and rate of firing. Polyphasic potentials of decreased size and short duration are characteristic. In lower motor neuron disease, the number and rate of unit firings are decreased. Low-voltage, long-duration polyphasic potentials during voluntary contraction are characteristic. Fibrillations at rest, although sometimes seen in myopathies, are most often associated with neurogenic atrophy.

Electromyography is helpful not only in diagnosis but also in defining involved muscles most likely to provide positive biopsy results.

Nerve conduction velocity determinations are a helpful adjunct in the differential diagnosis of myopathic and neuropathic disorders. They are particularly helpful in the diagnosis of local entrapment neuropathies such as the carpal and tarsal tunnel syndromes, and thoracic outlet compression. These studies are particularly useful in patients in whom objective neurologic findings are absent in the presence of subjective clinical disease manifestations. Although a range of normal values for various of the major nerves has been identified, it is well to compare conduction velocities in opposite extremities of the same patient. Not infrequently, a significant difference in velocities between the two sides gives the clue to diagnosis, in the face of values still within the normal range of either side.

Muscle Biopsy

Muscle biopsy studies are important in the diagnosis of muscle disorders. These studies are most likely to provide informative findings if performed on muscles that demonstrate involvement either by clinical symptoms or by positive electromyographic study. The physician should direct the surgeon to the specific muscle desired for biopsy and the surgeon should be well trained in the proper handling of the muscle specimen. All too often, specimens are so damaged in handling that a proper pathologic analysis of the tissue cannot be made. A needle-biopsy technique for obtaining specimens has been described but the specimens obtained are generally less adequate for diagnostic study. Frozen sections and sections fixed in formaldehyde should be obtained. Frozen sections are utilized for detailed histochemical studies. Electron microscopic examination is valuable when one of the more unusual disorders is suspected.

ROENTGENOLOGIC EXAMINATION

Roentgenologic examination of the joints is an important aid in differential diagnosis. In addition, it is valuable in the study of disease progress. Views other than the usual PA and lateral may be necessary to delineate subtle abnormalities. For example, skyline views of the knee will show pathologic changes in the patellofemoral joint more clearly than routine views (Fig. 2-8). Tunnel views taken with the knee in flexion outline abnormalities of intra-articular joint structure more clearly. Special techniques, such as spot films, laminograms, cineradiograms and myelograms, should be used when indicated. Cervical and lumbosacral spine studies require PA, lateral and oblique views for complete examination. Chest roentgenograms should be obtained from patients with any type of systemic disorder. Roentgenograms of other areas such as the gastrointestinal tract and kidneys should be ordered as the clinical picture dictates.

Figure 2-8.   Skyline view, patellofemoral joint. Joint space narrowing and spur formation clearly show in this patient with degenerative joint disease.

The indications for computed axial tomography (CAT scan) in patients with musculoskeletal disorders are expanding as the resolution of scanners improves. Computed tomography is already the procedure of choice for the diagnosis of spinal stenosis and lumbar facet joint disease. Preliminary studies suggest that it is effective in the diagnosis of intervertebral disk herniation.[93] Findings include displacement of the anterior epidural fat and dural sac by the prolapsed disc. Lack of specificity handicaps its use, since other soft tissue lesions such as epidural neoplasms or scar tissue cannot be differentiated. Examination of the spine at multiple levels may be required to exclude multiple lesions.

Radioisotope Scan

Joint scintigraphy is useful in the evaluation of inflammatory, ischemic and neoplastic changes involving diarthrodial joints and the bones of the body.[94,95] The two isotopes currently most used for joint scintigraphy are 99m Technetium pertechnetate and 99m Technetium diphosphonate. The pertechnetate form is utilized for studies of synovitis. Uptake is increased early due to increased vascular flow; delayed uptake represents binding of the nuclide to protein in the inflammatory exudate. Any inflamed joint may produce a positive scintiscan and, accordingly, abnormal findings are non-specific. The study may be of clinical use in demonstrating the presence of early inflammation in symptomatic joints that are negative to objective clinical examination. The increased uptake of the diphosphonate compound by inflamed joints is thought to result from their incorporation into hydroxy-apatite crystals of bone. Increased synovial vascularity likely contributes to the abnormal uptake. Studies with this nuclide are particularly useful in evaluating the presence of osteonecrosis or osteomyelitis. Its utility in the diagnosis of early ankylosing spondylitis is uncertain.[96-98] Bone scans are particularly useful in the delineation of bone disorders such as malignancy or Paget's disease. Technetium scans of the parotid glands, when carefully carried out, may aid in the diagnosis of patients with suspected Sjögren's syndrome.[99]

ARTHROGRAMS

Roentgenologic examination of joints following the instillation of contrast material, or air plus contrast material, helps to delineate a number of

Figure 2-9. Arthrogram of knee. A large popliteal cyst extends well into the calf.

joint disorders. These procedures are particularly useful in the diagnosis of tears of the meniscus or capsule of the knee, and in the demonstration of synovial cysts (Fig. 2-9). Ruptures of the rotator cuff of the shoulder can often be delineated. Double contrast arthrograms with air and contrast media generally provide more information than those using contrast media alone. False positive or false negative interpretations are not uncommon, especially in inexperienced hands.

SYNOVIAL BIOPSY

Synovial biopsy has its greatest value in the differential diagnosis of monoarticular or oligoarticular arthritis. In patients with more diffuse articular disease, the biopsy is likely to be nonspecific and less helpful, due to similarities in pathologic findings in these disorders. Special needles for closed synovial biopsy are available; their use is attended by minimal morbidity and complications. The knee is the most commonly biopsied joint

Figure 2-10.   Synovial biopsy needles. (A) Components of Jamshidi needle. (B) Components of Polley-Bickel needle.

because it lends itself most easily to this procedure. Closed biopsy should be strongly considered before open biopsy whenever possible. Smaller needles such as the Jamshidi needle (Kormed, Inc.) (Fig. 2-10, A) are usually utilized first. The Polley-Bickel needle (Fig. 2-10, B), a large-bore needle, requires a small skin incision and suture. It may be used initially or for repeat biopsy if the material obtained with a smaller needle is inadequate. Strict adherence to aseptic technique is vital. Synovial fluid is removed for analysis at the time of biopsy. Sufficient local anesthesia with 1% lidocaine is important to prevent discomfort. In addition, it is helpful to give meperidine, 50 to 75 mg IM, 20 to 30 minutes before biopsy. Specimens are obtained for culture and pathologic study. Tissue is taken from a number of sites to avoid missing localized isolated lesions. Following the biopsy, a compression bandage is placed around the knee and the patient is cautioned to avoid activity other than going to the bathroom or sitting quietly in a chair. Analgesics are prescribed to relieve postbiopsy pain. After a period of 24 hours, the compression bandage is removed and the patient may resume normal ambulation. Biopsy can be performed as an outpatient procedure when appropriate facilities are available. Complications of biopsy include infection and hemorrhage. These are rare when close attention to proper technique is carried out.

ARTHROSCOPY

Intra-articular endoscopic examination of joints can be performed by inserting an arthroscope through a small joint incision. The incorporation of fiber optics has allowed the development of instruments of decreased size and increased flexibility. Special operative arthroscopes have also been developed which allow limited definitive surgical procedures to be carried out if indicated. The procedure is performed in the regular operating room. Although local anesthesia can be utilized when the exam is limited, more complete evaluations require use of spinal or general anesthesia.

Arthroscopy has most often been used for studies involving the knee, but evaluation of other large joints such as the shoulder, elbow, and ankle has been carried out. Its greatest application is in the evaluation of patients with chronic knee symptoms for which no cause has been determined by other diagnostic procedures. The examination is particularly useful in identifying meniscal lesions, chondromalacia patellae, loose bodies, and other causes of mechanical derangements. Direct vision synovial biopsy can provide useful diagnostic data in various forms of inflammatory synovitis. Although a more extensive operative procedure than closed synovial biopsy, the added diagnostic potential of this procedure often makes it the choice over "blind" biopsy.

Diagnostic information obtained with this technique may prevent the need for exploratory arthrotomy in some patients. On the other hand, although postoperative morbidity is greater, open arthrotomy is still preferred by many because it allows the opportunity for more definitive treatment as well as diagnosis. Arthroscopy should not be carried out in the presence of a stiff joint or the presence of septic arthritis. Complications which are infrequent include infection and hemarthrosis.

REFERENCES

1. Postlethwaite, A. E., Bartel, A. G. and Kelley, W. N.: Hyperuricemia due to ethambutol. N Eng J Med 286:761, 1972.
2. Honda, H. and Gindin, R. A.: Gout while receiving levodopa for Parkinsonism. JAMA 219:55, 1972.
3. Gershon, S. L. and Fox, I. H.: Pharmacologic effects of nicotinic acid on human purine metabolism. J Int Clin Med 84:179, 1974.
4. Wyngaarden, J. J. and Kelley, W. N.: Gout and Hyperuricemia. Grune and Stratton, New York, 1976.
5. Ultmann, J. E.: Hyperuricemia in disseminated neoplastic disease other than lymphomas and leukemias. Cancer 15:222, 1962.
6. Ball, G. V. and Morgan, J. B.: Chronic lead ingestion and gout. Southern Med J 61:21, 1968.
7. Alepa, F. P., Howell, R. R., Klinenberg, J. R. and Seegmiller, J. E.: Relationships between glycogen storage disease and tophaceous gout. Am J Med 42:58, 1967.
8. Meyer, W. J., III, Gill, J. R., Jr. and Bartter, F. C.: Gout as a complication of Bartter's syndrome. A possible role for alkalosis in the decreased clearance of uric acid. Ann Int Med 83:56, 1975.
9. Cannon, P. J. et al.: Hyperuricemia in primary and renal hypertension. N Eng J Med 275:457, 1966.
10. Itskovitz, H. D. and Sellers, A. M.: Gout and hyperuricemia after adrenalectomy for hypertension. N Eng J Med 268:1105, 1963.
11. Mintz, D. H. et al.: Hyperuricemia in hyperparathyroidism. N Eng J Med 265:112, 1961.
12. Kirschner, D.: Hyperuricemia in hypoparathyroidism. Metabolism 5:703, 1956.
13. Leeper, R. D. et al.: Hyperuricemia in myxedema. J Clin Endocrinology 20:1457, 1960.
14. Franck, W. A. et al.: Rheumatic manifestations of Paget's disease of bone. Am J Med 56:592, 1974.
15. Dahlberg, P. J., Vandenberg, C. J., Kurtz, S. B., Wilson, D. M. and Smith, L. H.: Clinical features and management of cystinuria. Mayo Clin Proc 52:553, 1977.
16. Kaufman, J. M. and O'Brien, W. M.: Hyperuricemia in mongolism. N Eng J Med 276:953, 1967.
17. Postlethwaite, A. E. and Kelley, W. N.: Uricosuric effect of radio-contrast agents. Ann Int Med 74:845, 1971.
18. Ramadell, C. M., Postlethwaite, A. E. and Kelley, W. N.: Uricosuric effect of glyceryl guaiacholate. J Rheum 1:114, 1974.
19. Stein, H. B., Hasan, A. and Fox, I. H.: Ascorbic-acid induced uricosuria. Ann Int Med 84:385, 1975.
20. Nicholls, A., Snaith, M. L. and Scott, J. T.: Effect of oestrogen therapy on plasma and urinary levels of uric acid. Br Med J 1:449, 1973.
21. Kelley, W. N.: Inborn errors of purine metabolism—1977. Arthritis Rheum 20:S221, 1977.
22. Bishop, C., Zimdahl, W. J. and Talbott, J. H.: Uric acid in two patients with Wilson's disease (hepatolenticular degeneration). Proc Soc Exp Biol Med 86:440, 1954.
23. Cooper, D. S.: Oat-cell carcinoma and severe hypouricemia. N Eng J Med 288:321, 1973.

24. Bennett, J. S. et al.: Hypouricemia in Hodgkin's disease. Ann Int Med 76:751, 1972.
25. Michelis, M. F., Warms, P. C., Frisco, R. D. et al.: Hypouricemia and hyperuricosuria in Laennec's cirrhosis. Arch Int Med 134:681, 1974.
26. Schlosstein, L., Kippin, I., Bluestone, R. et al.: Association between hypouricemia and jaundice. Ann Rheum Dis 33:308, 1974.
27. Simkin, P. A., Hoover, P. L., Paxson, C. S. et al.: Uric acid excretion: quantitative assessment from spot, mid-morning serum and urine samples. Ann Int Med 91:44, 1979.
28. Wortmann, R. L. and Fox, I. H.: Limited value of uric acid to creatinine ratios in estimating uric acid excretion. Ann Int Med 93:822, 1980.
29. Bartfeld, H.: Distribution of rheumatoid factor activity in nonrheumatoid states. Ann N Y Acad Sci 168:30, 1969.
30. Moskowitz, R. W., Benedict, K. J. and Stouffer, R.: Serum antibodies to gamma globulin: inter-relationships of aging, disease and geography. J Chron Dis 20: 291, 1967.
31. Oreskes, I. and Siltzbach, L. E.: Changes in rheumatoid factor activity during the course of sarcoidosis. Am J Med 44:60, 1968.
32. Singer, J. M. et al.: Presence of antigamma globulin factors in sera of patients with active pulmonary tuberculosis. Ann Int Med 56:545, 1962.
33. Aho, K. et al.: Transient appearance of the rheumatoid factor in connection with prophylactic vaccinations. Acta Path Microbiol Scan 56:478, 1962.
34. Williams, R. C., Jr. and Kunkel, H. G.: Rheumatoid factor, complement, and conglutinin aberrations in patients with subacute bacterial endocarditis. J Clin Invest 41:666, 1962.
35. Oreskes, I. and Spiera, H.: Diabetes and rheumatoid factor. Ann Rheum Dis 32:431, 1973.
36. Oreskes, I. et al.: Rheumatoid factors in an acute psychiatric population. Ann Rheum Dis 27:60, 1968.
37. Vierucci, A.: Gm groups and anti-Gm antibodies in children with Cooley's anemia. Vox Sang 10:82, 1965.
38. Spiera, H., Oreskes, I. and Stimmel, B.: Rheumatoid factor activity in heroin addicts on methadone maintenance. Ann Rheum Dis 33:153, 1974.
39. Waller, M., Irby, R., Mullinax, F. and Loone, E. C., Jr.: Connective-tissue disease and rheumatoid factor in patients with renal transplants. N Eng J Med 273:12, 1965.
40. Bravo, J. F., Herman, J. H. and Smyth, C. J.: Musculoskeletal disorders after renal homotransplantation. A clinical and laboratory analysis of 60 cases. Ann Intern Med 66:87, 1967.
41. Aarden, L. A., DeGroote, E. R. and Feltkampe, T. E. W.: Immunology of DNA. III. Crithidia luciliae, a simple substrate for the determination of anti-dsDNA with the immunofluorescent technique. Ann N Y Acad Sci 254:505, 1975.
42. Crowe, W. and Kushner, I.: An immunofluorescent method using Crithidia luciliae to detect antibodies to double-stranded DNA. Arthritis Rheum 20:811, 1977.
43. Fritzler, N. J. and Tan, E. M.: Antibodies to histone in drug-induced and idiopathic lupus erythematosus. J Clin Invest 62:560, 1978.
44. Tan, E. M. and Kunkel, H. G.: Characteristics of a soluble nuclear antigen precipitating with sera of patients with systemic lupus erythematosus. J Immunol 96:464, 1966.
45. Winn, E. M., Wolfe, J. R., Lindberg, D. A., Fristoe, F. H., Kingsland, L. and Sharp, G. C.: Identification of a clinical subset of systemic lupus erythematosus by antibodies to the Sm antigen. Arthritis Rheum 22:1334, 1979.
46. Sharp, G. C., Irvin, W. S., Tan, E. M., Gould, R. G. and Holman, H. R.: Mixed connective tissue disease—an apparently distinct rheumatic disease syndrome associated with a specific antibody to an extractable nuclear antigen (ENA). Am J Med 52:148, 1972.
47. Alspaugh, M. A., Talal, N. and Tan, E. M.: Differentiation and characterization

of autoantibodies and their antigens in Sjögren's syndrome. Arthritis Rheum 19:216, 1976.

48. Kassan, S. S., Akizuki, M., Steinberg, A., Reddick, R. L. and Chused, T. M.: Antibody to a soluble acidic nuclear antigen in Sjögren's syndrome. Am J Med 63:328, 1977.

49. Scopelitis, E., Biundo, J. J. and Alspaugh, M. A.: Anti-SS-A antibody and other anti-nuclear antibodies in systemic lupus erythematosus. Arthritis Rheum 23: 287, 1980.

50. Catalano, M. A., Carson, D. A., Riederman, J. C. et al.: Antibody to the rheumatoid arthritic nuclear antigen. Its relationship to *in vivo* Epstein-Barr virus infection. J Clin Invest 65:1238, 1980.

51. Tan, E. M., Rodnan, G. P., Garcia, I., Moroi, Y., Fritzler, M. J. and Peebles, C.: Diversity of antinuclear antibodies in progressive systemic sclerosis. Arthritis Rheum 23:617, 1980.

52. Wolfe, J. F., Adelstein, E. and Sharp, G. C.: Antinuclear antibody with distinct specificity for polymyositis. J Clin Invest 59:176, 1977.

53. Hargraves, M. M., Richmond, H. and Morton, R.: Presentation of two bone marrow elements. The "tart" cell and the "LE" cell. Mayo Clin Proc, 1948.

54. Svec, K. H. and Veit, B. C.: Age-related antinuclear factors: Immunologic characteristics and associated clinical aspects. Arthritis Rheum 10:509, 1967.

55. Nagayo, H., Buckley, E. and Sieker, H. D.: Positive antinuclear factor in patients with unexplained pulmonary fibrosis. Ann Int Med 70:1135, 1969.

56. Kang, K. Y., Yagura, T. and Yammamura, Y.: Antinuclear factor in pneumoconioses. N Eng J Med 288:164, 1973.

57. Burnham, T. K.: Antinuclear antibodies in patients with malignancies. Lancet 2:436, 1972.

58. Matthews, L. J. and Troutman, J. R.: Clinical and serological profiles in leprosy. Lancet 2:915, 1965.

59. Hahn, B. H. et al.: Immune responses to hydralazine and nuclear antigens in hydralazine induced lupus erythematosus. Ann Int Med 76:365, 1972.

60. Blomgren, S. E., Condemi, J. J. and Vaughan, J. H.: Procainamide-induced lupus erythematosus. Am J Med 52:338, 1972.

61. Cannat, A. and Seligmann, M.: Possible induction of antinuclear antibodies by isoniazid. Lancet 1:185, 1966.

62. Jacobs, J. C.: Systemic lupus erythematosus in childhood. Report of 35 cases with discussion of seven apparently induced by anticonvulsant medication and of prognosis and treatment. Pediatrics 32:257, 1963.

63. Amrhein, J. A., Kenny, F. M. and Ross, D.: Granulocytopenia, lupus-like syndrome, and other complications of propylthiouracil therapy. J Pediatr 76:54, 1970.

64. Lee, S. L. and Chase, H. P.: Drug-induced systemic lupus erythematosus: a critical review. Sem Arth Rheum 5:83, 1975.

65. Sherman, J. D., Lover, D. W. and Harrington, J. F.: Anemia, positive lupus and rheumatoid factors with methyldopa. Arch Int Med 120:321, 1967.

66. Bole, G. G., Friedlander, M. H. and Smith, C. K.: Rheumatic symptoms and serological abnormalities induced by oral contraceptives. Lancet 1:323, 1969.

67. Fabius, A. J. M. and Gaulhofer, W. K.: Systemic lupus erythematosus induced by psychotropic drugs. Acta Rheum Scand 17:137, 1971.

68. Harpey, J. P. et al.: Lupus-like syndrome induced by D-penicillamine in Wilson's disease. Lancet 1:292, 1971.

69. Kendall, M. J. and Hawkins, C. F.: Quinidine-induced systemic lupus erythematosus. Postgrad Med J 46:729, 1970.

70. Howard, E. J. and Brown, S. M.: Clofibrate-induced antinuclear factor and lupus-like syndrome. JAMA 226:1358, 1973.

71. Reynolds, T. B. et al.: Chronic active and lupoid hepatitis caused by a laxative, oxyphenisatin. N Eng J Med 285:813, 1971.

72. Rubinstein, A.: LE-like disease caused by nalidixic acid. N Eng J Med 301:1288, 1979.

73. Grossman, J., Callerame, M. L. and Condemi, J. J.: Skin immunofluorescence

studies on lupus erythematosus and other antinuclear-antibody positive diseases. Ann Int Med 80:496, 1974.

74. Harrist, T. J. and Milm, M. C., Jr.: Review: the specificity and clinical usefulness of the lupus band test. Arthritis Rheum 23:479, 1980.

75. Michel, B., Milner, Y. and David, K.: Preservation of tissue-fixed immunoglobulins in skin biopsies of patients with lupus erythematosus and bullous diseases —a preliminary report. J Invest Derm 59:449, 1973.

76. O'Loughlin, S., Schroeter, A. L. and Jordan, R. E.: A study of lupus erythematosus with particular reference to generalized discoid lupus. Br J Dermatol 99 (1):1, 1978.

77. Burnham, T. K., Neblett, T. R. and Fine, G.: The application of fluorescent antibody technique to the investigation of lupus erythematosus and various dermatoses. J Invest Dermatol 41:451, 1963.

78. Prystowsky, S. D., Gilliam, J. N. and Tuffanelli, D. L.: Epidermal nucleolar IgG deposition in clinically normal skin. Arch Dermatol 114:536, 1978.

79. Franco, A. E. and Schur, P. H.: Hypocomplementemia in rheumatoid arthritis. Arthritis Rheum 14:231, 1971.

80. Glass, D. N. and Litvin, D. A.: Heterogeneity of HLA association in systemic onset juvenile rheumatoid arthritis. Arthritis Rheum 23:796, 1980.

81. Fink, C. W. and Stastny, P.: Results of serologic HLA-DR typing in juvenile arthritis and juvenile rheumatoid arthritis. Arthritis Rheum 23:673, 1980.

82. Tuffanelli, D. L.: False positive reactions for syphilis. Arch Derm 98:606, 1968.

83. McKenna, C. H. et al.: The fluorescent treponemal antibody absorbed (FTA-ABS) test beading phenomenon in connective tissue diseases. Mayo Clin Proc 48:545, 1973.

84. Vignos, P. J. and Goldwyn, J.: Evaluation of laboratory tests in diagnosis and management of polymyositis. Am J Med Sci 263:291, 1972.

85. Munsat, T. L. et al.: Serum enzyme alterations in neuromuscular disorders. JAMA 226:1536, 1973.

86. Cacace, L.: Elevated serum CPK after drug injections. N Eng J Med 287:309, 1972.

87. Demos, M. A. and Gitin, E. L.: Acute exertional rhabdomyolysis. Arch Int Med 133:233, 1974.

88. Schiavone, D. J. and Kaldor, J.: Serum CPK in brain damage. N Eng J Med 285:753, 1971.

89. Alias, A. G.: Serum transaminase and alkaline phosphatase in schizophrenia. Biological Psychiatry 4:89, 1972.

90. Hower, J. et al.: CPK activity in hypoparathyroidism. N Eng J Med 287:1098, 1972.

91. Calin, A.: Raised serum creatine phosphokinase activity in ankylosing spondylitis. Ann Rheum Dis 34(3):244, 1975.

92. Garcia, W.: Elevated creatine phosphokinase levels associated with large muscle mass. JAMA 228:1395, 1974.

93. Meyer, G. A., Haughton, V. M. and Williams, A. L.: Diagnosis of herniated lumbar disk with computed tomography. N Eng J Med 301:1166, 1979.

94. Dick, W. C.: The use of radioisotopes in normal and diseased joints. Seminars in Arth and Rheum 1:301, 1972.

95. Kirchner, P. T., and Simon, M. A.: Radioisotopic evaluation of skeletal disease. J Bone Joint Surg 63A:673, 1981.

96. Namey, T. C., McIntyre, J., Buse, M. and LeRoy, E. C.: Nucleographic studies of axial spondyloarthritides. I. Quantitative sacro-iliac scintigraphy of early HLA-B27 associated sacro-iliitis. Arthritis Rheum 20: 1058, 1977.

97. Ho, G., Sadovnikoff, N., Malkotra, C. M. and Claunch, B. C.: Quantative sacro-iliac joint scintigraphy: a critical assessment. Arthritis Rheum 22:837, 1979.

98. Esdaile, J. M., Rosenthall, L., Terkletaub, R. and Kloiber, R.: Prospective evaluation of sacro-iliac scintigraphy in chronic inflammatory back pain. Arthritis Rheum 23:998, 1980.

99. Daniels, T. E., Powell, M. R., Sylvester, R. A. and Talal, N.: An evaluation of salivary scintigraphy in Sjögren's syndrome. Arthritis Rheum 22:809, 1979.

CHAPTER 3

SYNOVIAL FLUID ANALYSIS

Synovial fluid analysis in the diagnosis of connective tissue disease should be considered equivalent to the use of urinalysis in the study of kidney disease. Studies may prove diagnostically specific as, for example, in septic or crystal-induced arthritis. In other cases, findings may be nonspecific but are still valuable in differentiating noninflammatory joint disease from inflammatory disorders. Complete examination of the fluid involves not only gross studies but also detailed microscopic, biochemical, and bacteriologic evaluations.

GROSS ANALYSIS

Normal synovial fluid is a light yellow straw color and sufficiently clear that large print can be read through it (Fig. 3-1). Turbidity increases with inflammation (Figs. 3-2, 3-3). The presence of gross blood or xanthochromia suggests a possible diagnosis of fracture, capsular or ligamentous tears, pigmented villonodular synovitis and other tumors or blood dyscrasias. Bleeding may also be seen sometimes in patients with rheumatoid arthritis, osteoarthritis and pseudogout. Bleeding secondary to the trauma of aspiration is generally uneven in distribution. Acute traumatic bleeding can also be differentiated from a bloody effusion by the fact that the latter exhibits little or no clotting. Normal fluid has a high viscosity similar to that of motor oil. It flows slowly from an inverted test tube and, when placed between the fingers, can be spread apart several inches before the fluid stream ruptures. In the presence of inflammation, the fluid becomes less viscous and more watery. Normal synovial fluid does not clot as it lacks a number of essential coagulation factors; conversely, pathologic fluids do clot and the rapidity of clotting increases with severity of inflammation.

An estimate of the degree of depolymerization of synovial fluid hyluronate which occurs in the presence of disease can be derived from the mucin

52

Figure 3-1. Normal synovial fluid (Courtesy, Dr. R. Gatter)

Figure 3-2. Synovial   fluid,   rheumatoid
arthritis. The fluid is slightly
cloudy.   (Courtesy,   Dr.   R.
Gatter)

clot test. When glacial acetic acid is added to normal synovial fluid, a tight
ropy mucin clot, white in color, is formed (Fig. 3-4). In the presence of
inflammation, the clot becomes friable and flocculent in increasing proportion to the degree of inflammation (Fig. 3-4). An alternative technique,
useful when the amount of synovial fluid is limited, is to add one part of
joint fluid (1 ml) to four parts (4 ml) of 2% acetic acid which has been
placed in a test tube or petri dish. Results of the test are classified as good,
fair or poor clot formation.

DETAILED ANALYSIS

Detailed studies of synovial fluid involve a total leukocyte count, a differential white blood cell count, sugar and protein determinations, ob-

Figure 3-3. Synovial fluid, septic arthritis. The fluid is grossly purulent. (Courtesy, Dr. R. Gatter)

Figure 3-4. Mucin clot test. A tight ropy clot forms when glacial acetic acid is added to osteo-arthritic synovial fluid (right). In contrast, a flocculent precipitate forms when the acetic acid is added to rheumatoid synovial fluid (left). (Courtesy, Dr. R. Gatter)

Table 3-1. Synovial Fluid Analysis in Arthritis

	Disease	Color	Clarity	Viscosity	Mucin Clot	WBC/mm³	% Polys	Sugar	Protein	Crystals	Bacteria, Fungi
Normal (Fig. 3-1)		Yellow	Clear	High	Good	< 200	25	± 10% of blood	2 g%	0	0
Group 1 Noninflammatory	Osteoarthritis Traumatic arthritis	Yellow*	Clear	High	Good	< 2,000	25	± 10% of blood	2 g%	0	0
Group 2 Mild to moderate inflammation (Fig. 3-2)	Rheumatic fever Rheumatoid arthritis Systemic lupus erythematosus Tuberculous and fungal arthritis	Yellow	Slightly cloudy	Variably decreased	Variably decreased	5,000 to 30,000	50 to 80†	20 to 50% less than blood	2.5 to 3.5 g%	0	0 (Except in tuberculosis or fungal infection)
	Gout Pseudogout	Yellow to milky	Slightly cloudy to cloudy	Low	Poor	20,000 to 80,000	60 to 90	20 to 50% less than blood	2.5 to 3.5 g%	+	0
Group 3 Severe inflammation (Fig. 3-3)	Gonococcal arthritis Septic arthritis	Yellow to purulent	Turbid to purulent	Low	Poor	50,000 to >100,000‡	75 to 100	More than 50% less than blood	3.0 to 4.0 g%	0	+

* May be bloody to xanthochromic if traumatic.
† 30 to 50% in rheumatic fever.
‡ May be lower in mild or early infection.

55

taining smears and culturing for organisms, and analysis for crystals (Table 3-1). The white cell count should be performed using saline as a diluent, because the usual white count diluent contains acetic acid, which will cause the synovial fluid to clot. The differential white blood cell count, performed after staining with Wright's stain, provides information about the relative number of monocytes and polymorphonuclear cells. Normally, the total leukocyte count is usually less than 200 cells per cubic mm, and the differential white cell count will reveal less than 25% polymorphonuclear cells. As inflammation increases, the total leukocyte count and percentage of polymorphonuclear cells progressively increase. Levels of 100,000 white cells per cubic mm with a differential count of 95% polymorphonuclear cells are not unusual in septic arthritis. Somewhat lesser elevations are seen in patients with crystal-induced inflammation.

Synovial fluid sugar determination is diagnostically important, especially if septic arthritis is suspected. The normal synovial fluid sugar varies within ± 10% of the fasting blood sugar. Synovial fluid and blood specimens should be drawn at the same time and with the patient in a fasting state, because it requires approximately four to six hours for the blood and synovial fluid sugar to equilibrate after food intake. Synovial fluid aspiration and analysis should not be delayed, however, if the clinical situation dictates the need for more immediate evaluation of other diagnostic synovial fluid studies. A low absolute value for synovial fluid sugar is diagnostically important regardless of when the specimen was obtained. Low synovial fluid sugar values are characteristic of severe septic arthritis. However, low values may also occur in patients with chronic rheumatoid or tuberculous arthritis that has been present for a long period of time.

It has been suggested that synovial fluid analysis for short chain fatty acids such as lactic and succinic acids, which serve as markers for bacteria in body fluids, may provide a supplemental diagnostic aid in the detection of septic arthritis.[1,2] In one study, synovial fluid lactic acid values were strikingly higher in nongonococcal septic arthritis, as compared to gonococcal or nonseptic acute disease.[1] In a subsequent study, however, lactic acid values were neither specific nor sensitive for septic arthritis.[2] Elevations of succinic acid were more helpful diagnostically, with a 100% sensitivity and 91% specificity for the presence of bacteria in synovial fluid.[2] These analyses require the availability of gas liquid chromatography, a procedure not routinely available at all hospitals.

Normal synovial fluid protein varies between 1.5 and 2.5 g%. The value progressively increases in proportion to the degree of inflammation. Measurement of total hemolytic complement (CH^{50}) may be helpful in diagnosis. Synovial fluid CH^{50} levels parallel the total protein in the same fluid and are accordingly one-third to one-half that in the patient's serum.

Obtaining smears and culturing for organisms should be routinely performed if infection is suspected. In patients in whom gonococcal infection is a consideration, the fluid should be plated immediately directly on blood agar and chocolate agar and taken at once to the laboratory for incubation. Repeated cultures of synovial fluid may be required for accurate diagnosis in any of the septic arthritides.

Analysis of synovial fluid for crystals is important in the diagnosis of gout and pseudogout. Initial studies are performed using an ordinary light microscope. For greatest accuracy, studies should be performed soon after joint aspiration. It is advantageous to add an anticoagulant so that the fluid can be re-examined later if necessary. Sodium heparin, EDTA (ethylenediamine tetra-acetic acid) or sodium citrate in solution can be used for this purpose. Lithium heparin anticoagulant should be avoided since it may yield crystals which resemble calcium pyrophosphate crystals of pseudogout.[3] Oxalate powder is also to be avoided because it provides a confusing source of crystal contamination. One or two drops of synovial fluid are placed on a glass microscope slide that has been thoroughly washed with alcohol and dried to remove contaminating particulate matter. A similarly washed cover slip is placed on top of the fluid and the edges of the slip are sealed with nail polish or Permount. The use of a sealant keeps the preparation from drying while under observation and also prevents motion of the fluid field. The crystals can often be seen at a magnification of $100\times$, but the $430\times$ magnification is usually required. Negative findings should be confirmed by study of synovial fluid cells and debris following mild centrifugation. Concentration of crystals in the sediment may yield positive findings in the absence of crystal identification in the routine wet smear. In acute attacks of gout or pseudogout, crystals are generally numerous and both intracellular and extracellular in location. These findings, properly interpreted, establish a diagnosis of crystal-induced synovitis.

Initial identification of crystals can be made on the basis of morphology. Monosodium urate (MSU) crystals are linear and needle-shaped (Fig. 3-5). Calcium pyrophosphate crystals are linear or rhomboid (Fig. 3-6, A). The linear form of the latter crystal is rod-like with blunt ends, in contrast to the more sharply pointed ends of urate crystals. Although the morphologic characteristics seen with ordinary light microscopy are helpful in differentiating the two types of crystals, polarizing microscopy is required for more specific diagnosis.[4,5] MSU crystals are strongly birefringent, in contrast to calcium pyrophosphate crystals, which are weakly or nonbirefringent. More specific identification can be obtained by using a first-order red plate compensator in the polarizing system. With this technique, urate crystals exhibit a strong negative birefringence. The crystals appear yellow when lying parallel to the axis of the line of slow vibration of the compensator and blue when lying at right angles to it. Calcium pyrophosphate dihydrate (CPPD) crystals, on the other hand, are nonbirefringent or weakly positively birefringent. They appear blue when lying parallel to the axis of the line of slow vibration of the compensator, and yellow at

Figure 3-5. Linear and needle-shaped monosodium urate crystals in synovial fluid. (Courtesy, Dr. A. Mackenzie)

Figure 3-6. Calcium pyrophosphate dihydrate crystals. (A) Rhomboid crystal, light microscopy. (B) Linear and rhomboid crystals, compensated polarized light microscopy. The large crystal lying at right angles to the axis of slow vibration is yellow, in contrast to the blue color of the crystals lying parallel to the axis. (Courtesy, the Arthritis Foundation)

right angles (Fig. 3-6, B). For practical purposes no further differential studies are usually necessary. Absolute identification of crystals requires more specialized techniques, such as x-ray or electron diffraction.

Crystals other than urates or calcium pyrophosphate may sometimes occur in synovial fluid. Calcium oxalate crystals may be present if oxalate anticoagulant has been used. As noted earlier, lithium heparin, used in some commercial vacuum tubes for plasma collection, may produce rod-like, rhomboid, or rectangular crystals with positive birefringence which resemble calcium pyrophosphate dihydrate crystals.[3] Dusting powders of starch used on sterile rubber gloves may be a contaminant. These crystals are ovoid-shaped and strongly birefringent. Steroid crystals are seen in fluid from joints recently injected with corticosteroid preparations for therapeutic purposes.[6] The appearance of these crystals varies, depending on the agent used. Some are identical in appearance to MSU crystals. Cholesterol crystals are not uncommon in chronic effusions. They have a characteristically flat plate-like appearance with notched corners. Xanthine crystals, seen in patients with xanthinosis, are strongly birefringent and negatively directed, similar to monosodium urate crystals. Fortunately, the rarity of xanthinosis makes diagnostic error unlikely. Other crystal populations related to arthritis have been described. Occasional cases have demonstrated the presence of dicalcium phosphate dihydrate crystals. These are strongly birefringent in a positive direction.

An association of apatite crystals as a cause of acute arthritis has been described.[7,8] Apatite crystals are rarely seen directly in the synovial effusion since they usually measure 1 μ or less in size. Certain light microscopic findings, however, suggest their presence. Shiny cytoplasmic coin-like inclusions result from clumps of crystals. Hematoxyphilic staining inclusions in cell cytoplasm seen on Wright's stained smears of synovial fluid may represent protein associated with clumps of crystals. Cytoplasmic inclusions of calcium appear dark brown with Von Kossa stain. Positively and negatively directed birefringent crystal chunks and rods which result from clumping of hydroxyapatite crystals are infrequently noted; these may be mistaken for monosodium urate or calcium pyrophosphate.

Some of the foregoing procedures for crystal identification can be performed in the physician's office with ordinary light microscopy. Studies of birefringence require polarizing disks, which are readily available and can simply be added to the ordinary microscope. Although a first-order red plate compensator requires a special microscope attachment, a reasonable substitute has been described that uses simple adhesive transparent cellophane tape.[5] One piece of tape is applied to the top of a glass slide, and then another piece of tape is applied over this. The cellophane-taped slide is placed over the polarizing disk and carefully rotated until the background is red. The long axis of the taped slide substitutes for the axis of slow vibration of the first-order red plate compensator. Not all adhesive

Figure 3-7. "RA cells," with protein inclusion bodies. (Courtesy, Dr. R. Gatter)

cellophane tape is equally effective and trials with various positions of tape may be required. Physicians whose practice includes a large number of patients with arthritis would do well to purchase a polarizing microscope with compensator attachment for ease and accuracy of diagnosis.

In addition to crystals, microscopic analysis may reveal protein inclusion bodies in the cytoplasm of polymorphonuclear cells (Fig. 3-7). These cells with their inclusions are called "RA cells," because they were first described in rheumatoid synovial effusions. Although they are seen most consistently and in highest number in rheumatoid arthritis, they are nonspecific and may occur in other rheumatologic disorders. Fragments of collagenous debris are not uncommonly observed during synovial fluid analysis. Although initially thought to be diagnostic of osteoarthritis, these fragments are a nonspecific finding associated with a number of arthritides. In osteoarthritis, these collagen fibers were shown to contain type II collagen, consistent with derivation from hyaline articular cartilage.[9] In inflammatory fluids, on the other hand, collagen types I and III were defined, suggesting a synovial membrane origin of these fragments. The collagen in these fibers may appear strongly positively birefringent; close attention to morphology and particle size usually allows ready distinction from crystals.

The presence of rheumatoid factor in synovial fluid tends to parallel positive findings in serum. Its presence in synovial fluid has limited diagnostic value, however, because a positive test may be seen in other rheumatic disorders.[10] Synovial fluid complement determinations provide some help in differential diagnosis. Low levels are characteristically seen in patients with systemic lupus erythematosus and seropositive rheumatoid arthritis but have also been observed in septic and crystal-induced arthritis. Elevated levels have been described in patients with Reiter's syndrome.

REFERENCES

1. Brook, I., Reza, M. J., Bricknell, K. S. et al.: Synovial fluid lactic acid: a diagnostic aid in septic arthritis. Arthritis Rheum 21:774, 1978.
2. Borenstein, D. G., Gibbs, C. and Jacobs, R. P.: Synovial fluid (SF) analysis by gas-liquid chromatography (GLC): succinic acid (SA) and lactic acid (LA) as markers for septic arthritis. Presented at Seventh Southeastern Regional Meeting, American Rheumatism Assn, Charleston, South Carolina, Dec., 1980.
3. Tanphaiachit, R. K., Spilberg, I. and Hahn, B. H.: Lithium heparin crystals simulating CPPD crystals. Arthritis Rheum 19:966, 1976.
4. Gatter, R. A.: The compensated polarized light microscope in clinical rheumatology. Arthritis Rheum 17:253, 1974.
5. Fagan, T. J. and Lidsky, M. D.: Compensated polarized light microscopy using cellophane adhesive tape. Arthritis Rheum 17:256, 1974.
6. Kahn, C., Hollander, J. and Schumacher, R.: Corticosteroid crystals in synovial fluid. JAMA 211:607, 1970.
7. Dieppe, P. A., Crocker, P., Huskisson, E. C. and Willoughby, D. A.: Apatite deposition disease: a new arthropathy. Lancet 1:266, 1976.
8. Schumacher, H. R., Smoylyo, A. P., Tse, R. L. and Maurer, K.: Arthritis associated with apatite crystals. Ann Int Med 87:411, 1977.
9. Cheung, H. S., Ryan, L. M., Kozin, F. and McCarty, D. J.: Identification of collagen subtypes in synovial fluid sediments from arthritic patients. Am J Med 68:73, 1980.
10. Huskisson, E. C., Hart, F. D. and Lacey, B. W.: Synovial fluid Waaler-Rose and latex tests. Ann Rheum Dis 30:67, 1971.

PART II

CLINICAL PRESENTATIONS

CHAPTER 4

ACUTE MONOARTHRITIS

Acute monoarthritis is a common form of joint disease. This problem frequently represents a medical semiemergency because pain and swelling can be severe and disabling, and also because infection, a common cause of this symptom, can result in rapid destruction of the involved joint.

DIFFERENTIAL DIAGNOSIS

Most likely causes to be considered:
Septic (infectious) arthritis
Gonococcal arthritis
Osteomyelitis
Crystal-deposition diseases (gout, pseudogout, calcium apatite)
Trauma
Mechanical internal derangement
Hemorrhage
Episodic rheumatoid arthritis
Palindromic rheumatism
Intermittent hydrarthrosis
Migratory osteolysis

Septic (infectious) arthritis due to acute infection is the most threatening cause of acute monoarthritis.[1-4] Gram-positive organisms such as streptococcus, staphylococcus, and pneumococcus are most frequently implicated in pathogenesis; gram-negative organisms such as the coliforms and salmonella are less frequently involved. Hemophilus influenzae is a common invader in infants and children up to age three years. Hematogenous spread from infections elsewhere, such as the skin, genitourinary tract, and lungs, is the most common mechanism of infection. Septic arthritis may result, however, from direct spread of organisms from structures contiguous to the joint or by direct penetration of the joint itself. Joints that are the site of prior disease, such as rheumatoid arthritis or osteoarthritis, are particu-

Figure 4-1.   Acute gonococcal arthritis, left ankle. A typical pustulovesicular lesion of the skin appears in the lower tibial area. (Courtesy, Dr. F. Bishko)

larly susceptible to secondary infection, much in the way that damaged heart valves are prone to develop subacute bacterial endocarditis. Septic arthritis is commonly seen in debilitated elderly patients, or in patients with chronic illness with low general resistance to infection. A diagnosis of septic arthritis should be strongly considered in patients with a disorder of the immune mechanism such as lymphoma and multiple myeloma. Clinically, large joints are more frequently involved. The joint becomes symptomatic over a relatively short period of time, usually measured in days. Pain, swelling, heat, redness and tenderness, the hallmarks of the inflammatory process, are present and increase in severity as the disease process advances.

Gonococcal arthritis, a form of septic arthritis, is discussed separately because it has characteristic clinical features not commonly seen in infectious arthritis due to other organisms.[5,6] Younger individuals are usually affected and a history of sexual experience can often be obtained. In males, symptoms of urethritis are frequently present prior to or at the time arthritis develops. Interestingly, gonococcal arthritis is now more frequent in females than males, probably because genitourinary gonococcal infection in the male is usually more obvious clinically than in the female and therefore more likely to be treated before joint infection develops.

Gonococcal arthritis occurs in two major clinical forms, systemic and localized. The systemic form is characterized initially by polyarthritis, high fever, rash and general malaise. Later, joint symptoms may become localized to one joint with persistent acute inflammation (Fig. 4-1). This clinical sequence can be likened to a burlesque show, in which the chorus girls step forth and then return to the line one at a time, after which the star finally comes out and stays! Large joints are more frequently involved, although small joints may be affected. The rash, usually seen best on the extremities, is the result of either hematogenous spread of infection to the skin with infectious angiitis or a systemic hypersensitivity reaction. It is most commonly characterized by pustulovesicular lesions that proceed to hemorrhage, ulcerate and crust (Fig. 4-1). Bullous lesions sometimes occur. The localized form of gonococcal arthritis is characterized by acute monoarthritis without the associated systemic manifestations just described. Prior involvement of other joints and cutaneous manifestations are absent; fever, if present, is low-grade. In both forms of the disease, tendinitis is common and most frequently involves the tendons over the dorsum of the hands and feet.

Acute osteomyelitis, an infection of the bony metaphysis, produces symptoms very much like those seen in septic arthritis and should be considered in the differential diagnosis of acute joint infection. A rapidly destructive disease, it occurs most frequently in infants and children. Although the infection may be initiated by introduction of bacteria from outside through a wound or from a neighboring infection of joints or soft tissues, hematogenous spread from a focus elsewhere is the most common inciting cause. Staphylococcus aureus is the most frequent infecting organism. In the usual hematogenous type, infection begins in the metaphysis of a long bone, most commonly the tibia, femur, or humerus. Bacteremia with septicemia are associated findings. Common constitutional manifestations include fever, chills, tachycardia, sweating and weakness. Locally, there is exquisite tenderness over the involved bone. The overlying skin is warm and the soft tissues are indurated. Laboratory studies reveal peripheral leukocytosis and an elevated erythrocyte sedimentation rate. Blood cultures are frequently positive. Roentgenograms may appear normal for several weeks. Later, bone destruction in the metaphysis is noted (Fig. 4-2). New bone formation is seen and the periosteum is elevated. Early diagnosis is important if severe bone destruction is to be avoided.

Most likely to be confused with monoarthritis of infectious origin are the crystal-induced arthritides. Gout and pseudogout (chondrocalcinosis) are the most common. More recently, acute arthritis related to calcium apatite deposition disease has been described.[7,8] *Gout* classically involves the metatarsophalangeal articulation of the great toes (podagra) (Fig. 4-3). Involvement of other areas, such as the tarsal joints, ankles (Fig. 4-3), and knees, is not uncommon, however. They may be the joints involved initially. Indeed, a significant number of patients may not show great toe involvement until after several years, if at all. Joint involvement is acute, often developing over a period of several hours. The average attack lasts three to five days, but prolonged symptoms lasting as long as several weeks may be present if the attack is untreated. The attack is related to precipitation of

Figure 4-2. Acute osteomyelitis, femur. Bony destruction appears as a radiolucent area in the metaphysis. (Courtesy, Dr. V. Goldberg)

Figure 4-3. Acute gouty arthritis. Acute inflammation of the first metatarsophalangeal joint. Acute gouty arthritis of the ankle was also present. (Courtesy, the Arthritis Foundation)

monosodium urate crystals with subsequent release of inflammatory mediators. Although an elevated serum uric acid is a characteristic finding in patients with acute gouty arthritis, normal levels may be seen in the initial stages of the disease. In some patients, elevated levels are noted only if the serum for study is drawn during the height of the acute attack. In other patients, for unexplained reasons, serum uric acid is normal during acute attacks, with elevations occurring during asymptomatic interval periods.[9]

Pseudogout, also known as chondrocalcinosis or CPPD (calcium pyrophosphate deposition disease), is also characterized by an inflammatory synovitis induced in response to deposition of crystals.[10,11] In this disorder, calcium pyrophosphate dihydrate crystals are deposited in articular hyaline and fibrocartilage and synovium, in contrast to urate crystal deposits in true gout. Symptoms are most frequently characterized by acute attacks; however, subacute and chronic symptoms characterized by low grade arthralgia or persistent swelling may occur. In some patients, a destructive, neurotrophic-like arthropathy may be seen, even in the absence of neurologic disorders.[12] The most common presentation is one in which calcium deposition is noted as a coincidental observation on roentgenograms involving asymptomatic joints. At times systemic reactions characterized by moderately high fever and, in older patients, a confusional state are noted. As in gouty patients, acute attacks of pseudogout may be precipitated by stress situations as after surgery or acute vascular accidents, or after marked diuresis in treatment of congestive heart failure. Precipitation of acute attacks following such illnesses may be related to a fall in serum and synovial fluid ionized calcium which results in dissolution of crystals from their cartilaginous matrix.[13]

The knees are the most frequently involved joints; podagra has been noted only infrequently. Other joints may be involved, including the wrists, elbows, shoulders, and ankles. Joint involvement may be monoarticular or polyarticular. Radiologic examination reveals characteristic calcifications in articular hyaline and fibrocartilage, which are seen with highest frequency in the knees (Fig. 4-4) and the wrists (Fig. 4-5). Although symptoms and roentgenographic evidence of joint cartilage calcification frequently correlate, joint calcification often occurs without symptoms. Conversely, symptoms may be present in absence of calcification on routine radiologic examination. In such cases, a diagnosis of pseudogout depends on finding calcium pyrophosphate crystals in synovial fluid or in synovial tissue at biopsy.

In most patients, pseudogout syndrome is idiopathic. Patients with hereditary forms of the disease have been described.[14–16] No definitive metabolic abnormality has been defined for any of these cases. Pseudogout has also been described in association with other disorders including hyperparathyroidism, hemochromatosis, Wilson's disease, hypophosphatasia, hypomagnesemia, hypothyroidism, and gout. It has been suggested that

Figure 4-4.   Knee, pseudogout syndrome. Meniscal calcification.

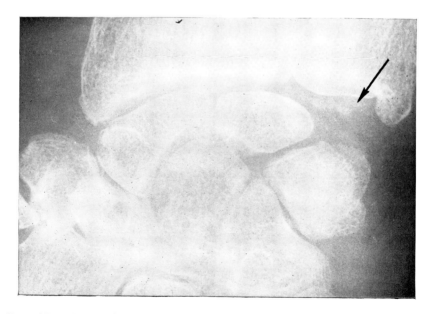

Figure 4-5.   Wrist, pseudogout syndrome. Note calcification of triangular cartilage at ulnar-carpal articulation (arrow).

inhibition of pyrophosphatase by calcium, ferrous and cupric ions may be related to the development of pseudogout in patients with hyperparathyroidism, hemochromatosis, and Wilson's disease, respectively. Absence of alkaline phosphatase, which possesses pyrophosphatase enzyme activity, and deficiency of magnesium, necessary for pyrophosphatase activity, are additional explanations for pyrophosphate deposition disease in some patients. A complete screening study for underlying associated diseases related to pseudogout would include serum calcium, phosphorous and alkaline phosphatase, serum iron studies, serum uric acid, serum magnesium and thyroxine levels. Calcium deposition disease secondary to hypomagnesemia and hypothyroidism are rare, however, and a practical screening study would include serum calcium, alkaline phosphatase, uric acid, and iron studies.

Recently, acute monoarthritis associated with calcium apatite crystals has been described.[7,8] Acute symptoms may occur in the absence of other articular disease, but associated osteoarthritis is not uncommon. The clinical presentation is similar to that seen in gout or pseudogout. Young as well as older patients are affected. Since apatite crystals are extremely small, they are rarely definable on light microscopic study of synovial fluid. Although periarticular calcification may occasionally be visible, roentgenograms of the involved joint are usually negative unless osteoarthritis is associated. Injection of apatite crystals into dog knees[8] and into rat intrapleural space and skin[7] demonstrate the phlogistic capabilities of these crystal materials. Specific identification of calcium apatite in synovial fluid or tissues from patients requires use of techniques such as electron probe or transmission electron microscopy studies.

Apatite crystal-induced inflammation may also be seen in patients with chronic renal failure.[17] Inflammatory symptoms may be articular, periarticular, or para-articular in location. A third syndrome related to apatite deposition disease is characterized by recurrent painful periarticular inflammation associated with roentgenographically demonstrable periarticular calcifications in multiple sites.[18,19] Common areas of involvement include the shoulder, greater trochanter of the hip, lateral epicondyle of the elbow, tendons about the wrists, and tendon attachments at the medial and lateral aspects of the knee. Material aspirated from the involved site often has a milky or cheesy consistency. Microscopic study of the material reveals typical globular bodies or "shiny coins" which likely represent clusters of apatite crystals. Disappearance of the calcific deposits noted on x-ray is not uncommon over a period of weeks or months following the acute inflammatory episode.

Acute trauma may cause acute joint swelling, with or without associated hemarthrosis. Pain, swelling and tenderness follow the trauma almost immediately. This is in contrast to the relationship of trauma to the precipitation of acute attacks of gout. In the latter situation, joint symptoms are usually delayed by 6 to 12 hours following injury, and the severity of joint manifestations is out of proportion to the extent of trauma itself. *Internal derangements of the knee,* such as tears of the menisci or cruciate ligaments, or loose bodies in the joint, are often associated with acute pain, swelling and limitation of motion. A history of trauma can often be elicited. The medial meniscus is most frequently involved and "locking" is common. Fracture in the area of a joint may simulate acute inflammatory arthritis as a result of tissue reaction to hemorrhage and damaged bone. A misdiagnosis of septic or gouty arthritis in patients with a fracture near a joint line is not uncommon! The chances for diagnostic error are augmented when the fracture is not associated with a specific traumatic event, as occurs in so-called fatigue *stress fractures* of bone. Patients with such fractures often show limited local pain and disability at first; later, pain increases and is accompanied by heat, edema, erythema and, at times, ecchymosis. Roentgenograms taken early are often negative; substantiation of the diagnosis is made only two or three weeks later when callous formation develops around the fracture site. Stress fractures are not uncommon in patients with osteoporosis but also occur in normal bones which have been subjected to repetitive, unconditioned stress activities. Frequent sites of involvement include the distal aspects of the metatarsal bones, proximal and distal tibia, and distal fibula.

Acute hemorrhage into a joint produces severe pain and tenderness. In addition to obvious swelling and warmth, the joint may become ecchymotic due to release of blood pigments. Joint hemorrhage may occur in normal persons following severe trauma. Patients with blood dyscrasias frequently develop hemarthroses, either spontaneously or following mild trauma.[20] Joint neoplasms such as synovial hemangiomas or malignant tumors must be strongly considered in diagnosis and appropriately excluded in patients who develop hemarthrosis in the absence of trauma or a known bleeding diathesis. Bleeding into the joint is a common complication of pigmented villonodular synovitis, a joint disorder of unknown etiology. Joint fluid in this disease is grossly bloody, or, more frequently, xanthochromic, as a result of previous hemorrhage. Pathologic study reveals a villous synovitis which, on histologic examination, shows synovial inflammation, distended synovial cells laden with lipid deposits, multinucleated giant cells and deposits of hemosiderin. Monoarthritis is the most common form of presentation, although sometimes two or three joints may be involved simultaneously.

Rheumatoid arthritis may occur as episodic attacks of acute monoarthritis (*episodic rheumatoid arthritis*). The patient's history reveals acute attacks of joint pain and swelling that begin abruptly and rapidly progress. Pain, often excruciating, is the initial symptom, and is followed in several hours by joint swelling, heat and redness. Interestingly, the pain may decrease in intensity as swelling ensues. The overall attack lasts several days to a week, and is followed by complete resolution. Small joints of the hands and feet, as well as larger joints, are involved. As the disease progresses, acute attacks become more frequent and prolonged, and complete remission no longer occurs. At this point, chronic joint changes characteristic of rheumatoid arthritis are noted. A similar clinical presentation occurs in patients with *palindromic rheumatism*.[21] Acute attacks of joint pain and swelling are similar to those described in episodic rheumatoid arthritis. Para-articular attacks of painful erythematous swelling of soft tissues are a frequent associated finding. Transient intracutaneous and subcutaneous nodules are seen. Chronic joint symptoms never develop, which differentiates this entity from episodic rheumatoid arthritis.

Intermittent hydrarthrosis, another form of intermittent joint disease, is characterized by acute, relatively painless, joint swelling.[22] This disorder usually involves one or both knees, although other joints may be affected. Attacks usually last two to four days. A true periodicity is noted, with attacks occurring at intervals of several weeks to months with almost clockwork repetitiveness.

An unusual cause of acute monoarthritis is *migratory osteolysis* (regional migratory osteoporosis, transient osteoporosis of the hip).[23] Patients are usually middle-aged men, and the hip, knee or foot is most frequently involved. Pain is often severe. Roentgenograms may be normal in the first several weeks, but osteoporosis becomes readily apparent later. Symptoms are self-limited, with symptoms disappearing and roentgenologic findings returning to normal after several months. Subsequent attacks in the same or other joints are not uncommon.

Although the foregoing disorders will account for the majority of patients with acute monoarthritis, almost any arthritic disease may occur in such fashion. Thus, in some patients, acute monoarthritis may be the initial manifestation of systemic lupus erythematosus, ankylosing spondylitis, the arthritis of ulcerative colitis or regional enteritis, Reiter's syndrome, necrotizing vasculitis and sarcoidosis. These latter illnesses are more likely to result in subacute or chronic polyarthritis, however, and associated clinical findings are usually sufficiently obvious to alert the physician to the correct diagnosis.

DIAGNOSTIC STUDIES

Synovial fluid analysis (see Chapter 3) is the most useful laboratory study available in the diagnosis of acute monoarthritis. Carefully performed, it often provides the diagnosis at the time of the first visit to the physician. Fluid from a septic joint is grossly opaque and cloudy and has a decreased viscosity. Frank pus is seen in severe cases. The addition of synovial fluid to acetic acid reveals a poor mucin clot, characterized by a loose flocculent precipitate. The white blood cell count is markedly elevated; counts of 90,000 to 100,000 white cells/mm³ are almost diagnostic. Polymorphonuclear leukocytes are the most prominent cells and comprise 75 to 100% of the cells seen on differential white count study. The offending organism may be seen on gram-stain study or will be identified by the next day following appropriate culture. Detection of bacterial antigens by counterimmunoelectrophoresis may be a helpful adjunct to diagnosis in the absence of routine identification of an offending organism.[24] In patients in whom *Staphylococcus aureus* septic arthritis is suspected but not confirmed by bacteriologic studies, assessment of acute and convalescent serum antibodies to teichoic acid in the bacterial cell wall may be diagnostically useful.[25,26] Elevated synovial fluid lactic acid has been described in patients with nongonococcal septic arthritis (see Chapter 3, p. 56). If gonococcal arthritis is suspected, the fluid should be cultured onto blood agar and chocolate agar immediately at the time of arthrocentesis. Simultaneous determinations of synovial fluid and blood sugar are important aids in the diagnosis. In septic arthritis, the synovial fluid sugar is markedly lowered, with the disparity between synovial and blood sugar paralleling the severity of the joint infection.

The synovial fluid in acute attacks of crystal-induced synovitis has many similarities to changes that occur in septic arthritis; the differences are mainly ones of degree. The fluid appears grossly opaque and cloudy, with decreased viscosity. The mucin clot test with acetic acid reveals a loose flocculent precipitate. The leukocyte count is most likely to range from 20,000 to 80,000 white cells/mm³, and the differential white count reveals 60 to 90% polymorphonuclear leukocytes. Characteristic crystals of monosodium urate or calcium pyrophosphate dihydrate can be seen, usually in large numbers (see Chapter 3). Gentle centrifugation of synovial fluid followed by examination of the sedimented material is a useful technique to follow when crystals are scanty.

A diagnosis of gout or pseudogout may be made by the identification of monosodium urate or calcium pyrophosphate crystals in asymptomatic first metatarsophalangeal joints.[27,28] As noted earlier (see Chapter 3), calcium apatite crystals can rarely be detected by light microscopy unless clusters of crystals are present, at which time they may resemble monosodium urate or pyrophosphate crystals. The presence of shiny cytoplasmic inclusions in wet preparations, purplish staining inclusions on Wright's stained smears, or dark brown cytoplasmic inclusions of calcium with von Kossa stain are strongly suggestive of the diagnosis.

Although a specific definition of crystal type is obviously important in final diagnosis, light microscopy alone is usually sufficient to determine that the patient has a crystal-induced synovitis. This information allows the institution of appropriate therapy for relief of symptoms, because these diseases respond to several similar therapeutic agents. The analysis of synovial fluid for crystals is most accurate if it is performed within several hours of arthrocentesis. If coagulation of the specimen has been allowed to occur, crystals can be best seen in white cells in the clot rather than in the supernatant. Although the finding of large numbers of crystals reassures one that the diagnosis is acute gout or pseudogout, septic arthritis may also be present on rare occasions; it is well to carry out appropriate cultures to complete the study.

Radiologic examination of the involved joint should be performed in all patients with acute monoarthritis. Loss of cartilage and bone demineralization are characteristic of septic arthritis, especially if diagnosis and treatment are delayed. Osteomyelitis reveals characteristic osteoporotic changes in the area of the metaphysis. Roentgenograms of the joint should be obtained at intervals of several days when osteomyelitis is suspected, because changes may not develop for a period of 7 to 14 days following onset of the disease. Evidence of fracture or chondrocalcinosis are other findings of value in the radiologic study of patients with acute involvement of a single joint.

Although clinical, synovial fluid and roentgenographic findings will lead to the correct diagnosis in many patients with acute monoarthritis, other laboratory studies may be necessary for diagnosis. Blood cultures are often positive in the presence of septic and gonococcal arthritis, and in patients with osteomyelitis. Gram-stains of material aspirated from cutaneous lesions in patients with gonococcal arthritis may reveal typical organisms. Interestingly, cultures from the same lesions are often negative. Uterine cervical and urethral cultures should be routinely performed if gonococcal infection is suspected. Rectal swab and pharyngeal cultures may be positive, particularly in patients infected by homosexual contact. It is imperative that all materials for culture for gonococcus be plated on culture media directly at the bedside, because the organism is very sensitive to temperature changes. Blood agar, chocolate agar and Thayer-Martin media should be utilized routinely for cultures from nonarticular areas.

Serum uric acid levels are valuable if gout is suspected, not only to provide diagnostic support but also to determine the severity of the biochemical abnormality prior to treatment. A needle can be used to demonstrate monosodium urate deposits if tophi are present. A 22-gauge needle is inserted directly into the tophus and rotated several times. Upon withdrawal of the needle, a small amount of urate material will be present at the needle tip. This is transferred gently to a clean glass microscope slide and studied as described in the crystal study of synovial fluid (p. 57). The tophaceous areas are usually avascular and bleeding is not a problem. Pain is usually minimal to absent. Serum calcium, phosphorus and alkaline phosphatase determinations, serum uric acid, and serum iron, iron-binding capacity and saturation levels should be performed routinely in patients with pseudogout to exclude associated disease states.

Studies of coagulation factors such as the platelet count, prothrombin time and partial thromboplastin time should be routinely performed if hemarthrosis is present. An elevated erythrocyte sedimentation rate militates against a mechanical etiology. A positive test in high titer for serum rheumatoid factor supports a diagnosis of episodic rheumatoid arthritis. Additional laboratory studies directed toward the diagnosis of less common causes of acute monoarthritis should be performed when these are suspected.

THERAPY

Patients with acute monoarthritis are often best managed by admission to hospital, especially if infectious arthritis is suspected or confirmed. Obvious cases of gout or pseudogout can usually be managed on an ambulatory basis. Even in these cases, however, severe discomfort may require a short period of hospitalization until symptoms are brought under control. Hospitalization allows expeditious institution of appropriate diagnostic studies and treatment. This is vital not only for relief of discomfort, but also to avoid rapid destruction of the joint in cases of infectious etiology.

In all forms of acute monoarthritis, pain relief is markedly aided by temporary immobilization. This can be most conveniently carried out by appropriate splinting. If a weight-bearing joint is involved, ambulation with its attendant stresses should be avoided until symptoms are under control. As symptoms subside, gentle joint range-of-motion exercises and power-building exercises for muscles should be instituted. Superficial applications of local heat may provide symptomatic relief. They pose some therapeutic hazard in the management of infectious arthritis because they may augment the inflammatory process; cold applications may be useful. Analgesic agents should be used as required. Although mild analgesics may be sufficiently effective, temporary use of narcotic agents may be necessary.

The specific management of septic and gonococcal arthritis and osteomyelitis requires the use of appropriate antibiotic agents directed toward the offending organism (see Chapter 19).

Acute gouty arthritis may be treated with any of a number of effective agents including colchicine, nonsteroidal anti-inflammatory agents, adrenocorticotrophic hormone, and adrenocortical hormone derivatives (see Chapter 19). Intra-articular corticosteroids may also be utilized once the diagnosis is made and septic arthritis excluded. Colchicine is the treatment of choice in patients whose diagnosis is questionable, since an excellent response supports the diagnosis. If the diagnosis based on clinical and laboratory findings is secure, the other agents outlined in management can be utilized. Acute pseudogout is similarly managed by one of several effective programs (see Chapter 19). Since the acute attack most commonly involves the knee, aspiration followed by intra-articular corticosteroid injection is feasible and effective. Symptoms in the knee and other joints also respond well to a short course of nonsteroidal anti-inflammatory agents. Response to colchicine is less predictable but this agent can be effective, especially when used intravenously.[29] Patients with acute arthritis or peri-arthritis secondary to calcium apatite crystals respond well to nonsteroidal anti-inflammatory agents. Response to colchicine is almost uniformly successful, in contrast to its relative unpredictability in pseudogout.

Joint rest is important in the management of acute monoarthritis due to trauma or internal derangement. Cold applications are advisable in the early stages, both to provide symptomatic relief and to prevent swelling. Warm applications are indicated later to reduce joint swelling. Isometric exercises help to prevent muscle weakness; elastic compression bandages are helpful. Surgical intervention may be indicated if ligament or cartilage injury is present.

Acute joint hemorrhage secondary to trauma usually responds to bed-rest, immobilization with splints to relieve pain, and appropriate analgesic agents. Cold applications used early help to diminish bleeding by inducing vasoconstriction. Warm applications are used later to speed resolution of swelling and resorption of clotted blood. The blood usually resorbs over a period of three to seven days and knee motion returns readily with appropriate physical therapy. In patients with blood dyscrasias, appropriate therapy for the underlying hemorrhagic disorder should be instituted to avoid further bleeding. If the hemorrhagic effusion is small, aspiration is not usually necessary. If there is a large, bulging effusion, aspiration is helpful to speed relief *after* the bleeding diathesis is systemically corrected.

Acute arthritides other than those of infectious, crystal-induced, traumatic or hemorrhagic origin can be treated initially with nonspecific anti-inflammatory agents; more definitive therapy can be instituted after the specific diagnosis has been ascertained (see Chapter 19).

CASE HISTORIES

History 4-1. Septic Arthritis

R. W., a 61-year-old black female, was well until January, 1973, at which time she noted dyspnea on exertion. Shortly thereafter, she developed muscle weakness that involved the proximal muscles of the upper and lower extremities. Joint symptoms were limited to the left knee. The latter symptoms had been present for many years and were characterized by pain in the knee on use, without swelling. Laboratory studies, including open lung biopsy and biopsy of the left deltoid muscle, were consistent with a diagnosis of polymyositis with pulmonary fibrosis. Left knee symptoms appeared unrelated to her primary diagnosis and were consistent with severe osteoarthritic changes seen on roentgenogram. The patient was placed on therapy with prednisone, 15 mg QID, to which both the muscle weakness and dyspnea responded well. Steroid therapy was gradually reduced to a maintenance dose of prednisone, 5 mg BID.

In June, 1973, the patient noted swelling and increased pain in the left knee. Symptoms became progressively worse over a two-week period. Analysis of synovial fluid aspirated from the knee revealed 55,000 WBC/mm³ with 78% polymorphonuclear leukocytes. Synovial fluid glucose:blood glucose values obtained with the patient in a fasting state were 30 mg/100 ml:96 mg/100 ml. No crystals were seen. Gram stain revealed gram-positive cocci. A culture of synovial fluid grew *Staphylococcus aureus*, coagulase positive. Antibiotic therapy with intravenous oxacillin was begun. Therapy with this agent was continued when sensitivity studies revealed that the organism was penicillin resistant. Oral oxacillin was substituted after four days, when clinical examination showed marked improvement in swelling, and synovial fluid analysis revealed a decrease in total white cell count and polymorphs. Therapy was continued for a period of six weeks, with successful resolution of acute findings.

Discussion: This patient with polymyositis and interstitial pulmonary fibrosis developed septic arthritis of an osteoarthritic left knee while on steroid therapy. Septic arthritis is more likely to occur in joints damaged by other arthritic diseases. Not infrequently, symptoms are attributed to a flare of the underlying disorder, rather than septic arthritis. A diagnosis of septic arthritis especially should be considered in patients on steroid treatment, because resistance to infection is diminished.

History 4-2. Acute Gonococcal Arthritis

E.L., a 29-year-old black, unmarried female, was seen in the outpatient clinic at University Hospitals on 9/22/80 with a history of pain in the right wrist beginning one day prior. Pain increased and was associated with acute swelling involving the right wrist and dorsum of the right hand. There was no history of trauma and the patient had been in good health. A history of sexual intercourse one week earlier was noted. Last menstrual period began 5 days prior to symptoms; there was no history of vaginal discharge nor dysuria. History was negative for fever, chills, or rash. Further inquiry revealed absence of history of Raynaud's phenomenon, sun-sensitivity, hair loss, dry eyes or mouth, or pleurisy. Past history was unremarkable.

On physical examination, the patient was noted to have acute inflammation involving the right wrist and dorsum of the right hand. The right wrist was swollen, grade II, erythematous and tender. There was similar swelling with inflammation involving the tendon sheaths over the dorsum of the right hand. Wrist motion was limited and painful. Joints elsewhere were normal to examination. Vaginal examination revealed normal external genitalia, normal vaginal mucosa without evidence of discharge, non-tender cervix, and a firm, non-enlarged and non-tender uterus. No masses nor tenderness were noted in the adnexa.

Laboratory studies revealed hematocrit 39%, white blood cell count 12,500/mm³, normal differential white cell count and an erythrocyte sedimentation rate of 35 mm/hour. Blood culture was negative. Culture of material obtained from the uterine cervix revealed *Neisseria gonorrhoeae*. Several drops of synovial fluid were obtained by arthrocentesis of the right wrist from a dorsal approach. Numerous polymorphonuclear leukocytes and a rare gram-negative diplococcus, not intracellular, were observed. *Neisseria gonorrhoeae* grew out in culture of this same material.

Although hospitalization for intravenous administration of penicillin was recommended, the patient requested outpatient treatment if at all possible. Accordingly, the patient was placed on a course of ampicillin, 500 mg QID p.o. (following a loading dose of 3.5 g administered with probenecid, 1 g) and was provided with a splint for relief of pain at the wrist. The patient was initially followed at daily intervals in the outpatient clinic and demonstrated good clinical improvement over the next several days to one week. Swelling, pain and tenderness of the right wrist and dorsal hand tendons rapidly improved and the patient was completely asymptomatic when seen in follow-up 16 days after the onset of her illness. Repeat culture of the cervix for gonococcal infection at that time was negative.

Discussion: This patient presented with characteristic manifestations of acute gonococcal arthritis manifested by acute monoarthritis and tenosynovitis. Rash, commonly seen as a result of either hematogenous spread of infection to the skin with infectious angiitis, or systemic hypersensitivity reaction was not noted, perhaps due to the rapid initiation of therapy following onset of her symptoms. Onset of acute gonococcal arthritis in close relationship to menses has been noted in previous descriptions of this disorder. Although high dose intravenous penicillin therapy is generally recommended to initiate treatment in this disorder, oral use of ampicillin or amoxicillin is reasonable when close follow-up can be maintained and the patient shows no evidence of systemic toxicity. Although the differential diagnosis must include other forms of septic arthritis, or acute onset of other connective tissue diseases, the clinical presentation was sufficiently characteristic to warrant a primary diagnosis of acute gonococcal arthritis by the house officer at the time of evaluation.

History 4-3. Gout

W. L., a 50-year-old white male, was first seen in consultation in October, 1973. Joint symptoms had begun approximately four years previously, at which time he noted acute onset of pain and tenderness in the left first metatarsophalangeal (MTP) joint. Serum uric acid studies performed at that time were elevated and a diagnosis of gouty arthritis was made. Joint symptoms resolved without specific therapy. An interval therapy program was not initiated. The patient had recurrent attacks of pain and swelling which separately involved the first MTP joints of both feet. Attacks were sudden in onset and lasted three to four days. Initially, episodes occurred at approximately six-month intervals; later, attacks became more frequent. Several months prior to evaluation he had noted acute pain and swelling in the third proximal interphalangeal (PIP) joint of the right hand. There was no known family history of gout and the patient had no history of renal stones. Colchicine was used for treatment of his last attack in the right first MTP joint, with excellent relief of symptoms. Six weeks prior to consultation, the patient had been placed on hydrochlorothiazide, 50 mg daily, for treatment of hypertension. System review was otherwise negative and past medical history was unremarkable. Social review revealed a moderately high intake of alcohol, with the patient consuming 6 to 8 ounces of whiskey per day.

On physical examination, blood pressure was 160/82 mm Hg. The third PIP joint of the right hand was slightly tender to palpation. Slight tenderness was also noted over the lateral epicondyle of the right elbow. No other physical abnormalities were noted. Laboratory studies revealed normal urinalysis, a hematocrit of 44%, a white blood cell count of 8400/mm³, and an erythrocyte sedimentation rate of 26 mm/hour (Wintrobe). Serum creatinine was 1 mg/100 ml. Serum studies for rheumatoid factor and antinuclear antibody were negative. Serum uric acid was 12 mg/100 ml. Roentgenograms of the chest, both hands and both feet revealed no abnormalities. A diagnosis of gouty diathesis with acute attacks of gouty arthritis was made. The patient was placed on colchicine, 0.6 mg BID. Laboratory studies were repeated several weeks later after hydrochlorothiazide therapy had been discontinued. Serum uric acid was 8 mg/100 ml and 8.6 mg/100 ml on repeat studies. Urinary uric acid excretion was 670 mg/24 hours. Creatinine clearance was normal. The patient was placed on probenecid, 0.5 g daily, with instructions to increase his dose at weekly intervals to a total of 0.5 g TID. Colchicine, 0.5 mg BID, was continued. Hydrochlorothiazide therapy was not reinstituted at that time. The patient was instructed to increase his daily fluid intake and to reduce or discontinue his alcohol consumption. On evaluation two months later, serum uric acid was 5.2 mg/100 ml on a dose of probenecid, 0.5 g TID. Blood pressure was 140/82 mm Hg. No acute attacks of gout had occurred during the period of followup.

Discussion: This patient had a typical history of acute gouty arthritis characterized by recurrent acute attacks involving the first MTP joints. Laboratory confirmation of the diagnosis was complicated by his diuretic therapy. Accurate evaluation of baseline uric acid metabolism required discontinuation of hydrochlorothiazide therapy. Colchicine, which does not affect uric acid metabolism, was given as prophylaxis against acute attacks while baseline laboratory investigations were being completed.

Should therapy for his hypertension be required in the future, several therapeutic approaches may be utilized. Mild hypertension may be treated with agents such as methyldopa, propranolol, hydralazine, or reserpine, which do not elevate the serum uric acid. Therapy with thiazides or other diuretics that elevate the serum uric acid may be utilized if appropriate increases in probenecid therapy are made to control the serum uric acid level.

History 4-4. Gout

H. M., a 59-year-old black male, was first seen in the hospital emergency room for evaluation of acute painful swelling of the left knee which had begun suddenly earlier that day. Symptoms had become progressively more severe and the patient had difficulty with ambulation. There was no prior history of joint symptoms, and no history of recent trauma. On physical examination, the left knee was acutely inflamed with marked swelling, heat and tenderness. Synovial fluid aspirated from the left knee was cloudy with a moderate decrease in viscosity. The mucin clot test was very abnormal. Detailed analysis of the fluid revealed 60,000 WBC/mm^3 with 92% polymorphonuclear cells. No bacteria were seen on gram stain. Further study showed numerous needle-shaped crystals with strong negative birefringence, both intracellular and extracellular in location. Subsequent laboratory studies revealed a serum uric acid of 11 mg/100 ml and a negative synovial fluid culture. The patient was placed on phenylbutazone, 100 mg QID, with instructions to gradually decrease the dose over a period of one week. Response to therapy was excellent. Repeat serum uric acid was 12.6 mg/100 ml, and daily urinary acid excretion was 540 mg. Interval therapy with probenecid and colchicine was begun. Probenecid, 0.5 g BID, was required to maintain the serum uric acid at a normal level.

Discussion: This case demonstrates the onset of acute gouty arthritis in a joint other than the great toe. Arthrocentesis and synovial fluid analysis allowed immediate diagnosis of the problem. Although the diagnosis of acute gouty arthritis appeared solid on the basis of synovial fluid findings, bacterial studies were performed to exclude septic arthritis, which may at times coexist. Phenylbutazone was used in the treatment of the attack. A trial of colchicine therapy would have been diagnostically valuable if the etiology of the patient's symptoms had been less certain. Newer less toxic nonsteroidal anti-inflammatory agents are effective in the treatment of acute gouty arthritis, and are currently generally preferable to the use of phenylbutazone.

History 4-5. Pseudogout Syndrome

W. T., a 62-year-old white male, was well until approximately six weeks prior to evaluation, at which time he noted acute onset of pain, swelling and tenderness of the left knee. There was no history of trauma or locking of the knee. Symptoms responded well to a short course of oral steroid therapy prescribed by his private physician. When seen at the time of referral, the patient was entirely asymptomatic. System review was essentially negative and past medical history was noncontributory. Specific inquiry revealed no prior history of joint symptoms. Physical examination was essentially normal with no evidence of joint swelling, tenderness or limitation. Presumptive differential diagnosis included gout, pseudogout, episodic rheumatoid arthritis or internal derangement of the knee. Laboratory studies revealed a normal complete blood count and urinalysis. Erythrocyte sedimentation rate was 23 mm/hour (Wintrobe). Serum studies for rheumatoid factor and antinuclear antibody were negative. Serum uric acid was 4.2 mg/100 ml. Serum calcium, phosphorus, and alkaline phosphatase values were normal. Roentgenograms of the knees showed calcification of the medial meniscus of the right knee and calcification of the medial and lateral menisci of the left knee. Joint spaces were well preserved. Roentgenograms of the wrist, feet and ankles were normal. A diagnosis of pseudogout syndrome as the probable cause of the patient's symptoms was made. No specific therapy was given and the patient was instructed to return for synovial fluid aspiration and analysis if acute joint swelling recurred.

The patient returned one month later when he had an acute onset of pain and swelling in the left knee similar to his initial episode. The left knee was grossly swollen; 50 ml of synovial fluid was removed. Analysis of the fluid revealed 32,000 white cells/mm^3 with 72% polymorphonuclear cells. Numerous linear and rhomboid-shaped crystals were noted, both intracellular and extracellular in location. Most of the crystals were nonbirefringent, but some crystals showed weak positive birefringence. The findings confirmed the initial diagnosis of pseudogout syndrome made earlier on the basis of clinical history and roentgenographic studies. The left knee was injected with local steroid and lidocaine, with good resolution of symptoms over several days.

Discussion: The clinical picture and laboratory findings in this patient were characteristic of pseudogout syndrome. Chondrocalcinosis of the menisci of the knees is not uncommon in older persons in the presence of few or no joint symptoms. It has also been described as a coincidental finding in patients whose joint manifestations are due to another underlying etiology, such as rheumatoid arthritis or gout. For this reason, pseudogout was initially considered a probable rather than definite cause of left knee symptoms in this patient when roentgenographic evidence of calcification was noted. Confirmation required demonstration of numerous crystals characteristic of calcium pyrophosphate in synovial fluid at the time of an acute attack.

In many patients with pseudogout syndrome, acute attacks are relatively infrequent and the disease can be managed effectively by joint aspiration and intra-articular injection of steroids at the time of an acute episode. When acute attacks are relatively frequent, prophylaxis may be attempted using various nonsteroidal anti-inflammatory agents on a regular daily basis.

History 4-6. Internal Derangement of the Knee

L. E., a 62-year-old white male, was in good health until 1964, at which time he sustained a twisting injury to the left knee when he fell from a golf cart. Slight swelling was noted and the patient was treated with ten days bed rest. Symptoms completely resolved. In 1967 and 1968 the patient had acute episodes of pain in the left knee associated with locking. Symptoms lasted for only several days each time and no swelling was noted. The patient was admitted to the hospital in November of 1972 for treatment of persistent locking of the left knee, which had developed two days previously. He was unable to achieve full extension of the knee without pain. No swelling was noted. System review was otherwise negative and the patient considered himself to be in good health. Past medical history was noncontributory.

Physical examination was completely normal except for findings involving the left knee. There was tenderness to palpation at the medial aspect of the joint line. Extension was limited to 15°. No swelling was noted. Laboratory studies revealed a hematocrit of 47%, a white blood cell count of 8100/mm³, an erythrocyte sedimentation rate of 4 mm/hour (Wintrobe), and a normal urinalysis. Serum uric acid was 4.9 mg/100 ml. Serum calcium, phosphorus and alkaline phosphatase determinations were normal. Routine serologic test for syphilis was nonreactive. Serum studies for rheumatoid factor and antinuclear antibody were negative. Chest roentgenogram was normal. Roentgenograms of the knees revealed narrowing of the medial joint space of the left knee with marginal osteophyte formation on the tibia and femur. An ovoid ossicle, 5 by 10 mm in size, appeared posterior to the tibial plateau, and seemed to represent a loose body. The right knee was normal. A double contrast arthrogram of the left knee was performed. The lateral meniscus appeared normal. The medial meniscus was shorter than normal and had a slight irregularity consistent with a tear. Arthrotomy of the left knee was carried out. There was an anterior tear of the medial meniscus, and two cartilaginous loose bodies were found. The lateral meniscus was badly scarred. The loose bodies were removed and the medial and lateral menisci were excised. The joint was carefully irrigated many times and a careful search was made for more loose bodies, but none were found.

Discussion: Monoarthritis in this patient was related to the presence of loose bodies and damaged medial and lateral menisci. Degenerative joint disease characterized by joint space narrowing and spur formation are frequent associated findings in patients with internal derangement disorders of the knee. Symptoms of locking are highly suggestive of the presence of loose bodies or meniscus injury. Recurrent acute effusions and, later, chronic persistent swelling are commonly seen. Similar symptoms are seen in patients with tears of the cruciate ligaments.

REFERENCES

1. Argen, R. J., Wilson, C. H. and Wood, P.: Suppurative arthritis. Arch Int Med 117:661, 1966.
2. Kelly, P. J., Martin, W. J. and Coventry, M. B.: Bacterial (suppurative) arthritis in the adult. J Bone Joint Surg 52A:1595, 1970.
3. Goldenberg, D. L., et al.: Treatment of septic arthritis. Comparison of needle aspiration and surgery as initial modes of joint drainage. Arthritis Rheum 18:83, 1975.
4. Goldenberg, D. L. and Cohen, A. S.: Acute infectious arthritis. A review of patients with nongonococcal joint infections with emphasis on therapy and prognosis. Am J Med 60:369, 1976.
5. Keiser, H. L. et al.: Clinical forms of gonococcal arthritis. N Eng J Med 274:234, 1968.
6. Partain, J. O., Cathcart, E. S. and Cohen, A. S.: Arthritis associated with gonorrhea. Ann Rheum Dis 27:156, 1968.
7. Dieppe, P. A., et al.: Apatite deposition disease: a new arthropathy. Lancet 1:266, 1976.
8. Schumacher, H. R., et al.: Arthritis associated with apatite crystals. Ann Int Med 87:411, 1977.
9. Hadler, N. M. et al.: Acute polyarticular gout. Am J Med 56:715, 1974.
10. Moskowitz, R. W. and Katz, D.: Chondrocalcinosis and chondrocalsynovitis (pseudogout syndrome): Analysis of 24 cases. Am J Med 43:322, 1967.

11. Moskowitz, R. W. and Garcia, F.: Chondrocalcinosis articularis (pseudogout syndrome). Arch Int Med 132:87, 1973.
12. Menkes, C. J., et al.: Destructive arthropathy in chondrocalcinosis reticulosis. Arthritis Rheum 19:329, 1976.
13. O'Duffy, J. D.: Clinical studies of acute pseudogout attacks. Comments on prevalence, predisposition, and treatment. Arthritis Rheum 19:349, 1976.
14. Zitnan, D. and Sitaj, S.: Natural course of articular chondrocalcinosis. Arthritis Rheum 19:363, 1976.
15. Regenato, A. J.: Articular chondrocalcinosis in the Chloe Islanders. Arthritis Rheum 19:395, 1976.
16. Van der Korst, J. K. and Geerards, J.: Articular chondrocalcinosis in a Dutch pedigree. Arthritis Rheum 19:405, 1976.
17. Moskowitz, R. W., et al.: Crystal-induced inflammation associated with chronic renal failure treated with periodic chemodialysis. Amer J Med 47:450, 1969.
18. Pinals, R. S. and Short, C. L.: Calcific periarthritis involving multiple sites. Arthritis Rheum 9:566, 1966.
19. McCarty, D. J. and Gatter, R. A.: Recurrent acute inflammation associated with focal apatite crystal deposition. Arthritis Rheum 9:804, 1966.
20. Kisker, C. T., Perlman, A. W. and Benton, C.: Arthritis in hemophilia. Seminars in Arth and Rheum 1:220, 1971.
21. Mattingly, S.: Palindromic rheumatism. Ann Rheum Dis 25:307, 1966.
22. Weiner, A. D. and Ghormley, R. K.: Periodic benign synovitis. Idiopathic intermittent hydrarthrosis. J Bone Joint Surg 38A:1039, 1956.
23. Duncan, H. et al.: Migratory osteolysis of the lower extremities. Ann Int Med 66:1165, 1967.
24. Dorff, G. J., Ziolkowski, J. S. and Rytel, M. W.: Detection by counterimmuno-electrophoresis of pneumococcal antigen and synovial fluid from septic arthritis. Arthritis Rheum 18:613, 1975.
25. Tuazon, C. U. and Sheagren, J. N.: Teichoic acid antibodies in the diagnosis of serious staph infections. Ann Int Med 84:543, 1976.
26. Mackowiak, P. A. and Smith, J. W.: Teichoic acid antibodies in chronic staphylococcal osteomyelitis. Ann Int Med 89:494, 1978.
27. Agudelo, C. A., et al.: Definitive diagnosis of gout by identification of urate crystals in asymptomatic metatarsophalangeal joints. Arthritis Rheum 22:559, 1979.
28. Ferraccioli, G. F., Manganelli, P. and Ambanelli, U.: Identification of pyrophosphate dihydrate crystals in asymptomatic metatarsophalangeal joints. Arthritis Rheum 23:1405, 1980.
29. Tabatabai, M. R. and Cummings, N. A.: Intravenous colchicine in the treatment of acute pseudogout. Arthritis Rheum 23:370, 1980.

CHAPTER 5

SUBACUTE AND CHRONIC MONOARTHRITIS

The diagnosis of subacute or chronic monoarthritis often represents one of the more difficult challenges in differential diagnosis in patients with rheumatic disease. This difficulty stems from the fact that subacute or chronic monoarthritis may be the presenting finding in a diverse number of rheumatic diseases, the clinical characteristics of which are often similar and at times indistinguishable. Fortunately, this form of arthritis usually does not represent a medical emergency. There is a reasonable period of time to elaborate the diagnosis, and nonspecific anti-inflammatory therapy is available for symptomatic relief until the diagnosis is made.

DIFFERENTIAL DIAGNOSIS

Most likely causes to be considered:

Rheumatoid arthritis
Degenerative joint disease (osteoarthritis)
Mechanical internal derangement
Plica syndrome
Osteochondritis dissecans
Avascular necrosis
Osteonecrosis
Chondrolysis
Chronic infection with Mycobacterium tuberculosis or fungi
Foreign body synovitis
Sarcoidosis
Pigmented villonodular synovitis
Synovial chondromatosis and osteochondromatosis
Joint neoplasms

Rheumatoid arthritis frequently appears in the monoarticular form, particularly in the juvenile form of the disease, in which monoarticular or oligoarticular involvement is common. The knee is particularly prone to

Figure 5-1.   Rheumatoid   arthritis,   right
knee. Joint space narrowing
is present. Bony erosions are
most marked at the lateral
aspect of the knee. (Courtesy,
The Arthritis Foundation)

this type of involvement, although any peripheral joint may be so affected. Swelling results from synovitis and accumulation of joint fluid. Other signs of inflammation, such as increased heat, redness and tenderness, are often present. Pain, even at rest, is a prominent complaint. These clinical characteristics are nonspecific and do not allow ready differentiation from other forms of monoarthritis. The erythrocyte sedimentation rate may be elevated only slightly; the test for serum rheumatoid factor is frequently negative. Roentgenographic examination reveals normal findings early in the disease. Later, osteoporosis, joint space narrowing and bony erosions appear (Fig. 5-1).

In *degenerative joint disease,* symptoms are slower and more insidious in onset. At first, pain occurs only with use; later, pain at rest is noted. Swelling, the result of proliferative changes in cartilage and bone, occurs late. Signs of inflammation are minimal unless an acute flare of disease is present. Acute inflammatory reactions secondary to associated calcium pyrophosphate or calcium apatite deposition disease are not uncommon. An exception to the usual lack of inflammation is seen in osteoarthritis of the hands. Here, osteoarthritis is often associated with a moderate inflammatory reaction in the distal and proximal interphalangeal joints. The erythrocyte sedimentation rate in degenerative joint disease is normal, and tests for serum rheumatoid factor are characteristically negative. Radiologic study reveals joint space narrowing, osteophytic spurs, subchondral bony sclerosis, and bony cyst formation (Figs. 5-2, 5-3).

Degenerative joint disease secondary to neuropathy, the so called Charcot joint, produces marked distortion of joint structures (Fig. 5-4). This florid form of osteoarthritis is associated with such disorders as tabes dorsalis, diabetes mellitus and syringomyelia, in which neuropathic changes affect normal pain and proprioceptive sensations in the joint. The joint is

Figure 5-2.   Degenerative joint disease, right knee, lateral and PA views.   Note joint space narrowing, extensive osteophyte formation and subchondral bony sclerosis.

Figure 5-3.   Degenerative joint disease, left hip.   Joint space narrowing, spurs, and bony cyst formation is evident.

Figure 5-4. Charcot joint, left knee. Valgus formation is severe. (Courtesy, Dr. A. Mackenzie)

readily overused, resulting in severe degeneration. The knee is involved most frequently, except in patients with diabetic neuropathy, in whom the joints of the feet are most frequently affected.[1]

Mechanical internal joint derangements most frequently involve the knee and usually result from tearing one of the menisci or cruciate ligaments. A history of trauma can usually be elicited, although the trauma is often so minor as to be overlooked. Pain occurs primarily with use; a history of locking is common. In contrast to rheumatoid arthritis, swelling at first is usually intermittent; persistent swelling follows if the disorder is left un-treated. Secondary degenerative joint disease is common. Loose joint bod-ies composed of fragments of cartilage, or cartilage and bone, produce similar symptoms.

Plica syndrome, due to persistent folds or bands of synovial membrane, is associated with symptoms similar to those described for mechanical in-ternal derangement.[2] Such folds or plica persist from early intra-uterine life. Inflammation of these plica may result from direct trauma or may be secondary to other mechanical disorders of the knee such as loose bodies or meniscal tears. Pain is increased with activity, particularly stair-climbing. Patients frequently complain of a sensation of snapping or clicking within the knee. Plain roentgenograms are usually normal; lateral pneumoarthro graphic views performed with the patient standing are diagnostically more definitive. Arthroscopy may be utilized to corroborate the diagnosis. Many patients respond to conservative management. Surgical release of the plica may be required.

Osteochondritis dissecans, a disease of unknown etiology, most frequently involves the knee and is usually monoarticular in distribution. It occurs most commonly in adolescents and young adults. This disorder is charac-terized by a separation of a section of cartilage and underlying bone from the larger bone to which it was attached. Although the lateral aspect of the medial femoral condyle of the knee is the most common site of occurrence, any diarthrodial joint may be involved. Pain, recurrent swelling, and lock-ing are typical clinical findings. Roentgenograms reveal a separation be-tween the involved segment of bone and cartilage and the bone to which it had been attached (Fig. 5-5). Early, the separated fragment lies in a

Figure 5-5. Osteochondritis dissecans, left knee. Roentgenogram reveals separation of a fragment of cartilage and bone.

relatively normal position within the bone. Later, there is a shallow exca-
vation at the articular surface and a fragment of cartilage and bone may
be seen lying free as a loose body. Secondary osteoarthritis is a common
complication when osteochondritis dissecans occurs after closure of the
epiphyseal lines.[3] Although the etiology of the disorder is unknown, several
mechanisms of pathogenesis have been postulated. An endarteritis that affects the blood supply to a segment of bone may result in necrosis and
subsequent detachment of the involved segment from its underlying bony
structure. On the other hand, detachment of a segment of cartilage and
bone may be a direct result of trauma, and ischemia of the fragment occurs
as a secondary phenomenon once the segment has separated. Endogenous
trauma such as repeated contact between an unusually prominent tibial
spine and the femoral condyle may at times be at fault.

Avascular (aseptic, ischemic) necrosis of bone results when an interrup-
tion occurs in its blood supply. Pain and disability in the involved joint
result. Lesions are most commonly monoarticular but multiple joints may
be involved. The head of the femur is a common site of involvement, but
the disease affects other joints as well. Symptoms of pain and joint limitation are slow in onset and localized. Roentgenograms reveal areas of bone
resorption in association with areas of increased bone density and frag-
mentation (Fig. 5-6). Bone scans may demonstrate abnormalities prior to
obvious roentgenographic change. Although the disorder may be idiopathic

Figure 5-6. Avascular necrosis, hip. A wedge-shaped area of bone resorption (arrow) is surrounded by areas of increased bone density.

in origin, underlying diseases that compromise the vascular supply of bone are often related.[4-8] Vascular impairment may follow trauma or may be associated with hematologic disorders such as hypercoagulability, polycythemia vera and hemoglobinopathy.[4] It occurs as a clinical complication of vasculitis in patients with systemic lupus erythematosus.[5] An increased frequency of avascular necrosis in patients on adrenocorticosteroid therapy[6] may be related to lipid changes in the blood, to fatty emboli from a fatty liver, or to marrow infarction from an increased fat cell volume. It is seen frequently in patients following renal transplantation,[7,8] in alcoholics, and in patients with cirrhosis or pancreatitis. Increased occurrence recently has been described in patients with hyperuricemia. An uncommon underlying cause is Gaucher's disease. Conservative therapy is designed to relieve pain and limit disease progression. Overuse of joints or excessive weight-bearing should be avoided. Analgesic agents provide pain relief. Intra-osseous pressure is elevated, even in early stages of the disease. Accordingly, core decompression by bone removal has been shown to be effective in symptomatic relief and, at times, in halting disease progression.[9,10] Other techniques of surgical management, including intramedullary bone grafting, osteotomy, arthroplasty, or prosthetic joint replacement have been utilized, depending on the stage of the disease. Management is most effective when diagnosis of the disorder is made early, when few or no radiologic changes are observed. Treatment of associated underlying disorders may prevent involvement of other joints.

Idiopathic *osteonecrosis* of the knee is a form of avascular necrosis.[11,12] It occurs in older patients and typically involves the weight-bearing surface of the medial femoral condyle. Pain is typically abrupt in onset; patients can often describe the onset of symptoms with unusual exactness. A history of injury is seldom elicited. Roentgenograms may be normal, especially early in the disease course. On the other hand, bone scintimetry shows a highly elevated uptake over the affected condyle even in the earlier stages of the process. Many patients with osteonecrosis respond to a conservative program with restricted weight-bearing, aspirin and other nonsteroidal anti-inflammatory agents, analgesics and straight leg raising exercises. Surgery, including osteotomy or total knee replacement, may be indicated in patients with continuous disabling symptoms and progressive osteoarthritic change.[12]

Osteonecrosis of the knee differs in several ways from osteochondritis dissecans. Osteochondritis dissecans is most commonly seen in a younger age group and a history of trauma is often present. The osteochondritic lesion is typically located on the lateral aspect of the medial femoral condyle; radionuclide uptake is usually only slightly elevated. Loose bodies are frequent with osteochondritis but rare with osteonecrosis.

Chondrolysis is an uncommon cause of monoarthritis of the hip joint.[13] Although most commonly associated with slipped capital femoral epiphysis in children, other associations such as lengthy immobilization have been described.[14] In some patients the disease is idiopathic. Symptoms consist of an insidious onset of hip pain and a limp. Roentgenographic examination demonstrates osteoporosis of juxta-articular bone, uniform reduction of the joint space and irregular blurring of the subchondral line of the femoral and acetabular surfaces. Conservative treatment with reduction of weight-bearing should be tried before surgery such as osteotomy or total joint replacement is considered.

Inflammatory monoarthritis due to *Mycobacterium tuberculosis* or various *fungi* may completely mimic rheumatoid arthritis. Pain and swelling are usually slow in onset. Systemic manifestations of the underlying disorder may be minimal or absent. Joint infection is usually secondary to primary infection elsewhere, such as in the lungs or genitourinary tract. Appropriate roentgenograms and culture studies directed to these common sites of primary involvement are essential in the complete evaluation of the patient. *Sarcoidosis* may similarly produce monoarthritis.[15] Synovial biopsy studies reveal either a nonspecific chronic inflammation that resembles that seen in rheumatoid arthritis, or may demonstrate noncaseating granulomas. Other manifestations of sarcoid, such as skin rash, parotid swelling and pulmonary symptoms, may be present.

Foreign body synovitis may follow the introduction of sharp, spiculated objects such as plant thorns,[16] wooden splinters,[17] or pieces of stone. The knee is the most common joint involved. Patients frequently present with a transient episode of acute synovitis following the injury; later, there is a variably long asymptomatic period followed by development of subacute and then chronic arthritis. Roentgenographic examination may be helpful if the foreign body is metallic. Thermography may delineate the inflammatory response surrounding the foreign object.[18]

The etiology of foreign body arthritis may remain obscure until the patient or family are directly questioned about a possible penetrating injury. Histopathologic examination of the synovium for vegetable tissue, seen particularly well with polarized light, is often essential to corroborating the diagnosis. Treatment is surgical. Because plant fragments may be too small to be seen grossly, all inflamed synovium as well as the entry track should be excised and examined carefully. If treated appropriately, complete return of joint function can be anticipated.

A rare cause of monoarticular disease, but one that should be considered in every such differential diagnosis, is *pigmented villonodular synovitis*.[19,20] This disorder has characteristics of both an inflammatory process and a benign neoplasm. Gross examination reveals a characteristic villous nodular synovitis. Histologic study reveals multinucleated giant cells, hemosiderin and distended synovial cells laden with lipid deposits. Pain and swelling are the principal clinical findings. Recurrent hemorrhage into the joint is common and accounts for the presence of grossly bloody or xantho-

Figure 5-7. Synovial osteochondromatosis, knee. Florid
ossification of synovium
is apparent.

chromic synovial fluid. Large joints such as the knees are most commonly affected but small joints may be involved. *Synovial chondromatosis,* another interesting entity, is characterized by metaplasia of synovium with replacement of synovial tissues by normal-appearing hyaline cartilaginous tissue. Ossification frequently follows with development of synovial osteochondromatosis (Fig. 5-7). This disease also occurs most commonly in the knee and presents as a chronic monoarthritis. Hips, elbows and shoulders may also be involved but to a lesser frequency.

Neoplasms of the joint, though relatively uncommon, must always be considered in the diagnosis of subacute or chronic monoarthritis. Lipomas and fibromas are seen but are quite rare. Synovial sarcoma (malignant synovioma) is a highly malignant disease of synovium with a low survival rate. Roentgenograms reveal a para-articular soft tissue mass, foci of calcification, and osteolytic defects in contiguous bone due to secondary invasion (Fig. 5-8). Metastatic neoplasms that involve bony structures close to joints may simulate chronic arthritis and should be excluded in differential diagnosis.

Figure 5-8. Synovial sarcoma. A soft tissue mass is interposed within the patello-femoral articulation. Lytic defects in the patella and femur are apparent. (Courtesy, Dr. V. Goldberg)

The preceding disease states will account for a high percentage of diagnoses in patients with chronic monoarthritis. Other etiologies must be considered, however, when the diagnosis is still unexplained. Chronic monoarthritis may be the presenting or major manifestation of any of the other connective tissue diseases, such as systemic lupus erythematosus, scleroderma or ankylosing spondylitis. Similarly, chronic monoarthritis may occur in psoriatic arthritis, the arthritis of ulcerative colitis and regional enteritis, and Reiter's syndrome. Finally, symptoms due to inadequately treated septic or gonococcal arthritis, gout or pseudogout may persist for many weeks and be the cause of subacute monoarticular disease.

DIAGNOSTIC STUDIES

As in the diagnosis of acute monoarthritis, synovial fluid analysis is helpful in differentiating the various causes of subacute or chronic monoarthritis. Findings characteristic of an inflammation (see Chapter 3) generally exclude degenerative joint disease as the cause of symptoms. Gross findings of xanthochromic or bloody fluid suggest a diagnosis of pigmented villonodular synovitis or joint neoplasm. Smear and culture of fluid should be performed routinely to exclude tuberculosis or fungal infection. Synovial fluid sugar is characteristically low in the presence of these latter chronic infections, but it may be similarly reduced in the presence of long-standing rheumatoid arthritis.

Peripheral blood studies should include a leukocyte count, differential white blood cell count, erythrocyte sedimentation rate and hematocrit, because abnormalities in these laboratory parameters are a clue to the presence of systemic disorders. Positive results for serum rheumatoid factor and antinuclear antibody are characteristic findings in rheumatoid arthritis and other related connective tissue diseases. It must be remembered, however, that positive tests for serum rheumatoid factor and antinuclear antibody are frequently seen in other disease states (see Chapter 2). Serum anti-DNA and "lupus band" study of the skin (see p. 34) should be obtained if systemic lupus erythematosus is suspected. Although gout is not a common cause of subacute or chronic monoarthritis, a serum uric acid determination helps to exclude this diagnosis. Abnormalities in the serum protein electrophoresis pattern support a diagnosis of a systemic disorder such as rheumatoid arthritis, tuberculosis or sarcoid. A broad elevation of the gamma globulin band is the most characteristic change observed.

Roentgenograms of the joint often have diagnostic value and should always be performed. Rheumatoid arthritis in its early stages is associated with a normal roentgenologic appearance of the joint. Later, osteoporosis of bone adjacent to the involved joint is seen. Advanced disease reveals loss of joint space due to cartilage erosion, bone cysts, and gross deformity of joint structures. Degenerative joint disease is characterized by loss of joint space, osteophyte spur formation, sclerosis of subchondral bone and bone cysts. It is important to note that osteoarthritis is a ubiquitous disease; degenerative changes may be present as a "red herring" and not be related to the clinical problem. Mechanical derangements of the knee usually do not produce radiologic changes unless they are chronic, at which time mild to moderate degenerative changes are noted. Double contrast arthrograms with air and opaque media are helpful in the diagnosis of meniscal tears, but experience is required for accurate interpretation. False negative and false positive reports are common. Roentgenographic changes similar to those described for rheumatoid arthritis are seen in patients with tuberculous or fungal infection, and in sarcoid arthritis. Pigmented villonodular synovitis produces characteristic large cystic erosions of cartilage and bone. Pneumoarthrograms may be needed to demonstrate the lesion at an earlier stage, particularly if small in size. Synovial chondromatosis is not visible on roentgenogram unless ossification with osteochondromatosis is present. In the latter condition, multiple bony opacities are observed within the confines of the joint. Erosive changes due to neoplasms are obvious when bone destruction occurs. Chest roentgenogram is helpful in delineating the presence of tuberculosis, fungal infection, sarcoid or primary neoplasm.

Joint scintigraphy may be helpful diagnostically, particularly in early stages of avascular necrosis or osteonecrosis. Unfortunately, in the later stages of chronic monoarthritis due to most of the disorders outlined, the radionuclide uptake will be nonspecifically increased and not helpful in differential diagnosis.

Skin testing for tuberculosis should be performed routinely. A negative test is reassuring evidence against tuberculosis but is consistent with a diagnosis of sarcoid. Cultures of sputum and urine should be considered if tuberculosis is strongly suspected. Appropriate serum serologic studies and skin tests should be performed if fungal infection is suspected.

When the diagnosis is not readily apparent, synovial biopsy should be considered. Closed synovial biopsy is attended by minimal morbidity and disability. Although the study can be performed on an ambulatory basis, it is often preferable to admit the patient to hospital for one or two days. Complications, which include infection and hemorrhage, are rare when the study is done properly. Tuberculous and fungal infections are characterized histologically by the presence of granulomas. The inciting organisms themselves are frequently demonstrable with appropriate staining techniques. Sarcoidosis is characterized by noncaseating granulomas; more commonly, however, nonspecific inflammatory changes of less diagnostic help are noted. Nonspecific inflammatory changes appear in rheumatoid arthritis and associated connective tissue diseases. Synovial findings in pigmented villonodular synovitis include multinucleated giant cells, hemosiderin and lipid deposits. Replacement of synovium by islands of hyaline cartilage, or cartilage and bone, are typical of synovial chondromatosis and osteochondromatosis respectively. Culture of synovium is helpful in the diagnosis of tuberculosis and fungi, since synovial fluid cultures may be negative even though infection of the joint is present.

Arthroscopy is diagnostically helpful, particularly when internal derangement disorders of the knee are suspected. This technique also allows localization of pathologic lesions for more accurate biopsy in patients with other local or systemic disorders. The availability of this diagnostic modality has decreased the need for open exploratory arthrotomy, a major surgical procedure which immobilizes the patient for several weeks until healing and physical therapy allow restitution of joint function.

Unfortunately, the diagnosis of the cause of chronic monoarthritis may remain obscure even after extensive evaluation utilizing all the above procedures. In most patients, however, careful diagnostic evaluation and long-term follow-up will usually lead to the appropriate diagnosis.[21]

THERAPY

Treatment of subacute or chronic monoarthritis usually involves two phases: treatment *prior to diagnosis* and treatment *after diagnosis*. Treatment prior to diagnosis is symptomatic and directed toward relief of pain, swelling, and limitation of motion. Adequate rest of the involved joint is important. The use of a cane or crutch in the hand opposite the involved joint is particularly beneficial if a weight-bearing joint is involved. Aspirin given in full dosage lessens inflammation and relieves pain. Further pain relief is provided by use of mild analgesic agents. Heat reduces inflammation and lessens pain; isometric exercises maintain tone and strength of involved muscles. In patients requiring additional therapy, other nonsteroidal anti-inflammatory agents can be utilized. When infection has been excluded, treatment with intra-articular corticosteroids may be considered. Use of the latter agent should be attended with appropriate caution; repeated injudicious use may result in secondary degenerative changes due to joint overuse and a direct deleterious effect of steroids on cartilage. In general, systemic corticosteroids are to be avoided even after infection has been excluded because their strong anti-inflammatory effect may obscure the diagnosis as the patient is observed in follow-up evaluation.

Specific forms of management including surgical considerations will vary depending on diagnosis. These measures can be instituted when the diagnosis becomes apparent (see Chapter 19).

CASE HISTORIES

History 5-1. Rheumatoid Arthritis

L.W., a 26-year-old white female, complained of left knee swelling beginning in August, 1972. Swelling and disability were gradual in onset. Pain was more severe in the morning and on stair-climbing. She was treated elsewhere with three intra-articular injections of local steroid into the knee, which gave relief for only short periods and was followed each time by recurrence of pain and swelling. There was no prior history of similar symptomatology and no history of trauma or locking. There were no joint symptoms elsewhere. System review and past medical history were noncontributory and she was in good general health. Physical examination at the time the patient was first seen in consultation in October, 1972 was negative except for moderate swelling of the left knee with slight limitation of flexion.

Laboratory studies revealed normal white blood cell count and differential, hematocrit, urinalysis, serologic test for syphilis and erythrocyte sedimentation rate. Latex fixation and antinuclear antibody studies of sera were negative, and serum uric acid was 4 mg/100 ml. Intermediate PPD and fungus skin tests were negative. Roentgenograms of the chest and left knee were normal. Synovial fluid aspiration studies of fluid from the left knee showed 3700 wbc/mm^3, with 43% polymorphonuclear leukocytes. Cultures for routine organisms, tuberculosis and fungi were negative. Initial diagnosis was monoarthritis of the left knee of indeterminate origin, possible monoarticular rheumatoid arthritis.

The patient was placed on therapy with aspirin, 960 mg QID, physical therapy, and avoidance of joint overuse. The patient had only moderate improvement and was admitted to hospital in January, 1973, for closed synovial biopsy. Repeat study of synovial fluid from the left knee showed no significant differences from the previous analysis. Tissue specimens obtained by closed synovial biopsy revealed mild synovial proliferation associated with a round cell inflammatory response and increased vascularity. No granulomas were seen. The patient was discharged on the same basic conservative program as previously outlined. Left knee swelling gradually improved, with only slight objective swelling noted nine months later.

Discussion: Findings in this case were consistent with monoarticular rheumatoid arthritis. No clinical or pathologic evidence of other causes of monoarthritis, such as tuberculosis, fungus infection, pigmented villonodular synovitis, osteochondromatosis, or internal derangement of the knee, were present. The patient did well clinically on a conservative program and showed no evidence of arthritis elsewhere. Roentgenographic examination and closed synovial biopsy were helpful in excluding other causes of monoarthritis.

History 5-2. Degenerative Joint Disease

R.K., a 74-year-old white female, was admitted to the hospital in December, 1973, for evaluation of pain and limitation of the left knee. Symptoms in the left knee had begun approximately ten years prior, when the patient noted onset of pain that was mild at first but became progressively more severe. Symptoms recently made ambulation difficult. Pain was aggravated by weight-bearing but was absent at rest. The patient complained of a grating sensation in the knee with use. There was no history of significant trauma or operative procedures to the knee. The patient denied symptoms in other joints and considered herself to be in generally good health. System review was otherwise negative and past medical history was noncontributory. Treatment with aspirin, indomethacin, physical therapy and use of a cane in the right hand gave only limited relief of symptoms.

On physical examination, there were no abnormal findings except for those noted in the left knee. Knee motion ranged from 5° extension to 100° flexion. There was no varus or valgus deformity. The knee was not tender and there was no evidence of effusion. A grating sensation was noted on palpation when the knee was moved through range of motion. Ligaments were stable. Laboratory studies revealed a hematocrit of 40%, a white blood cell count of 6400/mm^3, an erythrocyte sedimentation rate of 16 mm per hour (Wintrobe), and a normal urinalysis. Serum electrolytes, fasting blood sugar and serum calcium, phosphorus and alkaline phosphatase values were normal. Routine serologic test for syphilis was negative, as were serum studies for rheumatoid factor and antinuclear antibody. Serum uric acid was 4.2 mg/100 ml. Serum protein electrophoresis was within normal limits. Chest x-ray was normal. Roentgenograms of the knees revealed marked narrowing of the medial and lateral compartments of the left knee joint. Cystic changes were seen in the medial femoral condyle. Spur formation on both femoral condyles of the left knee was marked. The right knee joint appeared normal. Roentgenograms of the lumbosacral spine revealed moderately severe degenerative joint disease that involved the L1-2 and L2-3 intervertebral discs, and the apophyseal joints at L4-5. X-rays of the pelvis and the hips were within normal limits. A diagnosis of degenerative joint disease of the left knee and lumbar spine was made.

Due to the patient's severe pain and limitation of activity, a polycentric arthroplasty was performed on the left knee. At surgery, marked erosions of the cartilage of the medial plateau of the tibia and medial condyle of the femur were noted. The lateral femoral condyle revealed multiple small erosions. Large spurs were seen. Evidence of synovitis was minimal.

Discussion: In this patient, chronic monoarthritis was due to severe degenerative joint disease of the left knee. Treatment with aspirin, indomethacin, physical therapy and the use of a cane in the right hand was ineffective in controlling symptoms. The clinical features were consistent with a diagnosis of degenerative joint disease. Specifically, the patient had localized joint disease that was insidious in onset and slowly progressive. Systemic symptoms were absent. The pathologic findings noted on roentgenologic examination and at surgery were consistent with the degree of pain and limitation noted clinically.

History 5-3. Avascular Necrosis

J.M., a 37-year-old white male, was seen for evaluation in October, 1972. He had been well until a year prior, when he noted insidious onset of pain in the right hip. Symptoms gradually progressed, with increased pain and limitation of motion. Treatment with aspirin and short courses of phenylbutazone gave only mild relief. Crutch use was required to relieve increased distress associated with weight-bearing. No other joint symptoms were noted. System review was otherwise negative. Past medical history revealed a heavy intake of alcohol, up to 6 or 7 ounces of whiskey daily. On physical examination, the right hip was markedly limited and painful with motion. The remainder of his general physical examination and musculoskeletal system evaluation was negative.

Laboratory studies revealed a hematocrit of 46%, a white blood cell count of 6400/mm^3 with a normal differential, an erythrocyte sedimentation rate of 8 mm per hour (Wintrobe), and a normal urinalysis. Fasting blood sugar, serum alkaline phosphatase and protein electrophoresis studies were normal. Serum uric acid was consistently elevated with values ranging from 7.5 to 9 mg/100 ml. Twenty-four-hour urinary uric acid excretion on a normal diet was 830 mg. Creatinine clearance was normal. Serum studies for rheumatoid factor and antinuclear antibody were negative as were LE cell determinations. Chest x-ray was normal. Roentgenograms of the hips showed flattening of the right femoral head with preservation of joint space. The left hip appeared normal. Changes in the right hip were consistent with early avascular necrosis. Varus osteotomy and placement of a fibular bone graft into the right upper femur were performed.

Discussion: Avascular necrosis of the right hip developed over a relatively short period of time in this otherwise generally healthy male. Underlying etiologic factors that might have been related to the development of avascular necrosis in this patient included heavy alcohol intake and hyperuricemia. The patient was instructed to discontinue alcohol intake and was placed on an interval therapy program with probenecid for treatment of his hyperuricemia. No further evidence of avascular necrosis in other joints has been noted in subsequent followup.

History 5-4. Pigmented Villonodular Synovitis

S.D., a 73-year-old white female, first noted joint symptoms at age 72, at which time she developed intermittent pain and swelling of the right knee. Onset of attacks was subacute and symptoms lasted for periods of 7 to 21 days. There was no history of trauma or locking. Synovial fluid study during one of these clinical episodes revealed a grossly bloody effusion. The patient was in otherwise good health and no other joint symptoms were noted.

Physical examination was unremarkable except for the right knee, which was moderately swollen, slightly warm, and tender to palpation. Flexion was limited to 90°. Laboratory studies revealed a hematocrit of 36%, a white blood cell count of 6200/mm³ with a normal differential, and an erythrocyte sedimentation rate of 28 mm per hour (Wintrobe). Urinalysis, prothrombin time, partial thromboplastin time and platelet count were normal. Serum rheumatoid factor and antinuclear antibody studies were negative. Serum uric acid was 4.3 mg/100 ml. Skin test with intermediate strength PPD was minimally positive. Analysis of synovial fluid from the right knee showed normal color and viscosity. White cell count was 800/mm³ with 28% polymorphonuclear cells. Cultures for routine organisms, tuberculosis and fungi were negative. Chest roentgenogram was normal. Roentgenograms of the right knee showed degenerative spur formation and moderate narrowing of the femoral-tibial articulation. Severe narrowing and spur formation of the patellofemoral joint were also seen. Persistent severe symptoms were attributed to degenerative joint disease. Surgery of the knee was performed. Gross examination revealed moderate thickening of the synovial membrane and multiple erosions of joint cartilage. Histopathologic studies revealed changes characteristic of pigmented villonodular synovitis. A patellectomy and partial synovectomy were performed. The patient had moderate relief of symptoms and improvement in knee function.

Discussion: Pigmented villonodular synovitis most frequently presents as monoarticular arthritis. Xanthochromic or grossly bloody effusions are common. Etiology of this interesting entity is unknown. Symptoms may simulate those seen in monoarticular rheumatoid arthritis, severe degenerative joint disease, chondrocalcinosis, tuberculous arthritis, osteochondromatosis, internal derangements of the joint, or hemorrhagic blood dyscrasias. Definitive diagnosis depends on the demonstration of characteristic histopathologic findings on closed or open synovial biopsy.

REFERENCES

1. Sinha, S., Munichoodappa, C. S. and Kopak, G. R.: Neuro-arthropathy (Charcot joints) in diabetes mellitus: Clinical study in 101 cases. Medicine 51:191, 1972.
2. Hardaker, W. T., Whipple, T. L. and Bassett, F. H.: Diagnosis and treatment of the plica syndrome of the knee. J Bone Joint Surg 62A:221, 1980.
3. Linden, B.: Osteochondritis dissecans of the femoral condyles. J Bone Joint Surg 59A:769, 1977.
4. Tanaka, K. R., Clifford, G. O. and Axelrod, A. R.: Sickle cell anemia (homozygotes) with aseptic necrosis of the femoral head. Blood 11:988, 1956.
5. Ruderman, M. and McCarty, D. J.: Aseptic necrosis in systemic lupus erythematosus. Report of a case involving six joints. Arthritis Rheum 7:709, 1964.
6. Heinmann, W. G. and Freiberger, R. H.: Avascular necrosis of the femoral and humeral heads after high-dosage corticosteroid therapy. N Eng J Med 263:672, 1960.
7. Harrington, K. D. et al.: Avascular necrosis of bone after renal transplantation. J Bone Joint Surg 53A:203, 1971.
8. Ibels, L. S., et al.: Aseptic necrosis of bone following renal transplantation: experience in 194 transplant recipients and review of the literature. Medicine 57:25, 1978.
9. Zizic, T. M., Hungerford, D. S. and Stevens, M. B.: Medical versus surgical management of ischemic necrosis of bone in systemic lupus erythematosus. Arthritis Rheum 21:606, 1978.
10. Zizic, T. M., et al.: Occult ischemic necrosis of bone in systemic lupus erythematosus. Arthritis Rheum 23:767, 1980.
11. Lotke, P. A., Ecker, M. L. and Alavi, A.: Painful knees in older patients. Radio-

nuclide diagnosis of possible osteonecrosis with spontaneous resolution. J Bone Joint Surg 59A:617, 1977.

12. Rozing, P. M., Insall, J. and Bohne, W. H.: Spontaneous osteonecrosis of the knee. J Bone Joint Surg 62A:2, 1980.

13. Wenger, D. R., Mickelson, M. R. and Bonseti, I. V.: Idiopathic chondrolysis of the hip. J Bone Joint Surg 57A:236, 1975.

14. Hartman, J. T. and Gates, D. J.: Recovery from cartilage necrosis following slipped capital femoral epiphysis. Orthopaedic Review 1:33, 1972.

15. Spilberg, I., Siltzback, L. E. and McEwen, C.: The arthritis of sarcoidosis. Arthritis Rheum 12:126, 1969.

16. Sugarman, M., et al.: Plant thorn synovitis. Arthritis Rheum 20:1126, 1977.

17. Solomon, S. D.: Splinter induced synovitis. Arthritis Rheum 21:279, 1978.

18. Schenck, J. F. and Stosberg, J. M.: Use of thermography in the diagnosis of plant thorn synovitis. Arthritis Rheum 22:1037, 1979.

19. Smith, J. H. and Pugh, D. G.: Roentgenographic aspects of articular pigmented villonodular synovitis. Am J Roentgenol Radium Ther Nucl Med 87:1146, 1962.

20. Granowitz, S. P. and Mankin, H. J.: Localized pigmented villonodular synovitis of the knee. J Bone Joint Surg 49A:122, 1967.

21. Fletcher, M. R. and Scott, J. T.: Chronic monoarticular synovitis. Diagnostic and prognostic features. Ann Rheum Dis 34:171, 1975.

CHAPTER 6

ACUTE POLYARTHRITIS

Acute polyarthritis is a common manifestation of many rheumatic diseases. Relatively rapid diagnostic and therapeutic decisions are required by the physician to relieve the acute pain and limitation imposed on the patient. Hospitalization is frequently necessary to carry out appropriate diagnostic studies and to institute appropriate therapeutic measures for symptomatic relief.

DIFFERENTIAL DIAGNOSIS

Most likely causes to be considered:

> Acute rheumatic fever
> Rheumatoid arthritis
> Systemic lupus erythematosus
> Gonococcal arthritis
> Reiter's syndrome and other reactive arthritides
> Rubella and other viral arthritides
> Hepatitis-associated arthritis
> Arthritis associated with ulcerative colitis or regional enteritis
> Sarcoidosis
> Erythema nodosum
> Serum sickness
> Sickle cell anemia
> Intermittent arthritis syndromes

The arthritis of *acute rheumatic fever* is a characteristic prototype of acute polyarthritis. Classically, the arthritis is migratory, although a number of joints may be involved at one time. Although almost any peripheral joint may be affected, the rarity of involvement of the temporomandibular joints is a key diagnostic point. Fever, almost regularly present, may be as high as 103 to 104° F and is most frequently remittent in type. Clinical

101

evidence of carditis as manifested by congestive heart failure, pericarditic chest pain and murmurs secondary to endocarditis is common. Subcutaneous nodules occur primarily over bony surfaces, such as the subolecranon area of the elbow. Erythema marginatum, an evanescent nonpruritic pink or red rash, is a major manifestation of the disease. Lesions are characterized by peripheral erythema with central clearing. The margin of the rash frequently forms a ring, the so-called erythema annulare lesion. The rash usually affects the trunk and sometimes the limbs but never involves the face. Individual lesions appear and disappear rapidly over a period of a few hours. Evidence of prior streptococcal infection should be sought.

Rheumatoid arthritis may also begin as an acute polyarthritis. Onset may be strikingly abrupt with immobilizing joint manifestations developing over a period of 12 to 24 hours. More often, however, polyarthritic symptoms develop over a period of days. Systemic symptoms such as stiffness, fever, sweats and fatigue are prominent. Acute polyarthritis commonly occurs as the initial symptom in juvenile rheumatoid arthritis (JRA). Fever, a characteristic associated symptom, is high and intermittent in type; daily swings of 5 to 6° F are not unusual. At times, a remittent fever indistinguishable from that seen in rheumatic fever occurs. In contrast to the migratory arthritis seen in rheumatic fever, the arthritis in the JRA patient is persistent. Clinical diagnosis of JRA is aided by the presence of a typical rash that occurs in approximately one-third of patients. The eruption consists of pink or salmon-colored macular or maculopapular lesions that are rarely pruritic. Large lesions often exhibit central fading. Lesions tend to be evanescent and migratory and frequently develop concomitant with fever spikes. Involvement occurs chiefly on the limbs and trunk, but lesions may appear on the face, palms and soles.

Some adults may present as do children with a clinical picture typical of systemic juvenile rheumatoid arthritis (Still's disease).[1] Clinical manifestations are characterized by a spiking quotidian fever pattern, polyarthritis, and the characteristic evanescent, migratory salmon-colored macular or maculopapular eruption. Systemic symptoms are prominent and include fatigue, malaise, weight loss, and myalgia. Lymphadenopathy and hepatosplenomegaly are not uncommon.

Systemic lupus erythematosus may also begin as an acute polyarthritis. Other acute systemic manifestations such as fever, pleurisy and the characteristic facial butterfly rash (Fig. 6-1) are common associated symptoms. Additional symptoms, such as Raynaud's phenomenon, sun sensitivity and hair loss, may occur. Other of the so-called connective tissue diseases, such as polyarteritis nodosa, scleroderma, and dermatomyositis, may occasionally be associated with acute polyarthritis and simulate the joint manifestations of rheumatoid arthritis. In most of these diseases, however, the joint

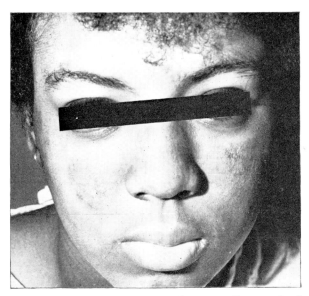

Figure 6-1. Facial butterfly rash, systemic lupus erythematosus. (Courtesy, Dr. B. Michel)

symptoms are limited and are overshadowed by other clinical manifestations.

Gonococcal arthritis often causes polyarthritis prior to localization to a monoarticular form of the disease. Low-grade fever and chills are frequently present. Tenosynovitis, although seen in other rheumatic disorders, is especially characteristic. A distinctive skin rash occurs: early, it is characterized by small maculopapular and vesicular lesions; later, the lesions become pustular and develop a dark necrotic center. A history of recent sexual exposure may be obtained. In the male, genitourinary symptoms such as penile discharge and dysuria are common; in the female, symptoms related to genitourinary gonococcal infection may not be obvious.

A not uncommon cause of acute polyarthritis in males is *Reiter's syndrome*. Clinically this disease state is characterized by a triad of arthritis, urethritis and conjunctivitis. Mucocutaneous lesions that involve the oral cavity and genitalia are common. In the mouth these lesions take the form of an aphthous stomatitis that is often painless. Genital lesions are characterized by superficial ulcerations of the penis that may coalesce to form a circinate balanitis. Cutaneous lesions most commonly occur on the palms and soles but may appear elsewhere. Small papules rapidly develop a pustular keratotic appearance. The lesions may become confluent and develop a thick keratotic crust, the so-called keratodermia blennorrhagica (Fig. 6-2). Skin lesions, although self-limiting, may last several weeks or months. Involvement of fingernails and toenails results in pitting and keratotic

Figure 6-2. Keratodermia blennorrhagica in a patient with Reiter's syndrome. (Courtesy, Dr. A. Mackenzie)

changes similar to those seen in psoriasis. Arthritis most frequently involves the large joints but the joints of the fingers and toes may also be swollen. The initial period of acute polyarthritis is usually followed by a more persistent inflammation, which may last from weeks to months. Urethral discharge or evidence of prostatitis is a characteristic finding. Although conjunctivitis is the classic manifestation in the eyes, iritis is frequently present. Up to 75% of patients are HLA-B27 positive, whether or not arthritis is present. The syndrome appears to be a "reactive arthritis" precipitated by various factors such as Salmonella or Shigella gastroenteritis or venereal contact in genetically predisposed individuals. Although considered at one time to be a relatively benign disorder, recurrent attacks and disability are not infrequent.

Infection with *Yersinia enterocolitica,* a gram-negative bacillus, may cause a syndrome similar, if not at times identical, to that seen in patients with Reiter's syndrome.[2] Infection with this organism most commonly causes a mild gastrointestinal illness characterized by abdominal pain, fever and diarrhea. Common non-gastrointestinal systemic manifestations include arthritis, urethritis, conjunctivitis, carditis and erythema nodosum-like cutaneous lesions. HLA-B27 antigen is found in up to 88% of patients with Yersinia arthritis. As with Reiter's syndrome, joint manifestations appear to represent a "reactive arthritis" in susceptible B27-positive patients.

Viral infections are not infrequently associated with acute polyarthralgia or polyarthritis. Amongst the best known and best studied of these syndromes are those that follow *rubella infection*[3] or *rubella vaccination*.[4] Joint symptoms are usually self-limited but attacks of brief duration may recur over a period of several years. The disease is more likely to affect adolescents or young adults, whether in association with spontaneously-occurring disease or after vaccination. Small joints of the hands are affected primarily, but large joints may also be involved. Articular symptoms usually occur synchronously with the typical maculopapular rash but may precede or follow it by a few days. Fever and suboccipital lymphadenopathy are common. *Erythema infectiosum,* "fifth disease," is a mild exanthematous illness, usually of childhood, which may simulate rubella infection causing a short-lived rash, fever, adenopathy, and arthritis.[5] The appearance of the bright red rash on the cheeks has led to its being called the "slapped cheek" syndrome. Joint symptoms occur most frequently in young adult females. Small and large joints may be involved.

An interesting form of acute polyarthritis occurs in association with *viral hepatitis*.[6] Studies suggest that joint symptoms are predominantly or uniquely associated with hepatitis B infection. Joint involvement is often symmetrical and polyarticular. Morning stiffness may occur. Hands, wrists, elbows and knees are involved most often. Urticarial, petechial and macular rashes are common. Tender erythematous subcutaneous nodules have been described. Joint symptoms often resolve as jaundice develops. Serum complement levels are characteristically low. Hepatitis B antigen (HB_sAg) is usually recoverable from blood when arthritis is present and has been detected in the synovial fluid as well. As the arthritis improves, HB_sAg usually disappears and the test for anti-HB antibody becomes positive. Cryoprecipitates derived from large circulating immune complexes have been described. This syndrome may be observed in patients with anicteric hepatitis,[7] in which case the diagnosis is frequently considered only late or not at all. Infection with hepatitis B virus may also be associated with clinical and pathologic findings of necrotizing vasculitis.[8]

Arthritis has been noted in association with a number of other viruses as well, including infection with arboviruses, adenoviruses, varicella, infectious mononucleosis, smallpox, and as a complication of vaccinia immunization. Viral arthritides often begin with nonspecific symptoms including fatigue and malaise, fever, sore throat, nausea, and vomiting. Mild fever and lymphadenopathy are not uncommon. Arthritis generally follows the prodrome although it may occur concomitantly. Rashes which vary with the particular infection are common. A diagnosis of viral arthritis should be considered in patients following recent immunizations, exposure during known viral epidemics and when joint symptoms are of short-lived duration without residua.

Articular symptoms associated with *ulcerative colitis* or *regional enteritis* are variable. The clinical spectrum includes arthralgias, chronic arthritis involving one or a few joints, erythema nodosum with subacute arthritis, and spondylitis. In addition, acute polyarthritis may be observed. Gastro-intestinal symptoms usually precede or occur simultaneously with joint symptoms. In certain cases, however, joint symptoms precede bowel symptoms by months or years.

Sarcoid is associated with variable joint manifestations, which include arthralgias or overt arthritis. Acute or chronic monoarthritis or polyarthritis may be seen. Other clinical evidence of sarcoid, such as fever, skin rash, iritis and parotid swelling, is frequently present. Hilar adenopathy and a negative tuberculin skin test support the diagnosis.

Erythema nodosum is a syndrome characterized by acute or subacute polyarthritis, hilar adenopathy, and tender, erythematous, nodular cutaneous swellings. This disorder may occur as a primary disease or secondary to other diseases including streptococcal infection, coccidioidomycosis, ulcerative colitis or regional enteritis, active tuberculosis and sarcoid. In addition, erythema nodosum is a manifestation of drug sensitivity, particularly to iodides, bromides and sulfonamides. More recently, its occurrence has been noted with the use of oral contraceptives. The nodular skin lesions appear most commonly on the anterior aspect of the lower extremities, especially the tibial areas (Fig. 6-3). Upper extremities are involved occasionally. The lesions are warm, tender and painful, and vary in size

Figure 6-3. Erythema nodosum. Erythematous nodular lesions are seen along both anterior tibial areas. (Courtesy, Dr. B. Michel)

from one-half centimeter to several centimeters in diameter. They frequently recur in crops and last for periods varying from days to weeks. The associated arthritis primarily affects large joints, such as ankles, knees and wrists.

Acute polyarthritis occurs as a manifestation of *serum sickness* or *drug sensitivity* reactions. Low-grade fever, urticaria and lymphadenopathy are associated symptoms. Large and medium-sized joints are usually affected, although any joint may be involved. The arthritis is often migratory and may resemble acute rheumatic fever or gonococcal arthritis.

Severe acute polyarthralgia or polyarthritis is seen in patients with *sickle cell anemia.*[9] Joint symptoms result from local sickling and thrombosis in synovial vessels. Variable degrees of joint swelling occur. Other symptoms of sickle cell disease, such as abdominal crises, are usually present. Diagnostic studies reveal anemia, sickling changes in peripheral red blood cells and the presence of hemoglobin S. Synovial fluid analysis often shows minimal deviations from the normal. Roentgenograms reveal widening of bony medullary cavities, cortical thinning and irregular trabecular markings. Other forms of joint involvement in the hemoglobinopathies include aseptic necrosis, gout, joint hemorrhage, osteomyelitis and septic arthritis.

Acute polyarthritis is also commonly seen in a group of arthritic syndromes characterized by their prominent intermittency of recurrence. Such syndromes include palindromic rheumatism, familial Mediterranean fever, Whipple's disease, relapsing polychondritis and arthritis associated with hyperlipidemia. These syndromes are discussed in more detail in Chapter 8.

Other diseases are associated with acute polyarthritis; these entities are interesting but fortunately relatively uncommon. *Behçet's syndrome,* a disease of unknown cause, is characterized by a clinical triad of oral and genital ulcers and iritis. In many cases, milder eye symptoms, such as conjunctivitis or episcleritis, are observed. Cutaneous lesions, phlebitis, colitis and central nervous system lesions are frequently present. Polyarthritis may be acute or subacute. *Henoch-Schönlein purpura* (anaphylactoid purpura) is characterized by arthralgias or arthritis, cutaneous purpura, abdominal pain, gastrointestinal hemorrhage and renal disease. It occurs mostly in children and young adults. Cutaneous lesions consist of erythematous urticarial papules and purpura (Fig. 6-4). Polyarthritis most frequently affects larger joints. Joint symptoms are transient and unassociated with deformity. Crampy abdominal pain and melena are common. Intussusception may complicate the clinical picture. Renal involvement may lead to proteinuria, hematuria and, at times, fatal renal failure. Prognosis is generally good if renal manifestations are mild.

Acute polyarthritis is occasionally seen in other diseases. These latter states do not represent a major problem in differential diagnosis, either because the disease itself or the appearance of joint symptoms as an acute

Figure 6-4.   Henoch - Schönlein (anaphylactoid) purpura, involving both lower extremities. (Courtesy, Dr. A. Mackenzie)

polyarthritis is relatively uncommon. For example, although gout classically initially appears as an acute monoarthritis, patients with acute polyarticular disease as an initial or early manifestation have been described.[10] Two or more joints may be involved. In other gouty patients, acute polyarthritis may occur after a prolonged period of disease when interval therapy has been inadequate. In the latter cases, a careful review of the history usually reveals previous recurrent attacks of acute monoarthritis for many years. Acute polyarthritis also occurs in patients with pseudogout syndrome (chondrocalcinosis). In most cases, however, joint symptoms are limited to one or a few joints at any given time.

Relatively acute polyarthralgia or polyarthritis is seen in patients with leukemia.[11] Joint symptoms and swelling result from leukemic infiltration of synovium, or from leukemic involvement of bone contiguous to the joint. Patients with pancreatic carcinoma or pancreatitis may develop subcutaneous fat necrosis and acute arthritis.[12] Involvement of other serosal surfaces leads to pleuritis with effusion, pericarditis, and ascites. Elevations of amylase and lipase are noted both in the serum and in involved body cavities. Although it is likely that the serositis and fat necrosis are strongly related to pancreatic enzyme activity, the finding of low complement levels in involved fluids suggests a possible immune complex pathogenesis for the disorder. Large joints of the lower extremities are most frequently affected. Although pauci-articular disease is most common, polyarticular disease may be seen.

Acute polyarthritis has been described in patients with Type II hyperlipoproteinemia,[13] in which case acute migratory arthritis may simulate rheumatic fever. Attacks last from a few days to one month. Large peripheral joints are usually affected. Episodic tendinitis of the Achilles tendon also occurs in this condition.[14] Associated clinical findings include xanthomatosis, xanthelasma, corneal arcus and early atherosclerosis. Laboratory studies reveal marked elevations of serum cholesterol with normal concentrations of triglycerides. Treatment of acute attacks is symptomatic. Rarely, acute polyarthritis may result from simultaneous involvement of several joints in patients with septic arthritis or hemorrhagic disorders.

DIAGNOSTIC STUDIES

A number of studies are frequently required in the search for the correct diagnosis in patients with acute polyarthritis. Initial studies should usually include a complete blood count, urinalysis, erythrocyte sedimentation rate, throat culture, antistreptolysin-O titer, electrocardiogram, serum protein electrophoresis, serum complement, and tests for rheumatoid factor and antinuclear antibody. A serologic test for syphilis (STS) is valuable because a false positive STS supports a diagnosis of systemic connective tissue disease. Serum glutamic oxaloacetic transaminase and hepatitis B antigen (Hb_sAg) and antibody determinations should be performed if viral hepatitis is suspected.

Roentgenograms of joints usually have limited diagnostic value, especially early in the course of the various diseases. Articular chondrocalcinosis is seen in pseudogout syndrome. Chest roentgenograms are helpful in the diagnosis of sarcoid or erythema nodosum. More specific diagnostic studies, such as sigmoidoscopy and roentgenograms of the large and small bowel, are indicated if one of the enteropathic arthritides such as regional enteritis or ulcerative colitis is suspected. Blood cultures are often positive in the presence of infectious polyarthritis. Joint fluid studies are especially helpful in delineating the presence of gonococcal or septic arthritis; they have lesser value in the differential diagnosis of other forms of acute polyarthritis because the findings are often similar and nonspecific. If gonococcal arthritis is suspected, a carefully performed culture from the uterine cervix should be obtained in women; in men, cultures of penile discharge or of penile secretions following prostatic massage are indicated. Gram-stain smear and cultures from cutaneous gonococcal lesions may be diagnostically helpful. Rectal swab and pharyngeal cultures are indicated, especially if homosexual contact is suspected.

Despite a carefully performed history and physical examination and detailed diagnostic studies, a specific diagnosis may remain elusive. When indicated, additional diagnostic studies such as barium enema, hemoglobin electrophoresis, clotting studies, immunoelectrophoresis, cryoglobulin determinations, and viral serologic studies should be pursued depending on the suspected diagnosis. In many cases, successful diagnosis usually depends on repeated and prolonged clinical observation and follow-up diagnostic studies.

THERAPY

As noted earlier, patients with acute polyarthritis usually require hospitalization in order to perform detailed extensive diagnostic studies and to institute nonspecific or specific therapeutic measures directed toward relief of symptoms. Bed rest and the appropriate use of splints for immobilization provide pain relief. High doses of aspirin reduce inflammation; in addition, its use may provide valuable clues to differential diagnosis. Rapid and complete resolution of fever and acute joint symptoms in response to high doses of aspirin supports a diagnosis of acute rheumatic fever. Doses of 100 mg/kg/day in small children and 960 mg every four hours in adults are utilized as a diagnostic test. Although aspirin induces some relief from symptoms and fever in other forms of acute polyarthritis, the response is considerably less complete and dramatic than that which occurs in acute rheumatic fever. Physical therapy should be limited to gentle range-of-motion exercises as tolerated. Local applications of superficial heat are usually beneficial, although some patients respond better to cold. Mild analgesic agents such as acetaminophen, propoxyphene HCl (Darvon), or ethoheptazine citrate (Zactane) are helpful; at times, short courses of mild narcotics such as codeine may be necessary. Overly aggressive nonspecific multiple therapeutic regimens should be avoided; symptoms may be temporarily relieved but often at the price of obscuring the diagnosis.

Other non-steroidal anti-inflammatory agents may be given when relief with aspirin is inadequate. The indiscriminate use of corticosteroids to treat acute polyarthritis should be avoided. They are hazardous if given in the presence of undetected infection; in addition, they may suppress symptoms and laboratory findings vital to diagnosis.

Definitive therapy directed to the various disorders is instituted when a specific diagnosis has been confirmed (see Chapter 19). In those cases in which the diagnosis remains uncertain, more aggressive therapeutic measures can be begun when infection has been excluded and a reasonable probable diagnosis has been made.

CASE HISTORIES

History 6-1. Acute Rheumatic Fever

S.C., a 13-year-old white male, was admitted to Babies and Children's Hospital with a two-day history of painful joints. The patient had been in good health until nine days prior to admission, when he developed a sore throat with "swollen glands." These symptoms cleared after one day and the patient was well until one week prior to admission when he sustained an injury to the left hip after a fall. The hip was painful for several days following. Three days prior to admission, the patient developed a fever and dry cough, worse at night. Two days prior to admission, the patient developed an erythematous rash which involved the umbilical area, lower trunk, and upper and lower extremities. Nodule formation was noted in the subolecranon area of the right elbow and occiput. One day prior to admission, the patient developed a painful swollen right ankle, followed by swelling and pain of the left ankle, left knee and left elbow. There was no history of diarrhea, dysuria, hematuria, chorea, dyspnea or orthopnea. Review for connective tissue disease symptoms revealed absence of pleurisy, sun-sensitivity, Raynaud's phenomenon or hair loss. Past medical history was essentially negative except for the usual childhood diseases.

On physical examination, blood pressure was 130/85, pulse 110/min, respirations 18/min, and temperature 39°C. There were multiple 2 $\times$ 4 cm wheal-like erythematous lesions with serpiginous borders over the skin of the trunk, arms and legs; these changed in appearance during the course of the examination. Cardiac examination revealed a hyperdynamic left ventricular impulse with an S_3 gallop at the apex. A grade II/VI systolic ejection murmur was heard at the left lower sternal border, a grade III/VI holosystolic murmur at the apex, and a grade II/VI diastolic decrescendo murmur at the left sternal border at the third intercostal space. The liver was enlarged to 3 cm below the costal margin and was slightly tender. There were 1 $\times$ 1.5 cm nodules at the right subolecranon area and at the occiput. Both ankles, the left knee and left elbow were swollen, painful, tender, red and slightly warm.

Laboratory evaluation revealed normal urinalysis except for 1+ albumin, BUN 16 mg/100 ml, normal blood sugar and serum electrolytes. White blood cell count was 15,700/mm³ with 67% segmented cells. Hematocrit was 38%. Erythrocyte sedimentation rate was 38 mm/hour, corrected. ASO titer was 333 Todd units. Monospot test for infectious mononucleosis was negative. Serum antinuclear antibody titer and rheumatoid factor studies were negative. Throat culture revealed a heavy growth of beta hemolytic streptococcus, group A. Chest roentgenogram showed slight prominence of the left border of the heart but otherwise normal configuration. Pulmonary vascular markings were normal and the parenchyma were free of infiltrates. Electrocardiographic study revealed low voltage with primary AV block. A diagnosis of acute rheumatic fever was made on the basis of 4 of 5 major criteria, including acute polyarthritis, subcutaneous nodules, erythema marginatum, and carditis with aortic and mitral regurgitation. Clinical examination supported a diagnosis of borderline congestive heart failure.

Therapy with prednisone, 20 mg q6h p.o., and penicillin-VK 250 mg q6h p.o. was begun, and digitalization initiated. The patient was placed on absolute bedrest and provided with a low salt diet. The patient became afebrile after 24 hours. Cardiac manifestations and joint symptoms were dramatically improved after 48 hours. Prednisone therapy was gradually reduced and full doses of salicylates substituted when the patient continued to exhibit good clinical response with respect to his subjective and objective manifestations of carditis, fever, rash and arthritis. The lesions of erythema marginatum and subcutaneous nodules resolved after a period of 7 days. No symptom rebound was noted when prednisone was discontinued after a period of two weeks and salicylates substituted. Penicillin therapy was discontinued after a 10-day course, and digoxin was stopped at hospital discharge. At discharge, cardiac murmurs had disappeared and there was no evidence of major manifestations of his rheumatic fever. Repeat throat culture was normal. He was begun on penicillin prophylaxis with penicillin G benzathine, 1.2 million units every 28 days and was to be followed in the Rheumatic Fever Clinic.

Discussion: This patient had classic manifestations of acute rheumatic fever with 4 of 5 major criteria. Although salicylates are effective in most patients in treating the inflammatory components of acute rheumatic fever, corticosteroid therapy is considered by some authorities of benefit in seriously ill patients, particularly when carditis with congestive heart failure is present. Although steroids are somewhat more potent than salicylates in suppressing acute exudative inflammation, their use in carditis has not been shown to decrease residual heart disease. Massive penicillin therapy has not been shown to alter course of the disease nor the frequency or severity of cardiac involvement, and the penicillin regimen usually recommended for treatment of streptococcal pharyngitis is adequate for use during the acute attack of rheumatic fever. Long-term prophylaxis with penicillin is indicated. The duration for which such continuous prophylaxis must be utilized will vary to some degree based on differences in risk related to factors such as age, interval from last rheumatic fever attack, and liability to exposure to streptococcal infection. (Case report kindly provided by Dr. Bernard Boxerbaum.)

History 6-2. Rheumatoid Arthritis

P.S., a 40-year-old white male, was in good health until December 2, 1972. At that time he noted sudden onset of chills and fever, followed over a period of several days by acute swelling of the left knee, left ankle, right elbow and several proximal interphalangeal (PIP) joints of both hands. Anorexia and malaise were noted. He was admitted to hospital elsewhere by his physician for study. The white blood cell count was 11,000/mm^3 with 78% polymorphonuclear cells. Erythrocyte sedimentation rate was 55 mm/hour (Westergren). Serum latex fixation study for rheumatoid factor was positive in a titer of 1:40. Serum antinuclear antibody titer and LE cell determinations were negative. Chest roentgenogram, electrocardiogram, serologic test for syphilis, protein electrophoresis and serum antistreptolysin-O titer were negative or normal. Fluid aspirated from the left knee revealed 8000 WBC/mm^3 with 52% polymorphonuclear cells. Synovial fluid, blood and urine cultures were negative. On system review the patient gave a negative history for urethritis, conjunctivitis, skin rash, pleurisy, Raynaud's phenomenon, hair loss or sun sensitivity. He denied extramarital sexual exposure. The patient was given aspirin, 960 mg QID, with only limited relief of joint symptoms. Low-grade temperature elevation persisted. Symptoms of acute polyarthritis, fever and malaise remained disabling despite an intensive program of conservative therapy using aspirin, 1280 mg QID, indomethacin, 25 mg QID, local heat, bed rest and physical therapy. Prednisone, 7.5 mg per day, was added, and several intra-articular injections of steroid were placed in the left knee, the site of greatest disability. He was discharged on this program of management only to be readmitted to hospital three weeks later when he had increased inflammatory swelling of the left knee and both ankles. Repeat evaluation showed persistently positive serum rheumatoid factor, weakly positive serum antinuclear antibody titer and negative LE cell preparations. No symptoms or signs of other connective tissue or systemic disease states were noted on full reinvestigation. A course of gold sodium thiomalate (Myochrysine) therapy was begun. Additional medications included aspirin, 1280 mg QID, and prednisone, 2.5 mg BID.

He was first seen in referral January 27, 1973, at which time he was afebrile and joint manifestations were limited to swelling of the left wrist and left knee. He had received a total of 200 mg of Myochrysine. Gold therapy was continued until proteinuria was noted at a total dose of 400 mg, at which time his joint symptoms had greatly improved. Gold was discontinued and the patient was placed on hydroxychloroquine (Plaquenil), 200 mg BID. Aspirin, 1280 mg QID, and prednisone, 2.5 mg BID, were continued in addition to a full physical therapy program. Hydroxychloroquine was reduced to 200 mg once daily after three months when the patient showed continued clinical improvement. When last seen in December, 1973, the patient was doing measurably better. Therapy consisted of aspirin, 1280 mg QID, prednisone, 2.5 mg once daily, and hydroxychloroquine, 200 mg per day. The left wrist and left knee were minimally swollen.

Discussion: This patient appeared initially with an acute onset of polyarthritis associated with systemic manifestations that included fever and chills, anorexia and malaise. Several diagnoses, such as acute rheumatic fever, acute gonococcal arthritis, and systemic lupus erythematosus, had to be considered. The clinical findings and laboratory studies were consistent with a diagnosis of rheumatoid arthritis of acute onset. The patient responded to a therapeutic regimen for rheumatoid arthritis with a great reduction of symptoms.

History 6-3. Gonococcal Arthritis

G.M., a 24-year-old black female, was first seen in consultation in hospital in August, 1973. She had been in good health until three days prior to admission when she developed migratory polyarthralgia associated with chills and temperature elevations to 39° C. Twenty-four hours later she noted swelling and tenderness in the left first metatarsophalangeal joint, both knees and both ankles. There was no past history of arthritis, sore throat, sun sensitivity, morning stiffness, skin rash, alopecia, Raynaud's phenomenon or pleurisy. She denied recent extramarital sexual intercourse. Menstrual periods were regular and there was no history of increased vaginal discharge. System review was otherwise negative and family history was unremarkable.

On physical examination, the patient's temperature was 37.5° C. There was no lymphadenopathy. Examination of the heart, lungs and abdomen was normal. Pelvic examination revealed a vaginal discharge but no tenderness and no palpable masses. Erythema, tenderness and swelling of both knees and ankles were noted. The right hip was painful on motion and the right shoulder was tender to palpation. Examination of the skin revealed several small erythematous papulovesicular lesions on the hands and forearms. Several lesions were slightly pustular in appearance.

The hematocrit was 36%, the white blood cell count was 5,000/mm³ with a normal differential, and the erythrocyte sedimentation rate was 32 mm/hour (Wintrobe). Urinalysis was normal. Serum studies for rheumatoid factor and antinuclear antibody were negative. No LE cells were seen. Liver function studies, routine serum electrolytes, chest roentgenogram and electrocardiogram studies were normal. Gram-stain study of material obtained from the uterine cervix revealed gram-negative diplococci in an intracellular location. Neisseria gonorrhoeae was identified on culture of the same material and on material obtained by rectal swab. Blood cultures were negative. A diagnosis of acute gonococcal arthritis was made.

The patient was treated with aqueous crystalline penicillin, six million units daily administered intravenously in divided doses. Joint symptoms resolved dramatically within a 48-hour period. Cutaneous lesions showed similar improvement. Penicillin therapy was continued by intramuscular and then oral routes for a total of 14 days, with complete resolution of symptoms.

Discussion: In this patient, gonococcal arthritis appeared as an acute polyarthritis. The presence of typical cutaneous lesions helped significantly in

5

clinical diagnosis. Bacterial studies confirmed the diagnosis and the patient had an excellent response to therapy. Gonococcal arthritis should be strongly considered in young people with acute arthritis, whether monoarticular or polyarticular in type. Associated manifestations of gonococcal arthritis, such as acute tenosynovitis and typical cutaneous lesions, are extremely helpful in diagnosis.

History 6-4. Rubella Arthritis

J.L., a 17-year-old white female, was first seen in consultation in September, 1970. History revealed acute onset of swelling of the proximal interphalangeal (PIP) and metacarpophalangeal (MCP) joints of the hands, both wrists, knees and ankles two weeks following rubella vaccination. Joint symptoms completely resolved after one week. A second attack of similar joint symptoms of lesser severity occurred several weeks later. Symptoms again remitted completely without therapy after approximately five days. The patient was seen when joint symptoms recurred a third time several weeks later. Symptoms were mild and involved primarily the PIP and MCP joints of the hands and the knees. There were no ancillary symptoms of connective tissue disease such as drug allergy, sun sensitivity, pleurisy, colitis, dry mouth or eyes, hair loss, or psoriasis. Past medical history was essentially negative. Joint examination revealed tenderness and slight swelling of PIP and MCP joints of both hands and the knees. General examination was otherwise normal.

The complete blood count and urinalysis were normal. Erythrocyte sedimentation rate was 5 mm/hour (Wintrobe). Serum studies for rheumatoid factor and antinuclear antibody were negative. Serum uric acid was 5.3 mg/100 ml. Serum glutamic oxaloacetic transaminase and routine serologic test for syphilis were negative. Antistreptolysin-O titer was less than 100 Todd units. EKG and chest x-ray were normal. A diagnosis of rubella arthritis was made.

The patient was placed on therapy with aspirin, 960 mg QID. Joint symptoms remitted after approximately one week. Her general health has been excellent and, on followup examination some years later, the patient remained in perfect health on no therapy.

Discussion: The sequence of events and the benign nature of the arthritis in this patient are consistent with a diagnosis of rubella arthritis following vaccination. In most cases symptoms are relatively mild and short-lived. The intermittent nature of the symptoms is not inconsistent with the diagnosis, because attacks of brief duration may recur for several years following vaccination.

History 6-5. Arthritis Associated with Ulcerative Colitis

K.P., a 25-year-old white female, had a history of ulcerative colitis beginning at age 23. Abdominal-perineal resection with removal of the colon and rectum was performed one year after the onset of her illness, when medical management with prednisone and salicylazosulfapyridine (Azulfidine) was ineffective in controlling symptoms. The patient did satisfactorily until July, 1973, when she appeared with pain, swelling and tenderness of the right wrist, left knee and left elbow. She denied abdominal pain, diarrhea, dysphagia, rash, photosensitivity, alopecia, pleurisy, dry eyes, or dry mouth. There was no prior history of joint disease. The patient had been taking no medications except diphenoxylate hydrochloride with atropine sulfate (Lomotil) and antispasmodics. Physical examination showed marked inflammation and swelling of the involved joints.

The hematocrit was 35%, the white blood cell count was 3600/mm³ with a normal differential, and the erythrocyte sedimentation rate was 38 mm/hour (Wintrobe). Serum electrolytes, glutamic oxaloacetic transaminase and creatine phosphokinase were within normal limits. Urinalysis revealed +1 albuminuria. Serum uric acid was 2.5 mg/100 ml. Serum rheumatoid factor and antinuclear antibody studies were negative, and serologic test for syphilis was nonreactive. Roentgenograms of the wrists, knees and elbows were unremarkable. Analysis of synovial fluid from the left knee revealed 12,000 white cells/mm³ with 55% polymorphonuclear cells. Synovial fluid glucose was 70 mg/100 ml when fasting blood sugar was 86 mg/100 ml. Mucin clot test was grossly abnormal. No crystals were noted. The fluid was negative for bacterial infection on smear and culture. The patient's symptoms responded well to a program of aspirin, 960 mg QID, in addition to bed rest and application of heat to involved joints. Joint swelling and pain responded sufficiently to allow discharge from hospital after ten days, and the patient was continued on salicylates and a physical therapy program.

Discussion: The presumptive diagnosis in this case is arthritis associated with chronic nonspecific ulcerative colitis. Although joint symptoms in such cases are frequently associated with active ulcerative colitis, joint symptoms may continue or sometimes begin when all evidence of colitis appears to have been removed.

History 6-6. Hepatitis-associated Arthritis

M.J., an 18-year-old white female, was admitted to hospital with a one-week history of pruritus of the legs and arms. Two days prior to admission she had noted painful swelling of the wrists and proximal interphalangeal (PIP) joints. Joint symptoms were intermittent and migratory and remained confined to the upper extremities. On physical examination, both wrists were tender and swollen, and the proximal interphalangeal joints were mildly tender to palpation. Urticarial lesions appeared on the arms and back. Malaise, nausea and anorexia were noted on the fifth hospital day. Clinical jaundice was absent.

The white blood cell count and differential, urinalysis, routine serologic test for syphilis, serum uric acid, heterophile antibody titer, and studies for serum rheumatoid factor and antinuclear antibody were normal or negative. Hematocrit was 34%. Initial serum glutamic oxaloacetic transaminase (SGOT) was 255 Henry units (normal, 9 to 25 units), and total serum bilirubin was 1.3 mg/100 ml. Serum alkaline phosphatase was 11 King-Armstrong units (normal, 3 to 13 units). Sulfobromophthalein retention was 10% at 45 minutes. Serum protein electrophoresis was normal. Serum complement was 35 CH⁵⁰ hemolytic units (normal control, 100 units). Antistreptolysin-O titer was 250 Todd units. LE cell studies were negative. Roentgenograms of the chest, hands, and wrists were unremarkable. Oral cholecystogram and liver scan were normal. Cultures of the blood, urine and uterine cervix were negative. Hepatitis-associated antigen (HBₛAg) was detected in the serum on the fifth hospital day. On the eighth hospital day, joint abnormalities disappeared. SGOT levels reached a maximum of 1200 units on the 18th day of hospitalization. The patient was discharged after 23 days, with no clinical symptoms and with normal liver function. One month later, she was completely asymptomatic and liver function studies remained normal. Hepatitis-associated antigen was no longer detectable.

Discussion: This patient had the characteristic clinical and laboratory findings of hepatitis-associated arthritis. Joint symptoms and an urticarial rash were noted. Abnormal laboratory results included abnormal liver function studies, a low serum complement and the presence of hepatitis-associated antigen in the serum. As noted in this case, hepatitis-associated arthritis may occur in patients with anicteric hepatitis. Accordingly, hepatitis as an etiology of arthritis may be readily overlooked in patients with this syndrome.

History 6-7. Gout

J.A., a 64-year-old black male, was seen in consultation in January, 1972. He gave a history of joint symptoms of 20 years duration, characterized initially by acute attacks of pain, swelling and tenderness involving the first metatarsophalangeal joints. Attacks lasted several weeks and cleared completely without therapy. Early in the course of his disease, attacks occurred at intervals of approximately one year. Later, attacks became more frequent and were often polyarticular with involvement of MTP joints, ankles, knees and wrists. Joint symptoms cleared completely over a period of one to two weeks, even when several joints were simultaneously involved. No joint symptoms or fibrositis were noted between acute episodes. Past treatment had included the use of aspirin and short courses of steroid therapy at the time of acute symptoms. The patient felt in good health otherwise and had no symptoms of Raynaud's phenomenon, pleurisy, hair loss, sun sensitivity, or skin rash. Past medical history was noncontributory.

Physical examination at the time the patient was first seen revealed marked tenderness and swelling of the right tarsal area and the right first MTP joint. No subcutaneous nodules or tophi were seen. A diagnosis of probable acute gouty arthritis was made and the patient was placed on therapy with phenylbutazone, 100 mg QID, and ACTH gel, 80 units IM. Clinical response was excellent.

Laboratory studies revealed normal urinalysis, hematocrit, white blood cell count and differential. Erythrocyte sedimentation rate was 36 mm/hour (Wintrobe). Serum uric acid was 11.2 mg/100 ml and serum latex fixation test for rheumatoid factor was positive at a titer of 1:40. Serum antinuclear factor study was negative. Diagnostic considerations included: (1) gout with associated positive serum rheumatoid factor of uncertain significance, (2) episodic rheumatoid arthritis with coincidental hyperuricemia, and (3) rheumatoid arthritis and gout. The patient was placed on an interval therapy program of probenecid, 0.5 g daily, with gradual increases to 0.5 g QID, which was required to maintain the serum uric acid at normal levels. Colchicine, 0.6 mg BID, was added. The patient had several episodes of acute arthritis involving the MTP joints, ankles, tarsal areas and knees over the subsequent six months. Analysis of synovial fluid removed from the right knee during one of these episodes revealed numerous needle-shaped crystals that were strongly birefringent in a negative direction. Attacks of joint pain gradually subsided and the patient has been essentially asymptomatic. Repeat studies for serum rheumatoid factor have been consistently negative.

Discussion: Gout characteristically appears initially as an acute monoarthritis. However, polyarthritis is not uncommon in later stages when inadequate or no treatment is given. The presence of polyarthritis and a positive test for serum rheumatoid factor when this patient was first seen made diagnosis more complex. The relationship of his symptoms to gout was confirmed later by the finding of crystals consistent with monosodium urate in synovial fluid and the clinical response to an interval therapy program for gout.

REFERENCES

1. Aptekar, R. G., et al.: Adult onset of juvenile rheumatoid arthritis. Arthritis Rheum 16:715, 1973.
2. Thomas, A. F., Solomon, L. and Rabson, A.: Polyarthritis associated with Yersinia entercolitica infection. S Afr Med J 49:18, 1975.
3. Yanez, J. E. et al.: Rubella arthritis. Ann Int Med 64:772, 1966.

4. Thompson, G. R., Ferreyon, A. and Brackett, R. G.: Acute arthritis complicating rubella vaccination. Arthritis Rheum 14:19, 1971.
5. Ager, E. A., Chin, T. D. Y. and Poland, J. D.: Epidemic erythema infectiosum. N Eng J Med 275:1326, 1966.
6. McCarthy, D. J. and Ormiste, V.: Arthritis and HB Ag-positive hepatitis. Arch Int Med 132:264, 1973.
7. Stevens, D. P. et al.: Anicteric hepatitis presenting as polyarthritis. JAMA 220: 687, 1972.
8. Gocke, D. J. et al.: Association between polyarteritis and Australian antigen. Lancet 2: 1149, 1970.
9. Schumacher, R. H., Andrews, R. and McLaughlin, G.: Arthropathy in sickle-cell disease. Ann Int Med 78:203, 1973.
10. Hadler, N. M. et al.: Acute polyarticular gout. Am J Med 56:715, 1974.
11. Silverstein, M. N. and Kelly, P. J.: Leukemia with osteoarticular symptoms and signs. Ann Int Med 59:637, 1963.
12. Potts, D. E., Mass, N. F. and Iseman, M. D.: Syndrome of pancreatic disease, subcutaneous fat necrosis and polyserositis. Am J Med 58:417, 1975.
13. Khachadurian, A. K.: Migratory polyarthritis in familial hyperlipoproteinemia (type II hyperlipoproteinemia). Arthritis Rheum 11:385, 1968.
14. Glueck, C. J., Levy, R. I. and Fredrickson, D. S.: Acute tendonitis and arthritis: a presenting symptom of familial type II hyperlipoproteinemia. JAMA 206:2895, 1968.

CHAPTER 7

SUBACUTE AND CHRONIC POLYARTHRITIS

Rheumatic diseases often occur initially as a subacute or chronic poly-arthritis. In other cases subacute or chronic polyarthritis follows mono-arthritis or acute polyarthritis as the articular involvement spreads or becomes more persistent.

DIFFERENTIAL DIAGNOSIS

Most likely causes to be considered:

> Rheumatoid arthritis
> Systemic lupus erythematosus
> Other connective tissue diseases (dermatomyositis, scleroderma, periarteritis nodosa, Sjögren's syndrome, mixed connective tissue disease)
> Degenerative joint disease (osteoarthritis)
> Psoriatic arthritis
> Reiter's syndrome and other reactive arthritides
> Arthritis of ulcerative colitis and regional enteritis
> Sarcoid arthritis
> Arthritis associated with malignant neoplasms
> Hypertrophic osteoarthropathy
> Chronic tophaceous gout; pseudogout

The most common cause of severe chronic polyarthritis is *rheumatoid arthritis*. Classically the proximal interphalangeal and metacarpophalangeal joints of the hands are affected, but all peripheral joints of the body may be involved at one time or another. Although joint involvement is frequently bilateral and symmetric, asymmetric involvement is not uncommon. In addition to the peripheral joints, such as the wrists, elbows, knees and ankles, the temporomandibular, sternoclavicular and cricoarytenoid joints may be affected. Weakness and atrophy of muscles contiguous to involved joints is common.

Systemic and extra-articular manifestations are frequent and diagnostically valuable. Generalized fibrositis characterized by stiffness and gelling of joints is most severe on awakening or after a period of inactivity during the day. Low-grade fever is common. Other extra-articular manifestations have prognostic as well as diagnostic importance in that they usually signify more severe disease. Subcutaneous nodules most often occur at the subolecranon areas of the elbows. They may be seen elsewhere, however, and are most apt to involve pressure areas such as the scapulae, buttocks and Achilles tendons. Lymphadenopathy may be striking. Splenomegaly is not uncommon; when associated with leukopenia the combination of symptoms is classified as Felty's syndrome.[1] Anemia may result from any of several causes, including chronic bone marrow depression, impairment of iron absorption, plasma dilution effect, hypersplenism, and drug-induced gastrointestinal blood loss. Eye manifestations may be severe. Band keratopathy is characterized by an equatorial corneal opacity caused by fibrosis of the cornea. Episcleritis may be localized or diffuse. Intense hyperemia of deep vessels is present. Iritis may occur. Scleritis may be acute, with widespread necrotizing sclerosis. In some cases, scleral involvement with nodular destruction is slow. The wall of the eye softens, and uveal tissue may herniate through the defect. This pernicious form of eye involvement is called scleromalacia perforans. Sicca syndrome with symptoms of dryness of the eyes and a sensation of scratchiness is common. Secondary glaucoma and cataracts are late sequelae of rheumatoid eye disease. Systemic necrotizing vasculitis, which fortunately occurs in only a small percentage of cases, is heralded by skin ulceration, subungual and paronychial infarcts, and neuropathy.

Joint symptoms in *systemic lupus erythematosus* are classically characterized as a non-deforming non-erosive arthritis. In many patients joint symptoms are limited to polyarthralgia of varying severity without significant objective changes. In approximately 10% of patients chronic polyarthritis identical to that seen in rheumatoid arthritis is observed, particularly in disease of long duration. Chronic polyarthritis in *other connective tissue diseases* such as dermatomyositis, scleroderma and polyarteritis nodosa is usually much more limited in extent and severity as compared to rheumatoid arthritis.

Sjögren's syndrome, which is a chronic inflammatory disease process characterized by diminished lacrimal and salivary gland secretion,[2,3] is usually classified with the connective tissue disorders. Joint symptoms consistent with those of classic rheumatoid arthritis occur in many patients. Clinical findings consistent with other connective tissue diseases, such as systemic lupus erythematosus, scleroderma, polymyositis or vasculitis, may also be noted. Chronic inflammatory changes are observed in the salivary and

Figure 7-1. Sjögren's syndrome. Note swelling of left parotid gland. (Courtesy, Dr. A. Mackenzie)

lacrimal glands, and in glandular components of the respiratory tract, gastrointestinal tract and vagina. Classic clinical features include dry eyes, dry mouth and parotid gland swelling (Fig. 7-1). Arthralgia and arthritis are common. Raynaud's phenomenon is seen in 20% of patients. Nonthrombocytopenic purpura related to serum hyperglobulinemia is seen most prominently over the lower extremities. Interstitial nephritis leads to renal tubular acidosis. Polymyopathy is common; proximal muscle weakness may be marked. Peripheral or cranial neuropathy including trigeminal neuropathy occurs. Primary biliary cirrhosis or chronic thyroiditis of the Hashimoto type may be seen. Chronic pulmonary disease leads to findings of chronic obstructive airway disease.[4] Immunoglobulin abnormalities produce cryoglobulinemia or macroglobulinemia. Proliferation of lymphoid tissues may become generalized producing "pseudolymphoma" in which the normal lymph node architecture is distorted but cellular changes do not meet histologic criteria for malignancy. In some patients, however, malignant changes do occur. The most common malignant lymphoproliferation is the highly undifferentiated reticulum cell sarcoma. A fall in serum IgM and rheumatoid factor titer which may precede the onset of malignant lymphoproliferation is an ominous prognostic sign.

Figure 7-2.   Schirmer test, filter paper strips in place. (Courtesy, Dr. A. Mackenzie)

Several supporting diagnostic studies are available.[5] Parotid salivary flow rates, measured following a stimulus such as lemon juice on the tongue, are diminished.[6] Involvement of the lacrimal glands can be measured by the simple Schirmer test, in which a strip of filter paper is folded and placed in the lower conjunctival sac (Fig. 7-2). Normally, after five minutes, the moistened portion of the paper measures 15 mm or greater. In Sjögren's syndrome, the moistened area usually measures 5 mm or less. Secretory sialography, performed by introducing a radiopaque contrast medium into the parotid duct orifice, reveals punctate, glandular or cavitary sialectasis (Fig. 7-3). Sequential salivary scintograms using technetium pertechnetate show decreased uptake, which correlates with impaired glandular function.[7,8] This technique serves as a noninvasive method to initially evaluate or to follow the course of Sjögren's syndrome. It is, however, a relatively expensive test and does involve some exposure to systemic radiation. Biopsy of labial minor salivary glands provides the most specific diagnostic criterion for the oral component of Sjögren's syndrome.[6] Disease severity generally parallels the number of foci of chronic lymphocytic inflammatory cellular infiltrates seen.

Immunologic abnormalities, such as hypergammaglobulinemia, positive tests for serum rheumatoid and antinuclear factors, and positive studies for LE cells, are common. Precipitating antibodies to the nuclear antigens, SS-A and SS-B have been reported in the sera of patients with Sjögren's syndrome. Anti-SS-A occurs in a broad spectrum of connective tissue diseases; antibody to SS-B, on the other hand, has a high specificity for patients with primary Sjögren's syndrome, or Sjögren's syndrome with systemic lupus erythematosus.[9,10]

Figure 7-3.   Sialogram,   Sjögren's   syndrome, showing globular and cavitary sialectasis. (Courtesy, Dr. A. Mackenzie)

Chronic polyarthritis may occur in patients whose clinical and laboratory findings represent a composite of several connective tissue disorders. For example, definitive evidence of systemic lupus erythematosus, polymyositis and scleroderma may be present in various combinations in the same patient. This overlapping has been given the name *mixed connective tissue disease* (MCTD).[11-15] Antibody to a specific nuclear ribonucleoprotein antigen (anti-nRNP) is characteristically present in the serum in high titer (frequently over 1:100,000). The typical overlapping clinical pattern associated with high titers of anti-nRNP has led to consideration of this syndrome as a specific entity. Not all investigators are in accord with this interpretation. Classically the patient demonstrates clinical and laboratory evidence of systemic lupus erythematosus, polymyositis and scleroderma. The clinical pattern is characterized by Raynaud's phenomenon, polyarthralgia or arthritis, swelling of the hands leading to a sausage appearance of the fingers, esophageal hypomotility and inflammatory myopathy. Pulmonary involvement is not uncommon. The arthritis may be typical of rheumatoid arthritis. Skin manifestations include scleroderma and lupuslike rashes. Proximal muscles are often tender and weak; elevated levels of muscle enzymes are noted. Electromyographic and biopsy studies are typical of inflammatory myositis. Esophageal changes simulate those seen in scleroderma. Renal disease is seen but is much less frequent than in patients with systemic lupus erythematosus. Lymphadenopathy and hepatosplenomegaly may occur.

Figure 7-4. Osteoarthritis of hands. (A) Clinical appearance. Knobby swelling of the distal and proximal interphalangeal joints is associated with horizontal joint deviation. Osteoarthritic changes of the first carpometacarpal joints cause a squared appearance in this area. (B) Radiographic appearance. Joint space narrowing and spur formation in involved joints.

Laboratory studies reveal a moderate anemia and leukopenia in up to 40% of the patients. As noted, high serum titers of anti-nRNP are present. Rheumatoid factor studies are frequently positive; high titers of antinuclear antibody with a speckled pattern are seen. Anti-DNA is surprisingly infrequent. Hypergammaglobulinemia may be striking.

Mild features of the disease such as polyarthralgia or mild arthritis may respond to nonsteroidal anti-inflammatory agents. Corticosteroid therapy is generally effective in the face of more severe symptomatology. In general, the scleroderma-like features of MCTD are least likely to respond. Overall prognosis is reasonably good.

Degenerative joint disease (osteoarthritis) is usually limited to involvement of one or a few joints. However, manifestations may sometimes be more widespread. Knobby involvement of the distal interphalangeal (DIP) joints of the hands (Fig. 7-4) (Heberden's nodes) is classic and common. This form of osteoarthritis occurs primarily in middle and older years, and affects women ten times more frequently than men. The lesions are usually insidious in development and associated with few or no symptoms. In other cases, however, onset is abrupt and inflammation relatively extensive. Osteoarthritic changes in the distal interphalangeal (DIP) joints are often followed by a similar involvement of proximal interphalangeal (PIP) joints (Fig. 7-4) (Bouchard's nodes). Involvement of metacarpophalangeal joints is relatively uncommon, an important differentiating point from rheumatoid arthritis. Other peripheral joints may be affected by osteoarthritis, often independently of DIP and PIP joint involvement. Particularly susceptible peripheral joints include the first carpometacarpal joint of the hands (Fig. 7-4), hips (Fig. 7-5), knees and first metatarsophalangeal

Figure 7-5. Osteoarthritis of hips. Changes are most marked in the left hip. Note joint space narrowing and bony cyst formation.

joints. The cervical and lumbar spine are frequently affected. Osteoarthritis rarely affects the wrists, elbows, shoulders and ankles unless secondary to some other disorder such as chronic trauma or injury.

The arthritis associated with *psoriasis* takes several forms[16,17] and may be difficult to differentiate from rheumatoid arthritis. The most typical form involves the distal interphalangeal (DIP) joints of the hands, usually in association with psoriatic changes in the fingernails. This has some diagnostic significance, because rheumatoid involvement of DIP joints early is uncommon. Of similar significance is involvement of the interphalangeal joints of the toes, which is also rare in patients with rheumatoid arthritis. A second form of psoriatic arthritis is characterized by extensive erosive changes in articulating bone. In the hand, these mutilating changes lead to the "main en lorgnette" or opera-glass hand, in which the fingers are highly mobile and are readily telescoped to shorter size. In the third form of psoriatic arthritis, joint changes may be similar to those seen in rheumatoid arthritis. However, the swelling of the small joints involved in psoriatic arthritis often appears sausage-shaped, which aids differential diagnosis (Fig. 7-6). Separation of the two disorders is aided by serum testing for rheumatoid factor—a positive result is supportive of rheumatoid arthritis. Moreover, spondylitis is common in psoriatic arthritis. Skin changes are usually characteristic and prominent but cases of psoriatic arthritis with minimal skin findings are not uncommon. Although skin and nail changes usually precede or occur simultaneously with articular disease, joint manifestations occasionally precede them by months or years. HLA-B27 occurs in up to 50% of psoriatic patients with sacro-iliitis or spondylitis, in contrast to the demonstrated lack of any relationship between B27 and peripheral psoriatic arthritis.

Subacute or chronic polyarthritis is a major component of the triad of ar-

Figure 7-6. Psoriatic arthritis. Sausage-shaped swellings of the interphalangeal joints of the toes.

thritis, urethritis and conjunctivitis seen in *Reiter's syndrome.*[18,19] Mucocutaneous lesions that involve the skin, oral cavity and genitalia are a common fourth component of the syndrome. More frequent in males, this syndrome is occasionally associated with extra-articular manifestations such as conduction abnormalities of the heart and neuropathy. Spondylitis is a common sequel; it often occurs late in the disease when peripheral joint symptoms are minimal or absent. Histocompatibility antigen, HLA-B27, is present in up to 96% of patients with this disorder.[20,21]

Subacute and chronic joint manifestations similar to those seen in Reiter's syndrome may occur in the reactive arthritis associated with infection with *Yersinia enterocolitica.* Systemic manifestations include urethritis, conjunctivitis, carditis, and erythema nodosum-like lesions. HLA-B27 antigen is found in up to 88% of patients with Yersinia arthritis.

Polyarthritis is a common associated symptom in patients with *ulcerative colitis* and *regional enteritis.* As in psoriatic arthritis and Reiter's syndrome, spondylitis is an important component of the joint manifestations. Joint symptoms usually occur simultaneously with or following gastrointestinal symptoms. Less frequently, arthritis precedes bowel manifestations. HLA-B27 histocompatibility antigen appears in approximately 75% of patients with ulcerative colitis or regional enteritis when spondylitis is present.[22]

Articular changes occurring in *sarcoid* are variable in type. Chronic polyarthralgia is common; in addition, acute, subacute or chronic monoarthritis or polyarthritis is seen. Joint symptoms may be difficult to differentiate from those of rheumatoid arthritis. Tuberculin skin reaction is usually negative.

Malignant neoplasms may be associated with chronic polyarthritis.[23,24] The clinical features of the joint involvement are similar to those seen in rheumatoid arthritis. This entity should be strongly considered in the differential diagnosis of chronic polyarthritis in older age groups. Although neoplasms in any organ can produce this syndrome, tumors of the genitourinary tract and lungs are particularly frequent. In many cases the offending neoplasm is occult when the patient is first seen. Rheumatoid factor study is usually negative but occasionally positive. Treatment of the neoplasm by surgical, radiologic or chemotherapeutic means may be associated with partial or complete resolution of joint symptoms. Non-steroidal anti-inflammatory agents provide symptomatic relief. Steroid therapy is sometimes indicated.

Hypertrophic osteoarthropathy is characterized by clubbing of the fingers, periosteal proliferation and synovitis. Large joints are involved most commonly. In some cases the syndrome is idiopathic or familial. More commonly, it occurs secondary to any of several other disorders, such as neoplasms, suppurative pulmonary disease, cyanotic congenital heart disease, subacute bacterial endocarditis, cirrhosis, chronic diarrheal states and following thyroidectomy for Graves' disease. Roentgenograms reveal subperiosteal new bone layering along the distal diaphyseal regions of long bones, especially of the legs and forearms. Involvement is usually symmetric. The diagnosis can also be suggested by ^{99}M Technetium scanning which reveals a linear accumulation of tracer along the involved long bones.[25] Nonsteroidal anti-inflammatory therapy provides symptomatic relief in many cases. Steroid therapy may benefit patients with severe joint manifestations. Treatment of underlying disorders such as empyema or bronchiectasis or resection of primary tumors may be associated with resolution of symptoms.

Chronic polyarthritis may be a manifestation of untreated or inadequately treated *gout* when large deposits of urate result in persistent synovitis and joint swelling (Fig. 7-7). Usually, a careful history reveals prior episodes of acute arthritis typical of the gouty diathesis. The other common form of crystal-induced synovitis, *pseudogout syndrome* (chondrocalcinosis),

Figure 7-7.   Monosodium urate deposits causing chronic polyarthritis in patient with tophaceous gout. (Courtesy, Dr. A. Mackenzie)

Figure 7-8. Behçet's syndrome. Mucosal ulcerations involve the tongue and
lower lip. (Courtesy, Dr. C. Denko)

may also produce chronic polyarthritis.[26,27,28] In most cases of pseudogout, joint manifestations are characterized by chronic polyarthralgia or by acute or subacute arthritis limited to one or a few joints. Chronic synovitis represents a chronic inflammatory response to synovial deposits of calcium pyrophosphate dihydrate crystals.

The foregoing entities will account for most diagnoses of patients with chronic polyarthritis. However, other disease states must be considered when the diagnosis remains elusive. These latter diseases occur less frequently or less commonly produce chronic polyarthritis as their major articular manifestation. For example, *Behçet's syndrome* is a relatively rare disease in which chronic arthritis may occur in association with the more classic symptoms of orogenital ulcerations (Fig. 7-8) and recurrent iritis.[29] Additional symptoms include phlebitis, colitis, inflammatory nodular skin lesions (which resemble erythema nodosum), pyoderma gangrenosum and central nervous system manifestations. Another rare cause of chronic polyarthritis is that associated with *shunting operations of the gastrointestinal tract,* including jejunocolic or jejunoileal procedures.[30-32] Large joints are most commonly involved. The arthritis may result from circulating immune complexes formed in response to absorbed bacterial antigens. Serum complement activation has been demonstrated. Articular symptoms may respond to nonsteroidal anti-inflammatory agents or corticosteroids. Lasting remissions of arthritis have followed re-anastomosis of the bowel.

Musculoskeletal manifestations including chronic arthritis have been described in patients with *subacute bacterial endocarditis.*[33] Arthralgias are the most common musculoskeletal symptom, although synovitis has been noted in almost one-third of cases reviewed. Joint symptoms are more often monoarticular but polyarticular disease may be present. Shoulder and lower extremity articulations are most commonly involved. Low back pain is a surprisingly common symptom; it may be the most prominent musculoskeletal complaint. Normal roentgenograms and absence of previous episodes of back pain are features that tend to distinguish these patients from those with other causes of low back pain. Myalgias are not uncommon, especially during episodes of high fever. Less common musculoskeletal manifestations include hypertrophic osteoarthropathy. Serum rheumatoid factor is noted in up to 50% of patients; positive results are more likely to be seen in disease of six or more weeks' duration. Antinuclear antibody test is positive in about 20% of patients. The presence of serum rheumatoid factor and antinuclear antibodies in patients with bacterial endocarditis suggests that immunologic mechanisms such as circulating immune complexes may be at fault in the induction of symptoms related to this entity.

Chronic polyarthritis has been described in patients with *hemochromatosis*.[34] Although large peripheral joints such as the hips and knees may be involved, chronic arthritis affecting the second and third metacarpophalangeal and proximal interphalangeal joints of the fingers is characteristic. Irregular joint space narrowing, osteoporosis and subchondral cyst formation appear on roentgenogram. Chronic polyarthralgia and symptoms resembling degenerative joint disease are common. This arthropathy frequently is associated with the radiologic findings of chondrocalcinosis and associated acute symptoms of pseudogout syndrome. Diagnosis is suggested by the typical clinical picture. Confirmation of the syndrome requires demonstration of elevations in serum iron and percent iron saturation of transferrin, and biopsy evidence of tissue deposits of hemosiderin. Articular symptoms of hemochromatosis may precede overt clinical presentation of other manifestations of the disease, such as skin pigmentation, diabetes mellitus and hepatic cirrhosis.[35]

Chronic polyarthritis may be observed in a small number of patients with *myxedema*.[36] Signs and symptoms of myxedema are usually present when rheumatic symptoms appear. Generalized stiffness is common. The most characteristic objective joint changes are marked synovial thickening and effusions in the knee and small joints of the hands and feet.

Chronic polyarticular symptoms occur in patients with familial type IV *hyperlipoproteinemia*.[37,38] Morning stiffness and arthralgias are common. Synovitis, when present, is mildly inflammatory and persistent rather than episodic. Disability is usually minimal. Large and small joints are involved; the disease tends to be oligoarticular. An increased incidence of positive serum rheumatoid factor tests has been noted.[38] Roentgenograms reveal generalized osteoporosis and juxta-articular or metaphyseal cystic lesions. In some patients with this disorder, dietary control of the hyperlipidemia has been associated with improvement in joint symptoms.[38]

Rheumatic symptoms have been described in patients with *primary biliary cirrhosis*.[39] Scleroderma and related syndromes in particular have been described. In addition, these patients may present with nondeforming erosive arthritis which is generally asymptomatic. Swelling and synovitis commonly involve the proximal and distal interphalangeal joints of the hands. Large joints may also be affected. Chondrocalcinosis may be an associated finding.[40]

Fever, paraspinal myalgias and periarthritis have been described in patients using *intravenous heroin*.[41] Continued heroin use is associated with progressive musculoskeletal symptoms, while discontinuation of such use results in complete recovery. The pathogenesis of this syndrome is unknown but may be related to an adulterant in the heroin mixture.

Although *tuberculous and fungal infections* may result in chronic polyarthritis, joint involvement is most commonly monoarticular or limited to two or three joints. Occasionally, more than three joints are involved and these diagnoses should be considered in the differential diagnosis of perplexing cases. Arthritis attacks in *Whipple's disease* are usually acute and relatively short-lived. Subacute or chronic joint manifestations occasionally appear.

DIAGNOSTIC STUDIES

In most cases of chronic polyarthritis, a well-performed history and physical examination will usually narrow the diagnostic field to a limited number of fairly common entities. In some cases, however, diagnosis is particularly difficult and less common diseases must be considered. Initial laboratory studies should include a complete blood count, erythrocyte sedimentation rate, urinalysis, serologic test for syphilis (to note false positive reactors), serum uric acid, serum latex fixation test for rheumatoid factor, serum antinuclear factor and serum protein electrophoresis.

Roentgenograms of the most severely involved joints should be obtained. They aid in differential diagnosis and, in addition, are valuable in delineating the degree of joint damage. Although radiologic findings are often nonspecific, they may be particularly valuable in certain diseases. Joint space narrowing, erosions and ankylosis of the distal interphalangeal joints are characteristic of psoriatic arthritis. Resorption of the terminal phalanges is common. A characteristic "pencil and cupping" deformity may be seen in which the sharply tapered end of the proximal bone of the joint fits into the flared end of the distal bony surface. Roentgenograms of affected joints show periosteal elevation and new bone growth in patients with hypertrophic osteoarthropathy. Calcification of fibrocartilages, particularly the menisci of the knees and the triangular cartilage of the wrist, is typical of pseudogout syndrome. Joint space narrowing, osteophyte formation, subchondral bony sclerosis and cyst formation are the classic changes of osteoarthritis. Chest roentgenogram may demonstrate pulmonary lesions characteristic of several connective tissue diseases, pulmonary sarcoidosis or neoplasms (see Chapter 12).

Additional diagnostic studies such as serum iron, binding and saturation, blood cultures, serum thyroxine levels, serum lipid studies, and sigmoid-oscopy and gastrointestinal roentgenograms should be performed when clinical suspicions suggest the presence of less common causes of chronic polyarthritis.

Synovial fluid analysis is less helpful diagnostically in this form of articular disease because the findings are often similar and nonspecific for the various disorders. Similarly, synovial biopsy is often nonspecific but may be diagnostically valuable in cases of arthritis due to sarcoid, chronic granulomatous infections, gout or pseudogout. Diagnostic studies should be repeated periodically because they might be negative when the patient is first seen but become positive over the ensuing months or years.

THERAPY

Management should remain conservative until the diagnosis has been established as definitely as possible. Rest and physical therapy relieve joint pain and maintain range of motion and muscle strength. Various forms of heat therapy help to relieve pain and muscle spasm. Canes and crutches should be utilized when lower extremities are severely involved. Aspirin given to maximal tolerance will usually relieve symptoms to some degree in most cases, whatever the etiology. Symptoms are further aided by the use of mild analgesic agents. Other non-steroidal anti-inflammatory agents can be considered for use in the more symptomatic cases; they usually will not obscure the diagnosis. Corticosteroid therapy should be considered only when diagnostic studies and observation have led to a reasonable probable diagnosis and to the exclusion of diseases in which their use would be contraindicated. The use of other agents and modes of therapy varies with the final diagnosis (see Chapter 19).

CASE HISTORIES

History 7-1. Rheumatoid Arthritis

M.F., a 52-year-old white female, was well until May, 1963, at which time she noted aching in the posterior cervical area and both shoulders. Shortly afterward she developed swelling and pain of both wrists, proximal interphalangeal (PIP) joints of the second and third fingers bilaterally, and both ankles and knees. Aspirin, 640 mg QID, provided mild relief. There was no past history of arthritis or rheumatic fever. System review was negative for Raynaud's phenomenon, pleurisy, sun sensitivity, psoriasis, diarrhea or alopecia. Additional symptoms included weight loss of ten pounds, prolonged morning stiffness, and easy fatigability. On physical examination, the palms were cool and moist. Swelling and tenderness of the second and third PIP and metacarpophalangeal (MCP) joints of the hands, both wrists, knees and ankles were noted. Pelvic and rectal examinations were normal.

Laboratory studies revealed normal urinalysis, hematocrit of 36%, white blood cell count of 7300/mm³, normal differential white cell count, erythrocyte sedimentation rate of 42 mm/hour (Wintrobe), negative serologic test for syphilis, slightly elevated serum gamma globulin, normal serum uric acid, and normal liver function studies. Chest roentgenogram was normal. Roentgenograms of the hands, wrists, knees and ankles showed periarticular bone demineralization. Serum latex fixation test for rheumatoid factor was positive in a titer of 1:1280. Serum antinuclear factor was weakly positive, but LE cell studies were negative.

Discussion: This patient represents a classic case of onset of rheumatoid arthritis. Several other connective tissue diseases that can simulate rheumatoid arthritis had to be excluded by appropriate clinical and laboratory evaluation. The patient was followed regularly over an extended period and unfortunately showed progressive changes of rheumatoid arthritis despite a full therapeutic program of aspirin, indomethacin, hydroxychloroquine, gold salt therapy and maintenance low-dose steroids. Bilateral total hip prostheses were required for therapy of severe hip involvement. However, the patient remained independent in activities of daily living despite persistent progression of her disease.

History 7-2. Systemic Lupus Erythematosus

D.K., a 60-year-old white female, was first seen in consultation in August, 1969. She was well until two years prior, at which time she noted swelling and pain in both wrists. Symptoms resolved completely after a period of one month with no specific therapy. In the fall of 1968 she noted fatigue associated with swelling of both wrists, proximal interphalangeal (PIP) joints of the hands, and both knees. Swelling persisted and other joints were subsequently involved. There was no history of hair loss, pleurisy, drug allergy, skin rash, dry eyes or dry mouth. She had a recent history of sensitivity to sun exposure, characterized by easy burning of the skin, and Raynaud's phenomenon. System review and past medical history were otherwise negative. On physical examination at the time of evaluation, no abnormalities were noted except for musculoskeletal findings. PIP and metacarpophalangeal (MCP) joints of the hands were mildly swollen and tender. The right elbow was swollen, with 15° limitation of extension. Both shoulders were limited to 50° abduction and both knees revealed mild swelling. Initial diagnosis was connective tissue disease, with a note to specifically exclude systemic lupus erythematosus on the basis of sun sensitivity and Raynaud's phenomenon.

Urinalysis, hematocrit, white blood cell count and differential, and routine serologic test for syphilis were normal or negative. Serum rheumatoid factor study was negative but serum antinuclear antibody was present in a titer of 1:1000. Anti-DNA titer in the serum was 1:80. LE cell study showed rosettes and several LE cells. In the absence of any overt major visceral manifestations of systemic lupus erythematosus, a conservative program of aspirin, 960 mg four times a day, mild analgesics and rest was instituted. Indomethacin, 25 mg TID with food, was added when joint symptoms remained mildly active. The patient did reasonably well on this conservative program of management, but in July, 1973, symptoms became more severe with increased swelling, pain and tenderness of numerous joints. Laboratory studies remained essentially unchanged. Due to the severe exacerbation of her joint symptoms and the economic necessity to remain active in her occupation, therapy with hydroxychloroquine (Plaquenil), 200 mg BID, and prednisone, 2.5 mg BID, was added. A baseline ophthalmologic evaluation was obtained for use in following hydroxychloroquine therapy, which was reduced to 200 mg daily after a period of four months. The patient did extremely well on her revised program.

Discussion: Arthritis was the major initial clinical manifestation of systemic lupus erythematosus in this patient. In the absence of evident involvement of critical visceral structures such as the kidneys, it was deemed reasonable to treat the patient with a conservative program of salicylates and indomethacin for a prolonged period of time following diagnosis. Increased joint symptoms prompted the addition of hydroxychloroquine and prednisone. Joint manifestations were identical to those seen in rheumatoid arthritis, and laboratory studies were required to substantiate the diagnosis of systemic lupus erythematosus.

History 7-3. Primary Generalized Osteoarthritis

J.B., a 42-year-old white female, first noted joint symptoms at age 40, at which time she developed pain in both hips with prolonged activity. Increased pain and limitation of motion of both hips was noted over the ensuing two years. One year prior to evaluation she developed pain and swelling of the distal and proximal interphalangeal joints of both hands and both first carpometacarpal joints. More recently, both knees had become painful with use, and locking of the left knee had occurred on several occasions. Treatment with aspirin, 640 mg QID, and indomethacin, 75 mg per day in divided doses, afforded some relief early in the course of her symptoms. More recently, this therapy was ineffective in controlling her distress. Mild morning stiffness lasting 15 to 30 minutes involved the knees, hips, and hands. There was no history of Raynaud's phenomenon, hair loss, dry eyes or mouth, dysphagia, sun sensitivity, psoriasis, colitis, or drug allergy. The patient considered herself to be in good health otherwise, and past medical history was noncontributory. Family history of documented severe degenerative joint disease in her father, a paternal uncle, and two paternal cousins was significant. Physical examination at time of consultation revealed bony swelling of the distal and proximal interphalangeal joints of the hands. First carpometacarpal joints bilaterally were tender and limited in motion. Hips were severely limited in range of motion in all directions, and movement was associated with severe pain. Knee swelling was absent but limitation of flexion to 90° bilaterally was evident.

The hematocrit was 43%, the white blood cell count was 8,000/mm³ with a normal differential, and the erythrocyte sedimentation rate was 22 mm/hour (Wintrobe). Serum electrolytes, calcium, phosphorus and alkaline phosphatase, and serum protein electrophoresis studies were within normal limits. Serum uric acid was 2.5 mg/100 ml. Fasting blood sugar was 90 mg/100 ml. Urinalysis was normal and serologic test for syphilis was negative. Urine study for homogentisic acid was negative. Serum studies for rheumatoid factor and antinuclear antibody were negative. Roentgenogram study of the chest was normal. Roentgenograms of the hips revealed significant degenerative changes bilaterally with narrowing of joint spaces, eburnation, and osteophytic spurring. Subchondral cyst formation was present in the femoral heads. Roentgenographic examination of the knees showed extensive degenerative changes bilaterally with narrowing of the joint spaces and spur formation. Multiple loose bodies appeared in the left knee. Roentgenograms of the hands and wrists revealed joint space narrowing and spur formation in numerous distal and proximal interphalangeal joints. A diagnosis of primary generalized osteoarthritis was made. Aspirin and indomethacin therapy was continued with inadequate relief of pain and disability. Multiple surgical procedures were indicated for management of the severe joint symptoms. Loose bodies were removed from the left knee and, at separate intervals, bilateral total hip replacements were performed.

Discussion: This patient had symptoms of severe generalized osteoarthritis at a relatively early age. A history of severe osteoarthritis occurring at an early age in other members of her family suggested a possible hereditary component to her disorder. Underlying disease states such as rheumatoid arthritis, hemophilia, and ochronosis, which are frequently associated with secondary osteoarthritis, were not evident.

History 7-4. Psoriatic Arthritis

R.P., a 34-year-old white male, was well until June, 1973, when he noted a pruritic dry scaly rash over the right temporal area. Shortly thereafter, similar lesions appeared on the scalp, the right ear and the lateral aspect of the right thigh. The lesions healed and itching decreased following therapy with local steroid cream. Approximately two months after onset of the rash, he developed insidious swelling and pain of the distal interphalangeal (DIP) joint of the left index finger and the interphalangeal joint of the third toe of the left foot. Morning stiffness lasted for 10 to 15 minutes. No ancillary symptoms of connective tissue disease were elicited.

Physical examination revealed dry scaly cutaneous lesions involving the scalp, right ear, and right thigh. Fingernails were slightly pitted. Fusiform sausage-like swellings of the DIP joint of the left index finger and the interphalangeal joint of the left third toe were noted. Both joints were warm and tender. Some tenderness of the second and fourth metatarsophalangeal (MTP) joints of the left foot was also observed.

Laboratory studies revealed normal complete blood count and urinalysis. Erythrocyte sedimentation rate was 23 mm/hour (Wintrobe). Serum uric acid was 5.9 mg/100 ml. Serum glutamic oxaloacetic transaminase, serologic test for syphilis, serum protein electrophoresis, electrocardiogram and chest x-ray were normal or negative. Roentgenograms of the involved joints were negative except for evidence of soft tissue swelling. A diagnosis of psoriasis with psoriatic arthritis was made.

The patient was placed on therapy with aspirin, 960 mg QID, with little relief of symptoms. Indomethacin, 25 mg QID, was helpful, but continued involvement of MTP joints caused moderate difficulty in walking. Local injections of steroid into the involved joints of the left hand and left foot provided considerable improvement. The patient remained on therapy with aspirin, 960 mg QID, and indomethacin, 25 mg QID, with only mild joint distress. Cutaneous lesions were kept under control with local applications of steroid cream.

Discussion: The clinical findings in this patient were consistent with the diagnosis of psoriatic arthritis. Fusiform sausage-like swellings of the joints, involvement of the distal interphalangeal joints of the hands and interphalangeal joints of the toes were characteristic. Although joint symptoms usually occur concomitant with or following the onset of psoriasis, arthritis may antedate psoriatic skin changes by months or years.

History 7-5. Mixed Connective Tissue Disease

Mrs. R.L., a 35-year-old white female was first seen in consultation on July 30, 1976. She gave a history of swelling of the small joints of the hands of 10 years' duration, and, over the past several years pain and slight swelling of the knees and the elbows. Raynaud's phenomenon had also been present for several years, characterized by white discoloration of the fingers followed by cyanosis. She took aspirin, 640 mg q4h prn for her symptoms. Recently she had been hospitalized elsewhere, and a diagnosis of systemic lupus erythematosus made. System review revealed a long history of classic migraine headaches. Sun exposure led to severe headaches and nausea. There was a history of pericarditis 3 years prior, but there was no history of pleurisy, hair loss, frequent canker sores in the mouth, iritis, or rash. The patient had never taken contraceptive medications. Past medical history revealed pericarditis, as noted above, but was otherwise non-contributory. Family history revealed that a maternal cousin had severe juvenile rheumatoid arthritis.

Physical examination revealed blood pressure 110/80, pulse 72/min, and normal temperature. The skin of the hands was thickened from the tips of the fingers to the metacarpophalangeal joints. Knees were swollen, grade I. No muscle weakness was noted. Hands and feet felt cool to palpation. There was no lymphadenopathy. Spleen and liver were not palpably enlarged. Initial differential diagnosis based on clinical findings, was 1) scleroderma, versus 2) systemic lupus erythematosus with secondary sclerodactyly, versus 3) mixed connective tissue disease with components of scleroderma and systemic lupus erythematosus. Laboratory findings revealed serum rheumatoid factor positive at 1:40 titer, a 3+ antinuclear antibody titer with rim pattern, and anti-DNA titer 1:20. The patient was hospitalized at University Hospitals for further evaluation. Additional laboratory studies at time of hospitalization revealed erythrocyte sedimentation rate 28 mm/hr, white blood cell count 4,400/mm^3, normal differential white cell count, hematocrit 40%, normal serum BUN, creatinine, electrolytes and normal urinalysis. LE cells were present in the peripheral blood. Coomb's test was negative. Serum creatine phosphokinase was normal as was the urinary creatine/creatinine ratio. Serum protein electrophoresis revealed elevated gamma globulin, 1.5 g/100 ml; serum immunoelectrophoresis revealed a polyclonal increase in IgG, IgM and IgA. Serum CH^{50} hemolytic complement was 50% of normal. Anti-nRNP titer was greater than 1:100,000. Serum cryoglobulin studies were negative. Skin biopsy study from dorsal forearm sun-exposed skin revealed absent basement membrane immunofluorescence, but positive epidermal nuclear staining. Electrocardiogram was normal. Roentgenograms of the chest, barium swallow, upper GI series and small bowel follow-through, and roentgenograms of the hands, wrists, elbows, shoulders, knees, and dental panorex were all normal. Pulmonary function studies were consistent with a minimal obstructive ventilatory defect which did not improve significantly after bronchodilators.

The patient was followed by her physician at home and was next seen in consultation in August 1978, at which time she was rehospitalized at University Hospitals for study. Joint symptoms with pain and swelling had spread to involve almost all peripheral joints. She continued to have moderately severe Raynaud's phenomenon which occurred even in warm summer weather. History also revealed intermittent malar butterfly rash and two interval episodes of pericarditis. The sclerodermatous changes in the hands were stable. On physical examination, a butterfly rash was present over the facial malar areas and several urticarial lesions were seen on the extremities. There was mild limitation of both shoulders and mild synovitis of numerous peripheral joints. Sclerodactyly changes of the hands were unchanged. Laboratory studies revealed hematocrit 40%, white blood cell count 3,700/mm^3, erythrocyte sedimentation rate 34 mm/hour, normal liver function studies, electrolytes and urinalysis. Chest roentgenogram and electrocardiogram revealed no changes and were considered normal. Echocardiogram was normal. Upper GI series and barium swallow revealed marked dilatation of the stomach with hypotonia involving the proximal duodenum. She was discharged on therapy with enteric-coated aspirin, 960 mg QID. Quinacrine, 100 mg/day, was initiated due to intolerance to hydroxychloroquine administration. Failure of symptomatic response to aspirin, and later, to various other nonsteroidal anti-inflammatory agents led to the institution of low-dose prednisone therapy, 5 mg/day.

The patient was followed subsequently in periodic consultation with satisfactory clinical response. When last seen on 6/2/81 she had mild sclerodermatous changes of the hands and minimal evidence of arthritis of peripheral joints. Therapy included prednisone 5 mg/day, quinacrine, 100 mg/day, taken six weeks on and two weeks off, rest and physical therapy.

Discussion. This patient exhibited clinical and laboratory findings consistent with a diagnosis of Mixed Connective Tissue Disease. Clinical manifestations included elements of scleroderma, systemic lupus erythematosus and rheumatoid arthritis. There was, however, no clinical or laboratory evidence of myositis commonly seen in this syndrome. Anti-nRNP antibody was present in high titer. Epidermal nuclear staining, seen on immunofluorescent study of the skin biopsy specimen, has been shown to correlate with anti-nRNP antibody; it does not appear to be specific for Mixed Connective Tissue Disease, being noted as well in patients with systemic lupus erythematosus, scleroderma and rheumatoid arthritis. Hypotonia of the bowel was consistent with the scleroderma component of her illness, and abnormal pulmonary function studies have been described in patients with Mixed Connective Tissue Disease. Patients with this disorder generally respond well to a conservative therapeutic program, although low-dose steroid therapy may be required for control of symptoms. Antimalarial therapy appeared helpful in treating various components of her symptom complex.

REFERENCES

1. Barnes, C. G., Trumbull, A. L. and Vernon-Roberts, B.: Felty's syndrome. Ann Rheum Dis 30:359, 1971.
2. Mason, A. M. S., Gumpel, J. M. and Golding, P. L.: Sjögren's syndrome—a clinical view. Semin Arthritis Rheum 2:301, 1973.
3. Whaley, K., Chisholm, D. M., Mason, D. K. et al.: Sjögren's syndrome. Quarterly J Med 42:279, 1973.
4. Newball, H. H. and Brahim, S. A.: Chronic obstructive airway disease in patients with Sjögren's syndrome. Am Rev Resp Dis 115:295, 1977.
5. Cummings, N. A. et al.: Sjögren's syndrome. Newer aspects of research, diagnosis and therapy. Ann Int Med 75:937, 1971.
6. Daniels, T. E., et al.: The oral component of Sjögren's syndrome. Oral Surgery 39:875, 1975.
7. Alarcon-Segovia, D. et al.: Salivary gland involvement in diseases associated with Sjögren's syndrome. 1. Radionuclide and roentgenographic studies. J Rheumatology 1:159, 1974.
8. Daniels, T. E. et al.: An evaluation of salivary scintigraphy in Sjögren's syndrome. Arthritis Rheum 22:809, 1979.
9. Kassan, S. S. et al.: Antibody to a soluble acidic nuclear antigen in Sjögren's syndrome. Am J Med 63:328, 1977.
10. Scopelitis, E., Biundo, J. J. and Alspaugh, N. A.: Antibody and other antinuclear antibodies in systemic lupus erythematosus. Arthritis Rheum 23:287, 1980.
11. Sharp, G. C. et al.: Mixed connective tissue disease—an apparently distinct rheumatic disease syndrome associated with specific antibody to an extractable nuclear antigen (ENA). Am J Med 52:148, 1972.
12. Reichlin, M.: Problems in differentiating SLE and mixed connective tissue disease. N Eng J Med 295:1194, 1976.
13. Sharp, G. C.: Mixed connective tissue disease—current concepts. Arthritis Rheum 20:S181, 1977.
14. Halla, J. T. and Hardin, J. G.: Clinical features of the arthritis of mixed connective tissue disease. Arthritis Rheum 21:497, 1978.
15. Ramos-Niembro, F., Alarcon-Segovia, D. and Hernandez-Ortiz, J.: Articular manifestations of mixed connective tissue disease. Arthritis Rheum 22:43, 1979.
16. Moll, J. M. H. and Wright, V.: Psoriatic arthritis. Semin Arthritis Rheum 3:55, 1973.
17. Roberts, M. E. T., Wright, V., Haill, A. G. S et al.: Psoriatic arthritis: follow-up study. Ann Rheum Dis 35:206, 1976.
18. Ford, D. K.: Reiter's syndrome. Bull Rheum Dis 20:588, 1970.
19. Lassus, A. and Karnoven, J.: Reactive arthritis, Reiter's disease and psoriatic arthritis. In Clinics in Rheumatic Diseases. W. B. Saunders Co., Philadelphia, 1977, p 281.

20. Morris, R. et al.: HLA-W27—a clue to the diagnosis and pathogenesis of Reiter's syndrome. N Eng J Med 290:554, 1974.
21. Woodrow, J. C.: Histocompatibility antigens and rheumatic diseases. Semin Arthritis Rheum 6:257, 1977.
22. Morris, R. I. et al.: HLA-W27—a useful discriminator in the arthropathies of inflammatory bowel disease. N Eng J Med 290:1117, 1974.
23. Lansbury, J.: Collagen disease complicating malignancy. Ann Rheum Dis 12:301, 1953.
24. Mackenzie, A. H. and Scherbel, A. L.: Connective tissue syndromes associated with carcinoma. Geriatrics 18:745, 1963.
25. Donnelly, B. and Johnson, P. M.: Detection of hypertrophic pulmonary osteoarthropathy by skeletal imaging with 99M-tc-labeled diphosphate. Radiology 114:389, 1975.
26. Moskowitz, R. W. et al.: Chronic synovitis as a manifestation of calcium crystal deposition disease. Arthritis Rheum 14:109, 1971.
27. Moskowitz, R. W. and Garcia, F.: Pseudogout syndrome. Arch Int Med 132:87, 1973.
28. McCarty, D. J.: Calcium pyrophosphate dihydrate crystal deposition disease—1975. Arthritis Rheum 19:275, 1976.
29. O'Duffy, J. D., Carney, J. A. and Deodhar, S.: Behçet's disease: a report of ten cases, three with new manifestations. Ann Int Med 75:561, 1971.
30. Shagrin, J. W., Frame, B. and Duncan, V.: Polyarthritis in obese patients with intestinal bypass. Ann Int Med 75:377, 1971.
31. Fernandez-Herlihy, L.: Arthritis after jejuno-ileostomy for intractible obesity. J Rheum 4:135, 1977.
32. Zapanta, M., et al.: Arthritis associated with jejunoileal bypass. Arthritis Rheum 22:711, 1979.
33. Churchill, M. A., Geraci, J. E. and Hunder, G. G.: Musculoskeletal manifestations of bacterial endocarditis. Ann Int Med 87:754, 1977.
34. Dymock, I. W. et al.: Arthropathy of haemochromatosis. Ann Rheum Dis 29:469, 1970.
35. Gordon, D. A. and Little, H. A.: The arthropathy of hemochromatosis without hemochromatosis. Arthritis Rheum 16:305, 1973.
36. Bland, J. and Frymoyer, J.: Rheumatic syndromes in myxedema. N Eng J Med 282:1171, 1970.
37. Goldman, J. A. et al.: Musculoskeletal disorders associated with type IV hyperlipoproteinemia. Arthritis Rheum 14:384, 1971.
38. Buckingham, R. B., Bole, G. G. and Bassett, D. R.: Polyarthritis associated with type IV hyperlipoproteinemia. Arch Int Med 135:286, 1975.
39. Clarke, A. K., Galbraith, R. N., Hamilton, E. B. D. and Williams, R.: Rheumatic disorders in primary biliary cirrhosis. Ann Rheum Dis 37:42, 1978.
40. Marx, W. J. and O'Connell, J.: Arthritis of primary biliary cirrhosis. Arch Int Med 139:213, 1979.
41. Pastan, R. S., Silverman, S. L. and Goldenberg, D. L.: A musculo-skeletal syndrome in intravenous heroin users. Ann Int Med 87:22, 1977.

CHAPTER 8

INTERMITTENT ARTHRITIS SYNDROMES

In some patients, joint symptoms are characterized by acute attacks that are frequent, recurrent, and intermittent with variable periods of complete remission. Sometimes the recurrences have a periodic character. A limited number of rheumatic diseases produce such a clinical picture, in contrast to numerous arthritic diseases in which articular symptoms are cyclic but exacerbations are usually long in duration and remissions, unfortunately, are limited and incomplete. For example, rheumatoid arthritis, systemic lupus erythematosus and rheumatic fever frequently demonstrate remissions and exacerbations but usually would not be classified as "intermittent arthritis syndromes."

Diseases characterized as intermittent arthritis syndromes include:

Gout
Pseudogout
Episodic rheumatoid arthritis
Palindromic rheumatism
Intermittent hydrarthrosis
Familial Mediterranean fever
Whipple's disease
Relapsing polychondritis
Arthritis of hyperlipidemia

DIFFERENTIAL DIAGNOSIS

Gout is classically characterized by attacks of acute arthritis abrupt in onset. The usual attack lasts three to seven days followed by variable periods of complete remission during which the joint is normal. Early in the disease, remissions may be prolonged, lasting for months or years. Later, as the disease progresses, acute attacks become more frequent until they recur as often as several times a month. The first metatarsophalangeal joint is most frequently involved (podagra) (Fig. 4-3), but other joints such as the tarsal area, ankle and knee are commonly involved. At times, peripheral joints of the upper extremities are affected. Acute attacks occur spontaneously or may be precipitated by such factors as trauma, surgery, overindulgence in alcohol, intake of high purine foods or diuretic therapy. Acute inflammation results from precipitation of monosodium urate crystals in synovial fluid with subsequent release of various inflammatory mediators. Finding urate crystals in synovial fluid removed from the joint is specific for the diagnosis.

Pseudogout syndrome (chondrocalcinosis) is similarly characterized by acute attacks of joint inflammation that are abrupt in onset. Attacks tend to be less frequent than those seen in true gout. Clinically, the joint most frequently involved is the knee. Other large joints may be involved; podagra occurs but is relatively uncommon. As in true gout, surgery or diuretic therapy may precipitate attacks. Often, there is a background symptomatology of low-grade chronic arthralgia upon which acute attacks are superimposed. Acute symptoms are related to the activation of inflammatory mediators by calcium pyrophosphate dihydrate crystals in synovial fluid. Roentgenograms reveal typical calcifications of articular hyaline and fibrocartilage (Figs. 4-4, 4-5).

Rheumatoid arthritis may occur as an episodic disease, so-called *episodic rheumatoid arthritis,* which is difficult to differentiate from gout and pseudogout. Abrupt onset of acute attacks over a period of several hours is characteristic. Attacks last 36 hours to several days and are followed by complete remission. As the disease progresses, acute attacks become more frequent and prolonged, and complete remission no longer ensues. A similar clinical picture is characteristic of *palindromic rheumatism.*[1] This interesting entity of unknown etiology is also characterized by acute, abrupt attacks of joint inflammation. Symptoms often develop within a period of hours. Severe pain occurs early, followed by joint redness, tenderness and swelling. Any peripheral joint may be affected. Interestingly, joint pain may decrease when swelling is maximal. Duration of attacks varies from a few hours to as long as a week; attacks lasting only several days are most common. One or a limited number of joints are involved at a time. The interval between attacks varies from several days to months. The pattern of attacks with respect to area and frequency of joint involvement may be characteristic in a given patient. Para-articular inflammation characterized by variably-sized painful erythematous swellings in soft tissues adjacent to joints is common. Transient intracutaneous and subcutaneous nodules may be seen. Prognosis is excellent with respect to crippling because, by definition, chronic joint changes do not evolve. On the other hand, control of disease symptoms may be difficult with considerable distress and limitation occurring during the periodic recurrent attacks.

The similarities between palindromic rheumatism and episodic rheumatoid arthritis may cause appreciable diagnostic confusion. It has been suggested that palindromic rheumatism is a prodromal or atypical form of rheumatoid arthritis.[2] Many cases originally diagnosed as possible palindromic rheumatism eventually manifest themselves as rheumatoid arthritis as attacks become more frequent and remissions less complete. The presence of rheumatoid factor in high titer in the serum supports a diagnosis of rheumatoid arthritis. Low titers of rheumatoid factor are less helpful; such findings have been reported in palindromic rheumatism.[2] Serum complement studies during and following acute episodes of palindromic rheumatism failed to show reduction in any of a variety of complement components.[3] Accordingly, attacks do not appear to be precipitated by systemic activation of the complement system. In these studies the authors were unable to differentiate episodic rheumatoid arthritis from palindromic rheumatism by laboratory or clinical evaluation.[3] It was their impression that many if not all cases will "convert" to rheumatoid arthritis if followed for a sufficiently long period of time.

Intermittent hydrarthrosis is characterized by acute recurrent attacks of joint swelling of predictable periodicity.[4] Joint effusions are notable for their lack of local inflammatory change and relatively little pain. Systemic signs and symptoms are absent. Usually, symptoms completely resolve and attacks abate in two to four days. Knees are involved most commonly. Although attacks are usually monoarticular, polyarticular involvement does occur. The interval between attacks varies from one week to one month, with intervals of one to two weeks being most common. Attacks at monthly intervals are likely to be related to menstruation in women. In some patients, effusions cease after many years; other patients, unfortunately, will have the syndrome as a life-long condition. There are no characteristic laboratory findings.

Familial Mediterranean fever is an inherited disorder of people from the Eastern Mediterranean area, chiefly Sephardic Jews, Levantine Arabs, Turks and Armenians.[5] The disease is characterized by recurrent acute or subacute attacks of arthritis, frequently associated with fever and with abdominal and chest pain due to polyserositis. Symptoms are usually short-lived, lasting several days to one or two weeks. In some cases, however, arthritis persists for months. Knees, ankles and hips are involved most frequently. Fortunately, functional joint recovery between attacks is usually complete. Many patients develop an erysipelas-like erythema and tenderness around the ankles. Amyloidosis, a dreaded manifestation of the disease, is a common cause of death.

Whipple's disease[6] is characterized by fever, abdominal pain, diarrhea, cutaneous hyperpigmentation, adenopathy and arthritis. Joint symptoms are frequently acute in onset, episodic and transient, lasting only for several hours or days. Residual joint changes are uncommon. In many cases, articular manifestations precede abdominal symptoms by years. Large joints, such as the knee and the ankle, are involved most often, but smaller joints are also affected.

Relapsing polychondritis is a systemic disorder characterized by inflammation of cartilaginous tissue, involvement of organs of special sense such as the eye and ear, and cardiovascular structures.[7,8] Classically, involvement of the cartilaginous portions of the ears (pinnas) is associated with marked swelling, tenderness and purplish-red discoloration. Inflammation of laryngeal and tracheal cartilages leads to hoarseness, cough and, when severe, occlusion of respiratory passages which at times necessitates emergency tracheostomy. Involvement of the bridge of the nose produces a characteristic saddle-nose deformity. Middle and inner ear involvement results in hearing impairment or acute attacks of vertigo. Episcleritis, conjunctivitis or iritis are common. Aortic regurgitation occurs due to involvement of the aortic ring with progressive dilatation. Articular symptoms are seen in up to 75% of cases. They may be the presenting manifestation in up to one-third of patients. Large joints are usually involved, in an asymmetric migratory pattern. Joint symptoms are frequently episodic, lasting several days to weeks usually followed by spontaneous resolution to an asymptomatic state. In some patients, however, chronic oligoarticular or polyarticular disease may develop, with acute attacks of arthritis developing on a background of well-established chronic disease. Involvement of costochondral junctions not infrequently leads to parasternal pain and tenderness, and a flail chest wall.

Acute, subacute and chronic arthritis has been described in patients with *hyperlipidemia*. Familial hypercholesterolemia (type II hyperlipoproteinemia) is associated with a migratory form of acute polyarthritis which simulates acute rheumatic fever.[9] Large joints are most frequently affected and attacks are typically migratory in nature. Achilles tendinitis and tenosynovitis are occasionally noted.[10] The overall disorder is characterized clinically by associated cutaneous xanthomatosis, xanthelasma, arcus senilis of the cornea, and premature atherosclerosis. Patients with type IV hyperlipoproteinemia most frequently have joint manifestations which are limited in distribution and subacute in presentation.[11] In some patients, however, acute attacks of arthritis which occur in episodic fashion develop. Attacks last a few days to weeks and may be moderately severe.

Other diseases, such as Behçet's syndrome, ulcerative colitis, and Henoch-Schönlein purpura, may be associated with intermittent joint manifestations. Articular symptoms are usually overshadowed by serious abnormalities related to other organ systems.

DIAGNOSTIC STUDIES

Clinical similarities may make it extremely difficult to differentiate the foregoing diseases not only from one another but from other forms of rheumatic disease. Close attention to subtle details of the history and physical examination is vital. Diagnosis often depends on carefully considered laboratory investigation. Initial laboratory studies should include a complete blood count, erythrocyte sedimentation rate, urinalysis, serologic test for syphilis, serum latex fixation test for rheumatoid factor, serum antinuclear factor, serum protein electrophoresis, synovial fluid analysis and x-ray of involved joints. Synovial fluid analysis is particularly helpful in the diagnosis of gout or pseudogout, because the finding of intracellular and extracellular crystals of monosodium urate or calcium pyrophosphate dihydrate respectively is diagnostic. Joint fluid examination should be performed early in the acute attack if possible, because crystals are often few or absent during remissions. Although serum uric acid determinations are helpful in corroborating a diagnosis of gout, some studies suggest an increased frequency of coincidental hyperuricemia in pseudogout patients. Serum calcium, phosphorus and alkaline phosphatase and serum iron, iron-binding capacity, and iron saturation studies should be performed in patients with pseudogout to exclude the presence of hyperparathyroidism and hemochromatosis.

A high-titer positive test for serum rheumatoid factor supports a diagnosis of episodic rheumatoid arthritis. Low or negative titers are consistent with rheumatoid arthritis or palindromic rheumatism. Increases in erythrocyte sedimentation rate are common during acute attacks in both diseases. Final differentiation depends on the development of more prolonged attacks and incomplete remissions in patients with episodic rheumatoid arthritis.

There are no specific diagnostic laboratory studies for intermittent hydrarthrosis. The clinical finding of periodic attacks of acute swelling of the knees associated with little or no pain is fairly characteristic, however, and differentiation from the other syndromes described previously usually is not difficult.

Familial Mediterranean fever should be strongly considered in the differential diagnosis of acute intermittent arthritis in patients of Mediterranean origin. Although several abnormal laboratory findings are frequently noted, they are unfortunately nonspecific. The erythrocyte sedimentation rate and the plasma fibrinogen level are elevated during attacks and may even remain slightly elevated during intercritical periods. Massive proteinuria often develops if amyloidosis intervenes. Serum gamma globulin elevations are common. The serum latex fixation test for rheumatoid factor is usually negative. Synovial fluid analysis reveals nonspecific evidence of mild inflammatory disease.

The diagnosis of Whipple's disease depends on demonstrating PAS-positive inclusion bodies in macrophages of the small intestinal mucosa or mesenteric nodes. Jejunal biopsy is performed by peroral approach. Rod-shaped organisms infiltrating the lamina propria of the intestinal mucosa appear on electron microscopic study.

The diagnosis of relapsing polychondritis is based on the clinical presentation, since there are no specific laboratory diagnostic studies. In many patients, disease manifestations do not occur in co-existent fashion; the diagnosis is suspected only after long-term follow-up when multiple clinical components of the disease become evident. Not infrequently, polychondritis involving the ear and nose is diagnosed as a nonspecific cellulitis until recurrences with involvement of other systems alerts the physician to the correct diagnosis. An elevated erythrocyte sedimentation rate and mild leukocytosis are not uncommon during acute disease activity. Nonspecific anemia may be seen. False-positive serologic tests for syphilis and circulating immune complexes have been described. Serum protein electrophoresis abnormalities are nonspecific. Roentgenograms are helpful mainly in demonstrating complications of the disease. Calcification of cartilages of the ear, nose or lower respiratory tract, although not specific, may be diagnostically useful.

Acute intermittent arthritis as a result of abnormalities in plasma lipoproteins may be suggested by the finding of cutaneous xanthomas or premature atherosclerosis. Studies of serum cholesterol and triglycerides, and lipoprotein electrophoresis should be carried out as a screening measure in patients with atypical acute polyarthritis of otherwise undefined diagnosis.

Radiologic studies are helpful in the diagnosis of pseudogout and familial Mediterranean fever. In the former, characteristic calcifications of articular hyaline and fibrocartilage are seen. In familial Mediterranean fever, joints involved for a long period of time show coarse trabecular osteoporosis and pseudocyst formation. Swelling of the knee is associated with enlargement of the femoral condyles. In a few patients, a characteristic "eggshell line" may be found on both sides of the radiolucent osteoporotic zone at the distal femur. This double contoured line may persist after osteoporosis resolves as the attack abates. Roentgenographic studies of patients with type IV hyperlipoproteinemia may reveal juxta-articular osteoporosis and cystic lesions of the metaphyseal area.

THERAPY

Acute attacks of gout or pseudogout may be treated effectively with varius therapeutic agents (see Chapter 19). Acute attacks of episodic rheumatoid arthritis of mild severity may respond to high-dose salicylate therapy. In more severe cases, full doses of alternative newer nonsteroidal anti-inflammatory agents may be useful. In patients who fail to respond to these agents, prednisone in a dose of 5 mg q.i.d. is often effective. Acute attacks can often be aborted or lessened in severity by instituting anti-inflammatory therapy at the first sign of pain, before the attack reaches a significant degree of intensity. Continuous prophylaxis with nonsteroidal anti-inflammatory agents may afford long-term suppression when recurrent attacks are frequent. More frequently beneficial for this purpose is long-term therapy with antimalarial agents, such as hydroxychloroquine (Plaquenil), gold or D-penicillamine. Hydroxychloroquine is given in a dose of 200 mg twice a day for three to four months, following which the dose usually can be decreased to 200 mg daily. Periodic eye evaluation should be performed to avoid toxicity occasionally associated with long-term use of this agent. Gold therapy, carried out as in the usual case of rheumatoid arthritis, has equal or greater effect. D-penicillamine may be similarly useful. Treatment and prevention of acute attacks of palindromic rheumatism is similar to that described for episodic rheumatoid arthritis. Continuous prophylaxis with hydroxychloroquine or gold is particularly effective in many patients and should be considered if attacks are frequent and severe. Preliminary studies suggest that D-penicillamine may be helpful for these patients as well.[12]

No satisfactory treatment is presently available for intermittent hydrarthrosis. Daily salicylate therapy during attacks may ameliorate the swelling and is attended by little hazard. Fortunately, pain is usually not a problem and more aggressive therapy is not required. In patients with familial Mediterranean fever, aspirin, other analgesic agents and local heat may provide partial relief for acute attacks. Corticosteroid agents are surprisingly ineffective. More recently, full therapeutic doses of colchicine used early in the onset of acute attacks have been found beneficial in the management of acute episodes in some patients.[13] Colchicine, 0.6 mg TID, administered on a regular daily basis, has been shown to be effective in prophylaxis of recurrent attacks.[14] Other agents reported to have therapeutic value include conjugated estrogens[15] and indomethacin.[16]

The response of Whipple's disease to antibiotics is highly successful. A program that includes procaine penicillin G, 1.2 million units, and streptomycin, 1 g daily for two weeks, followed by tetracycline, 250 mg QID for 10 to 12 months, is currently recommended.

Joint manifestations of relapsing polychondritis can frequently be controlled by use of aspirin or other nonsteroidal anti-inflammatory agents administered at time of acute attacks. Chronic administration of these agents may be indicated in patients with more continuous joint symptomatology. *Investigational* trials of colchicine in doses of 0.6 mg b.i.d. or t.i.d. have been shown successful in controlling not only some of the systemic manifestations of polychondritis, but in prevention of recurrences of arthritis as well.[17] Acute attacks of arthritis have been similarly successfully treated by use of full therapeutic doses of this agent. In patients with serious systemic manifestations, or in whom arthritis is disabling, consideration may be given to the use of corticosteroid agents. Long term administration of corticosteroids or immunosuppressive agents, necessary in some patients for control of life-threatening disease manifestations, is rarely needed to control articular symptoms alone. Dapsone, a sulfone drug, has been described as an effective agent in treatment of this disorder,[18,19] although its use at present remains *investigational*. Hemolysis, with associated methemoglobinemia is a frequent side-reaction, particularly in patients with G-6PD deficiency. Bone marrow suppression and hepatotoxicity are further toxic effects which must be monitored.

In patients with arthritis due to lipoprotein abnormalities, therapy directed at reduction of abnormally elevated lipids may at times diminish articular manifestations. Acute and subacute attacks of arthritis not infrequently respond to nonsteroidal anti-inflammatory agents.

CASE HISTORIES

History 8-1. Gout

N.V., a 42-year-old white male, first noted joint symptoms at age 32, at which time he developed sudden onset of acute pain and swelling of the first metatarsophalangeal (MTP) joint of the right foot. Symptoms resolved after five or six days without specific treatment and the patient was essentially asymptomatic. Recurrent acute attacks of monoarthritis were noted at intervals of approximately six months. Symptoms were acute in onset, extremely painful, and lasted for four to seven days. Right and left first MTP joints and the tarsal areas of the feet were involved. Complete remission occurred after each attack. After approximately six acute episodes, a diagnosis of gout was made on the basis of the clinical picture, the presence of a serum uric acid level of 9.2 mg/100 ml, and a family history of gout in his brother and paternal grandfather. Treatment with probenecid, 0.5 g daily, was instituted. The patient continued to have similar attacks at intervals of six to nine months. Acute symptoms were treated with short courses of phenylbutazone, but no changes were made in his interval therapy program.

The patient was first seen in consultation in December, 1973, after he had been admitted to the urology service with a history of acute right flank and right lower abdominal pain. Intravenous pyelogram was normal but the patient passed a uric acid stone after two days in the hospital. Serum uric acid on admission, while the patient was still on probenecid, 0.5 g daily, was 8.6 mg/100 ml. Probenecid therapy was discontinued to study baseline uric acid metabolism. Colchicine, 0.6 mg BID, was given as prophylaxis against acute gouty attacks until studies were completed on an outpatient basis. Laboratory studies performed two weeks after discharge from hospital revealed serum uric acid levels of 9.8 and 10.6 mg/100 ml, and daily urinary uric acid excretions of 1120 mg and 1360 mg on a normal diet. Hematocrit, white blood cell count and differential, urinalysis, and creatine clearance studies were normal. Colchicine, 0.6 mg BID, was continued, and allopurinol (Zyloprim) was begun in a dose of 300 mg daily. Serum uric acid level, rechecked after a period of four weeks on his new therapeutic regimen, revealed a serum uric acid of 4.8 mg/100 ml. His clinical course was uncomplicated and the patient was free of recurrent attacks of acute gouty arthritis or renal stones for a period of prolonged follow-up.

Discussion: The clinical history in this patient was characteristic of gouty arthritis. Attacks of monoarthritis were acute in onset, lasted four to seven days in duration, and were followed by complete remission. Involvement of first MTP joints was prominent. Inadequate therapy with probenecid was associated with continued symptomatology. The presence of hyperuricosuria and uric acid stone formation prompted use of allopurinol rather than probenecid for treatment of his articular and renal manifestations.

History 8-2. Episodic Rheumatoid Arthritis

H.R., a 56-year-old white male, was first seen in consultation in March, 1971. Joint symptoms had begun approximately one year prior, at which time he developed recurrent acute attacks of pain and swelling that separately involved the left and right knees. Attacks began over a period of hours and resolved in 24 to 36 hours without specific therapy. Acute episodes recurred at intervals of two to six weeks. Especially severe attacks of pain were treated with short courses of phenylbutazone or intramuscular injections of steroids. In January, 1971, he noted similar intermittent acute attacks of pain that involved, at various times, the ankles, proximal interphalangeal (PIP) and metacarpophalangeal (MCP) joints of the hands, and the tarsal areas. Attacks became somewhat more frequent. Remission of symptoms was less complete and attacks were more prolonged. System review was negative for skin rash, sun sensitivity, colitis, iritis, renal stones or hair loss. There was no family history of gout. Past medical history was significant in that the patient had severe urticaria and headaches with use of coal tar products. Therapy consisted of prednisone, 2.5 mg QID.

On physical examination there was acute swelling of the right wrist and the right second MCP joint. Serum rheumatoid factor and antinuclear antibody studies were negative. Serum uric acid was 5.4 mg/100 ml. Hematocrit, white blood cell count and differential, and urinalysis were normal. Serum protein electrophoresis was within normal limits. Roentgenograms of the chest, both knees, and both hands and wrists were negative except for evidence of soft tissue swelling about the right wrist joint. A diagnosis of probable episodic rheumatoid arthritis was made. The patient was maintained on therapy with prednisone, 2.5 mg QID, with instructions to increase the dose temporarily at the onset of acute attacks in the hope of aborting the symptomatic episodes. Hydroxychloroquine (Plaquenil), 200 mg BID, was added to the program. Symptoms improved only minimally on this regimen and hydroxychloroquine was discontinued after a six-month trial. Gold sodium thiomalate therapy was begun. The patient noted great improvement in symptoms at a total dose of 275 mg of gold salt. Shortly thereafter, on a program of 50 mg of gold salt weekly, the patient developed severe stomatitis and generalized pruritus; gold was discontinued. After one month, gold therapy was reinstituted, beginning with a trial dose of 5 mg of gold salt. The dose was gradually increased and weekly maintenance injections of 20 mg were given. The patient tolerated this dose without complication and continued to do well. The interval of gold administration was gradually increased to once a month.

The patient did satisfactorily until December, 1972, when he had a generalized flare of arthritis with extensive swelling and pain of the PIP and MCP joints, both wrists, both knees and ankles. Subcutaneous nodules were noted over both subolecranon areas. Serum rheumatoid factor study, which had been negative on prior repeated testing, was now positive in a titer of 1:256. An increase in the dose of gold salt to 25 mg weekly was not associated with notable clinical improvement. Prednisone, which had been reduced to 2.5 mg BID, was increased to 2.5 mg QID. Further increase in gold therapy to 30 mg weekly was associated with stomatitis and skin rash. The patient was hospitalized in January, 1973, for therapy of his severe uncontrolled joint symptoms. Gold therapy was discontinued and, with the advised consent of the patient, therapy with chlorambucil (Leukeran), 2 mg BID, was begun because of his lack of response to gold therapy in the maximal tolerated dose. The patient continued to have severe, persistent joint symptoms until April, 1973, when he noted a significant progressive improvement. Prednisone intake was gradually reduced to 2.5 mg BID. Rheumatoid arthritis symptoms stabilized over a period of several years follow-up and chlorambucil was discontinued. The patient continued to do satisfactorily on a program consisting of prednisone 2.5 mg b.i.d. with no additional therapy. Joint symptoms were characterized by only mild swelling of both wrists and elbows; occasional acute flares responded to intermittent use of intramuscular injections of triamcinolone acetonide.

Discussion: This patient had acute episodes of arthritis lasting 24 to 36 hours in duration. Attacks became progressively more frequent and severe with less complete remission. Eventually, joint symptoms were chronic and persistent and characteristic of the joint involvement in rheumatoid arthritis. Subcutaneous rheumatoid nodules and a positive test for serum rheumatoid factor eventually appeared. Good control of symptoms was obtained with gold therapy but toxicity necessitated consideration of other therapeutic measures. The patient subsequently appeared to respond well to the use of chlorambucil. Although immunosuppressive agents have been reported as useful in the treatment of rheumatoid arthritis, their utilization in general remains investigative at this time. Immunosuppressive therapy was discontinued in this patient after a period of several years since his overall response was reasonably satisfactory with maintenance therapy on low doses of prednisone alone.

History 8-3. Intermittent Hydrarthrosis

L.S., a 39-year-old white female, was first seen in consultation in November, 1972. She was well until approximately four years prior when, approximately one month after the birth of her third child, she noted acute onset of relatively painless swelling of the left knee. Symptoms receded spontaneously after two days. Since that time she had been afflicted with recurrent episodes of acute attacks of joint swelling that involved the right knee, the left knee or both knees simultaneously. Swelling was relatively painless, lasted two or three days, and resolved without specific therapy. Attacks initially occurred at intervals of one month, beginning several days before the onset of menses. Later, attacks continued to occur on a regular basis, but at intervals of eight or nine days. There were no other joint symptoms. System review was otherwise completely negative and past medical history was unremarkable. On physical examination, performed several days after the onset of one of her attacks in the right knee, a small amount of fluid was noted on palpation and there was a positive bulge sign. No tenderness or increased warmth was noted.

Urinalysis, white blood cell count and differential, hematocrit, and serologic test for syphilis were normal or negative. Erythrocyte sedimentation rate was 22 mm/hour (Wintrobe). Serum studies for rheumatoid factor and antinuclear antibody were negative. Serum uric acid was 3.1 mg/100 ml. Roentgenograms of both knees showed no calcifications or other abnormalities. Differential diagnostic considerations included benign idiopathic intermittent hydrarthrosis, and intermittent hydrarthrosis secondary to rheumatoid arthritis. The patient was advised to use aspirin, 960 mg QID, for mild acute attacks, and short courses of phenylbutazone for more severe episodes. A trial of hydroxychloroquine (Plaquenil), 200 mg BID, was to be added later in an effort to diminish or eliminate the frequency and severity of attacks. She was asked to return at the time of one of the attacks so that synovial fluid could be obtained for analysis. Shortly thereafter, the patient moved to another area of the country and was lost to follow-up.

Discussion: The clinical picture of acute episodes of relatively painless knee swelling occurring on an intermittent regular basis and resolving spontaneously is consistent with a diagnosis of benign idiopathic intermittent hydrarthrosis. A diagnosis of rheumatoid arthritis could not be completely excluded, because a similar pattern of joint manifestations may be seen in early cases. The increased frequency of attacks prompted concern in this regard. Synovial fluid analysis would have been helpful to exclude crystal-induced synovitis, a less likely diagnostic consideration. Prolonged observation is generally necessary to substantiate a diagnosis of benign idiopathic intermittent hydrarthrosis.

REFERENCES

1. Mattingly, S.: Palindromic rheumatism. Ann Rheum Dis 25:307, 1966.
2. Williams, M. H. et al.: Palindromic rheumatism. Clinical and immunological studies. Ann Rheum Dis 30:375, 1971.
3. Wajed, M. A., Brown, D. L. and Currey, H. L. F.: Palindromic rheumatism: clinical and serum complement study. Ann Rheum Dis 36:56, 1977.
4. Weiner, A. D. and Ghormley, R. K.: Periodic benign synovitis. Idiopathic intermittent hydrarthrosis. J Bone Joint Surg 38A:1039, 1956.
5. Sohar, E. et al.: Familial Mediterranean fever. A survey of 470 cases and review of literature. Am J Med 43:227, 1967.
6. Kelly, J. J. and Weisiger, B. B.: The arthritis of Whipple's disease. Arthritis Rheum 6:615, 1963.
7. O'Hanlin, M. et al.: The arthropathy of relapsing polychondritis. Arthritis Rheum 19:191, 1976.
8. McAdam, L. P. et al.: Relapsing polychondritis: prospective study of 23 patients and review of the literature. Medicine 55:193, 1976.
9. Khachadurian, A. K.: Migratory polyarthritis and familial hypercholesterolemia (type II, hyperlipoproteinemia). Arthritis Rheum 11:385, 1968.
10. Shapiro, J. R., et al.: Achilles tendinitis and tenosynovitis. A diagnostic manifestation of familial type II hyperlipoproteinemia in children. Am J Dis Child 128:486, 1974.
11. Buckingham, R. B., Bole, G. G. and Bassett, D. R.: Polyarthritis associated with type IV hyperlipoproteinemia. Arch Int Med 135:286, 1975.
12. Huskisson, E. C.: Treatment of palindromic rheumatism with D-penicillamine. Br Med J 2:979, 1976.
13. Wright, D. G. et al.: Efficacy of intermittent colchicine therapy in familial Mediterranean fever. Ann Int Med 86:162, 1977.
14. Dinarello, C. A. et al.: Colchicine therapy for familial Mediterranean fever: a double-blind trial. N Eng J Med 291:934, 1974.
15. Bodel, P. and Dillard, G. M.: Suppression of periodic fever with estrogen. Arch Int Med 131:189, 1973.
16. Kats, B. A.: Indomethacin in familial Mediterranean fever. Lancet 2:1202, 1972.
17. Askari, A.: Personal communication.
18. Martin, J. et al.: Relapsing polychondritis treated with Dapsone. Arch Dermat 112:1272, 1976.
19. Ridgeway, H. B., Hausotia, P. L., Schorr, W. F.: Relapsing polychondritis: unusual neurological findings and therapeutic efficacy of Dapsone. Arch Dermat 115:43, 1979.

CHAPTER 9

SYNDROMES OF MUSCULAR PAIN OR WEAKNESS

Diseases in patients whose chief complaint is directed primarily to muscles can usually be divided into three major clinical categories:

Muscular pain without weakness
Muscular pain with associated weakness
Muscular weakness without pain

MUSCULAR PAIN WITHOUT WEAKNESS

Fibrositis (Myofascitis)

Fibrositis is a clinical syndrome characterized by low-grade aching and stiffness of muscles and the connective tissues with which they are intimately related. Stiffness tends to be maximal in the morning or following periods of physical inactivity during the day. Symptoms are worse in cold damp weather and, conversely, are often relieved by heat. Patients may describe symptoms somewhat vaguely, but the term "gelling" is commonly used. Fibrositis is often associated with muscle tenderness and a feeling that the muscles are "knotted up." It may be generalized or local.

Localized Fibrositis. This extremely common entity is usually benign in origin. It may follow a recent nonspecific infection or occur spontaneously in otherwise healthy people. Symptoms are localized to limited, focal anatomic areas. The patient complains of tightness of muscles associated with pain of variable intensity. Movement accentuates the pain, which may become lancinating. The areas of involvement are described as trigger areas of pain from which more diffuse aching radiates. The posterior cervical region, areas around the scapulae, and mid to lower lumbar areas are most often involved. Palpation of tender areas reveals evidence of severe muscle spasm.

Generalized Fibrositis. Generalized fibrositis may be primary (idiopathic) or may be a secondary manifestation of generalized disease. The fibrositis syndrome may be the first manifestation of any of the connective tissue diseases, such as rheumatoid arthritis, systemic lupus erythematosus, scleroderma and polymyositis. Generalized fibrositis also occurs in other systemic diseases, such as hypothyroidism. Symptoms of secondary fibrositis may precede objective findings of underlying systemic disease by many months or years.

A diagnosis of primary fibrositis should be entertained only when typical symptoms occur in the absence of systemic disease or other demonstrable causes.[1,2] Aching and stiffness are generally diffuse, and not localized to specific joint areas. Symptoms are worsened by tension, physical inactivity and weather changes. Localized points of deep muscle tenderness, so-called trigger points, are a characteristic finding. The patient's pain is readily reproduced upon trigger point palpation. Disturbed sleep patterns are common.[3] Sleep is frequently not restful, and the patient may awaken more fatigued in the morning than at bedtime. Studies have demonstrated disturbances in non-rapid eye movement (non-REM) sleep; it is uncertain whether such abnormalities are causal in their relationship to fibrositis, or occur as a secondary response.[3] Patients with fibrositis tend to be tense with compulsive, perfectionistic personalities. Laboratory studies such as routine blood counts, erythrocyte sedimentation rate, and serum antibodies seen in connective tissue diseases such as rheumatoid arthritis and systemic lupus erythematosus are characteristically normal. Primary fibrositis may be diagnosed when clinical features are consistent, and when possible underlying diseases have been excluded by a critically performed history and physical examination, appropriate laboratory studies and prolonged observation.

Polymyalgia Rheumatica

This syndrome, seen primarily in patients over 50 years of age, is characterized by severe pain and stiffness in the shoulder and pelvic girdle areas.[4] Associated symptoms include weight loss, sweating and sometimes depression. Physical examination frequently reveals limitation of shoulder and hip motion but no real muscle weakness. Laboratory studies usually show an elevated erythrocyte sedimentation rate, with values as high as 90 to 100 mm/hour. A normochromic, normocytic anemia is frequently present. Elevated alpha-2 globulins and plasma fibrinogen are often present. Circulating immune complexes have been described.[5] Abnormal liver function tests, including alkaline phosphatase elevation, occur in up to one-third of patients. These determinations may be of diagnostic value especially when sedimentation rates are normal or only slightly elevated.

Polymyalgia rheumatica syndrome may be idiopathic or associated with several underlying disorders. Many cases are associated with active temporal arteritis[4] (Chapter 13). Occasionally, cases are associated with carcinoma or lymphoma. In some patients, the syndrome represents an early manifestation of rheumatoid arthritis. In those cases related to temporal arteritis, inflammation of the temporal vessels may be relatively asymptomatic and not obvious; the diagnosis is made only by temporal artery biopsy, with or without preceding arteriograms. A thorough search for underlying associated disorders should be carried out before a diagnosis of idiopathic polymyalgia rheumatica is made. Failure to diagnosis the presence of temporal arteritis may be particularly hazardous to the patient, because sudden blindness as a result of occlusion of the ophthalmic artery or nutrient vessels to the optic nerve is a common complication. Although polymyalgia rheumatica is commonly considered to be a benign disease, visual and cerebral complications due to occult associated temporal arteritis may occur long after disease onset.[6] Close follow-up and appropriate management are indicated in all cases. Fortunately, in the majority of patients, early treatment of associated temporal arteritis with corticosteroids can usually prevent serious complications, in addition to providing relief of generalized symptoms of myalgia.[7-9]

Trichinosis

Infestation of muscles with larvae of Trichinella spiralis causes severe disabling muscle pain. History may reveal mild diarrhea preceding larval deposition in the muscle, but this symptom is often absent or so mild and transient as to be overlooked. Other findings include fever and characteristic periorbital edema. Laboratory studies reveal leukocytosis and significant eosinophilia. Serum complement fixation studies for trichina are valuable. Finding larvae in muscle biopsy specimens is diagnostic.

Necrotizing Vasculitis

Polyarteritis nodosa frequently causes muscle pain without weakness. Associated systemic findings such as fever, night sweats and weight loss are common. Symptoms that reflect vascular involvement of organ systems other than the muscles are present, although only muscles are involved for long periods in some cases. Cutaneous involvement leads to a multiplicity of lesions including purpura, urticaria, maculopapular lesions, vesicles, blebs and bullae. Subungual splinter hemorrhages are common. Ulceration, perforation or hemorrhage of any part of the gastrointestinal system causes a wide spectrum of abdominal symptoms. Renal involvement is associated with hypertension and renal failure. Central nervous system lesions produce hemiparesis, cranial nerve abnormalities and convulsions. Involvement of vessels to peripheral nerves causes various forms of peripheral neuropathy.

Figure 9-1. Polyarteritis nodosa. Histologic study of involved artery reveals fibrinoid necrosis of vessel wall and diffuse inflammatory infiltrate. (Hematoxylin and eosin) (Courtesy, Dr. A. Mackenzie)

The most characteristic of these is mononeuritis multiplex, in which impairment of several large nerves, such as the median, radial and peroneal, is prominent. Coronary arteritis results in ischemia with symptoms of angina and infarction. Pulmonary lesions include transient or progressive necrotizing pneumonitis.

Laboratory studies reveal leukocytosis, elevated erythrocyte sedimentation rate and, frequently, eosinophilia. Abnormal urine findings include albuminuria, red cells, white cells and various casts. Electromyograms may demonstrate myopathic abnormalities due to vascular lesions in muscle. In patients with ischemic neuritis, electromyographic study shows neurogenic patterns and slowed nerve conduction velocities.

Muscle biopsy, performed from involved areas, shows evidence of vasculitis. Histopathologic lesions are characterized by fibrinoid necrosis of the vessel wall and infiltration with polymorphonuclear leukocytes, eosinophils, plasma cells and mononuclear cells (Fig. 9-1). Later, healing and fibrosis are evident. In polyarteritis nodosa, small and medium-sized muscular arteries are involved.

In patients with allergic (hypersensitivity) angiitis, vascular lesions involve small arteries, veins and capillaries.[10] In addition, pulmonary artery involvement and extravascular focal necrosis and granulomas are common. Allergic granulomatous angiitis, as described by Churg and Strauss,[11] is seen in patients with a long history of asthma who develop granulomatous angiitis and diffuse extravascular granulomas. Eosinophilia is characteristic. Wegener's granulomatosis, a variant form of vasculitis, is associated with granulomatous inflammation of the upper respiratory tract, granulomatous disease of the lungs and necrotizing glomerulonephritis.

Although a specific etiology of polyarteritis nodosa has not been established, studies have linked this disease in some patients to infection with hepatitis B virus (HB_sAg).[12,13] The detection of HB_s antigen in involved muscular arteries, together with the presence of serum immune complexes and diminishd complement, suggest that the arteritis may be an immune complex disease initiated by hepatitis viral antigen.[14,15] In another series of cases, polyarteritis was associated with drug abuse.[16] Methamphetamine was the one drug taken in common by persons so affected.

Arteriograms of renal or mesenteric vessels may be diagnostically helpful in patients with vasculitis because they frequently reveal areas of narrowing and aneurysmal dilation.[17,18] Although characteristic of vasculitis, similar aneurysms may be seen in patients with atrial myxomas,[19] and this diagnosis should be excluded when clinically indicated.

Polymyositis

The first symptoms of polymyositis may be muscle aching and tenderness, with minimal weakness early in the course of the disease. Later, more profound weakness usually follows (see following section) and allows differentiation of this entity from the preceding syndromes.

Miscellaneous Diseases

Muscle aching may be a major manifestation of metabolic disorders such as hypothyroidism and subacute thyroiditis. In other patients, symptoms simulating diffuse muscle pain may result from involvement of other tissues such as the bones in patients with multiple myeloma or metastatic carcinoma.

MUSCULAR PAIN WITH ASSOCIATED WEAKNESS

Polymyositis (Dermatomyositis)

Polymyositis is often characterized by both muscle aching and weakness. Weakness usually involves the proximal hip and shoulder girdle muscles (Fig. 9-2). Other muscles involved relatively soon in the course of the disease are the cervical and abdominal flexors. As the disease pro-

Figure 9-2.   Dermatomyositis, illustrating weakness of the shoulder girdles (Courtesy, Dr. A. Mackenzie)

Figure 9-3.   Dermatomyositis. Dusky erythematous discoloration of the eyelids is associated with swelling. (Courtesy, the Arthritis Foundation)

Figure 9-4. Calcinosis universalis. Calcium deposition in subcutaneous soft tissues is extensive. (Courtesy of Dr. A. Mackenzie)

gresses, distal muscles are also involved. The term dermatomyositis is used to define this severe condition when skin manifestations are present. Dusky erythematous lesions appear most frequently on the eyelids (Fig. 9-3) and over extensor surfaces such as the knuckles of the hands, the knees, the malleoli and elbows (see Chapter 10). Cutaneous swelling and induration occur over involved muscles in acute cases. Muscle tenderness may be a prominent finding. Dysphagia results when skeletal muscles in the pharyngeal and upper esophageal regions are involved.

Organ systems other than muscle are frequently affected. Raynaud's phenomenon is common and may precede overt evidence of muscle disease. Polyarthralgia or polyarthritis is seen. Although chronic disabling joint changes are uncommon, articular findings sometimes simulate rheumatoid arthritis. Pulmonary fibrosis occurs and can lead to major disturbances in pulmonary function. Chronic polymyositis may be associated with calcinosis universalis, in which calcium deposits are noted in subcutaneous tissue, deep connective tissue and muscle (Fig. 9-4). Fever, ranging from 101 to 102° F, anorexia, fatigue and weight loss are seen in acute severe cases. The incidence of associated malignant neoplasms is increased in patients with these disorders.[20] Although more frequently associated with dermatomyositis, neoplasms may be seen in patients with polymyositis as well. For this reason, a thorough physical examination and appropriate diagnostic studies to exclude malignancy are indicated in all patients over age 40 with myositis. The neoplasm may be occult and undetectable when the patient is first seen. Repeat studies may be indicated at one- to two-year intervals for several years following onset of the disease, depending on clinical response. In some patients, polymyositis is associated with other connective tissue diseases, such as systemic lupus erythematosus and scleroderma.

Inclusion Body Myositis

Inclusion body myositis (IBM) is a recently described inflammatory disease of skeletal muscle which may simulate polymyositis,[21] but lacks the associated connective tissue disease features characteristic of the latter entity. The disease has a relatively benign and protracted course. Distal as well as proximal muscles are involved; pain occurs but is not prominent. Serum muscle enzymes are often normal or only slightly elevated. Electromyographic studies reveal both neurogenic and myopathic abnormalities.

Pathologic changes are characterized by vacuoles in muscle fibers lined by a hematoxylinophilic layer of small basophilic granules. Mononuclear inflammatory infiltrates and necrosis of muscle are variably present. Atrophic fibers are suggestive of neurogenic disease. Characteristic lesions may be dissolved out on routine paraffin-prepared sections; accordingly, cryostat sections should be performed. Definitive diagnosis is made by electron microscopy which reveals masses of abnormal filaments and membranous whorls. Corticosteroid treatment has, in general, been unsatisfactory.

Myoglobinuria

Muscle breakdown with release of myoglobin in the serum and urine results from several diverse causes. In some patients, it follows extreme exercise. Other causes include prolonged muscle ischemia, crush injury and seizure. It may be an associated finding in patients with severe polymyositis. Myoglobinuria is also seen in patients with drug intoxication with phenobarbital, narcotics or alcohol. In these cases, it may result from crush or postural injury to muscle, although a direct toxic effect has also been postulated. A rare cause of myoglobinuria is cobra venom poisoning. Myoglobinuria following strenuous activity is a frequent concomitant of muscle disease associated with hereditary disorders of glycogen and lipid metabolism (see following).

Clinically, the patient with myoglobinuria complains primarily of severe muscle cramps and pain and passes darkly discolored urine. Serum levels of muscle enzymes such as creatine phosphokinase, aldolase and glutamic oxaloacetic transaminase are elevated. Increased levels of serum potassium result from both muscle breakdown and renal impairment due to pigment casts. Urinalysis reveals proteinuria due to the presence of myoglobin and to tubular dysfunction. A positive urine benzidine test is supportive but not specific of the diagnosis, because hemoglobin gives similar findings. More specific tests for myoglobin include those based on gel electrophoresis, spectrophotometric study, or immunologic methods. Fortunately, most cases are associated with full clinical recovery.

Hereditary Disorders of Glycogen and Lipid Metabolism

These myopathies are due to deficiency states which result in defective metabolism of fuel needed for muscle activity; they represent a small group of neuromuscular disorders in clinical practice.[22-25] Glycogen-related abnormalities of muscle have been described in patients with deficiencies of muscle phosphorylase (McArdle's disease), muscle phosphofructokinase,[23] acid maltase, debrancher, and brancher enzymes.[24] Patients with muscle phosphorylase or phosphofructokinase deficiencies have exercise intolerance, with development of painful cramps and weakness after variable periods of exertion. Myoglobinuria is common. The infantile form of disease associated with acid maltase deficiency is characterized by cardiomyopathy plus generalized muscle weakness and hypotonia. Late onset disease manifests as insidious limb-girdle weakness. Debrancher enzyme deficiency begins in adult life and leads to slowly progressive proximal weakness, with or without distal wasting. Lack of brancher enzyme is rare; muscle hypotonia is overshadowed by severe hepatic disease. In patients with enzyme deficiencies affecting glycogen metabolism, venous blood drawn from the arm during muscle use reveals decreased production of lactic acid as an end product of glycogen metabolism. Studies of muscle biopsy specimens show excess amounts of glycogen, and partial or complete absence of affected enzymes.

Two disorders of muscle lipid metabolism have recently been biochemically identified. Carnitine deficiency is associated with progressive muscle weakness, proximal more than distal.[25] Deficiency of carnitine palmityl transferase results in symptoms similar to the glycogen storage disorders, in which patients have recurrent episodes of muscle pain and myoglobinuria after exercise.[22] Venous lactic acid production after exercise is generally normal. Abnormal deposits of lipids and deficiency of carnitine or carnitine palmityl transferase enzyme are noted on study of muscle biopsy specimens.

Hypothyroidism

Progressively severe hypothyroidism results not only in muscle aching but eventually in muscle weakness. Patients with this combination of findings are frequently overtly myxedematous, and diagnosis is usually not too difficult.

MUSCULAR WEAKNESS WITHOUT PAIN

Muscle weakness without pain may originate in the nerves or muscles. Accordingly, initial diagnostic efforts in these patients should center upon determining whether the etiology is neurologic or myopathic. Neurologic weakness results from involvement of anterior horn cells, nerve roots or peripheral nerves. Involvement of anterior horn cells causes characteristic fasciculations of muscle and loss of deep tendon reflexes in the involved area. Peripheral neuropathy is also associated with loss of deep tendon reflexes, but fasciculations are not seen. In myopathic disorders, deep tendon reflexes are not lost until late when severe atrophy ensues, and fasciculations are not seen.

Neurologic Causes

Primary spinal atrophy, a disease of lower motor neurons, is characterized by severe muscle weakness. Older persons are usually affected. Upper extremity symptoms usually precede involvement of the lower extremities. Muscle atrophy is prominent and fasciculations are pronounced. Weakness usually involves distal muscles early; later, proximal extremity and trunk muscles are affected. Loss of deep tendon reflexes occurs as the disease progresses. Primary spinal atrophy can be considered a variant of *amyotrophic lateral sclerosis,* which affects not only lower motor neurons but lateral corticospinal tracts as well. In this disease, weakness and atrophy of distal muscles of the upper extremity occur first; trunk and lower extremity muscles are affected later. Early in the disease, deep tendon reflexes are overactive; later, these reflexes are lost as anterior horn cell involvement advances. A Babinski sign and ankle clonus are common. In primary spinal atrophy and amyotrophic lateral sclerosis, muscle biopsy shows neurogenic atrophy and electromyography shows denervation changes. Giant potentials and fasciculations are characteristic. Nerve conduction velocities are normal.

One form of spinal atrophy is particularly interesting because it usually begins in early childhood and may simulate muscular dystrophy. This disease, known as *juvenile muscular atrophy* (Kugelberg-Welander disease), affects proximal muscles of the lower extremities first, with resultant weakness of the pelvic girdle. Fasciculations are common but may be absent. Muscle atrophy is prominent. Mildly increased levels of serum creatine phosphokinase may be noted. Muscle biopsy usually shows neurogenic atrophy; electromyography shows denervation changes.

Peripheral neuropathies produce muscle weakness and loss of deep tendon reflexes. Pain is usually defined only vaguely. Frequently, the patient may complain of numbness and paresthesia. The common peripheral neuropathies are diffuse and symmetric, involving both lower and upper extremities. Distal aspects of the limbs are primarily involved. The more common underlying etiologies include diabetes mellitus, alcoholism, nutritional deficiencies, ingestion of various toxins such as lead and arsenic, and carcinoma. Porphyria, though an uncommon disorder, frequently manifests peripheral neuropathy. Involvement of peripheral nerves may be a prominent symptom of various connective tissue diseases, such as systemic lupus erythematosus, necrotizing vasculitis, and Sjögren's syndrome.

Certain distinct forms of peripheral neuropathy have been described. *Guillain-Barré syndrome* (infectious polyneuropathy) causes muscle weakness abrupt in onset. Progression of the disease leads to weakness of numerous muscles of the upper and lower extremities. Distal muscles are usually involved first. Muscles of respiration and deglutition, as well as those supplied by cranial nerves, may be affected. Sensory changes occur but usually are not prominent. Spinal fluid studies characteristically reveal an elevated protein with normal cell count (albuminocytologic dissociation). *Charcot-Marie-Tooth disease* (peroneal muscular atrophy) is an heredofamilial form of peripheral neuropathy. Peripheral nerves demonstrate degeneration of myelin sheaths and axis cylinders, and proliferative changes in Schwann cells. Spinal roots may also be involved. Motor symptoms are prominent and characterized by atrophy and weakness of foot and leg muscles. Peroneal muscles and toe extensors are affected most. Secondary equinovarus is common. Atrophy of the calves and lower thighs leads to an appearance of the lower extremities resembling "inverted champagne bottles." Upper extremities are usually involved late. Sensory disturbances are common; superficial sensation is affected most. A similar disorder, which may be closely related to Charcot-Marie-Tooth disease, is *hypertrophic interstitial neuropathy of Déjérine-Sottas*. Distal atrophy and weakness usually begin in the lower extremities; upper extremities are involved later. Deep tendon reflexes are diminished or absent. Palpable enlargement of involved peripheral nerves is distinctive. Degenerative changes affect the myelin of peripheral nerves; spinal roots may also be involved. In the presence of peripheral neuropathy, nerve conduction velocities are characteristically slowed. Electromyography reveals neurogenic potentials and fibrillation.

Myasthenia gravis often causes distinctive muscle weakness. Early in the disease, weakness is most prominent following activity. Patients with severe progressive disease are chronically weak, with further accentuation of weakness following activity. Involvement of muscles of the eyes, tongue and deglutition leads to symptoms of ptosis, diplopia and difficulty in chewing and swallowing. Improvement in strength with cholinesterase-inhibitors, e.g., neostigmine bromide and edrophonium chloride, confirms the diagnosis. Thymomas are frequent in adults with this disease. Appropriate radiologic studies of the chest and mediastinum should be performed in all cases. A similar syndrome, *myasthenic syndrome of Eaton-Lambert,*[26] is associated with underlying malignancy, most commonly intrathoracic neoplasms. Clinical findings characterized by fatigue, weakness, and muscle wasting are related to a defect in neuromuscular transmission. Ptosis, diplopia, dysarthria and dysphagia may occur. Muscle power may temporarily increase after brief exercise.

Myopathic Causes

The differential diagnosis of the primary myopathies requires strict attention to various facets of the clinical history, such as sex, age at disease onset, pattern of muscle involvement and rapidity of disease progression. Physical examination late in the course of these diseases, when muscle involvement is diffuse, no longer reveals characteristic patterns and provides limited diagnostic help.

Polymyositis, as noted earlier, may cause muscle pain with minimal weakness in its early stages, or sometimes both weakness and pain. However, many cases are characterized by progressive weakness with little or no pain. Although this latter symptomatology occurs primarily in cases that are subacute in onset and slowly progressive, weakness without pain is sometimes observed in patients with rapidly advancing disease.

Duchenne's dystrophy (pseudohypertrophic muscular dystrophy) begins in early childhood, usually before age six. It is characterized early by weakness of proximal muscle groups of the hip and shoulder girdles. As the disease progresses, muscle weakness becomes more diffuse and peripheral areas are involved. This disease, the most common of the dystrophies, is inherited by males as a sex-linked recessive. Early symptoms include slowness in walking and difficulty in climbing stairs. There is visible pseudohypertrophy of muscles, especially of the calf and thigh. Myocardial involvement can frequently be identified on electrocardiographic study.

Limb-girdle muscular dystrophy affects both sexes. It tends to begin before the age of five and is characterized initially by weakness in the muscles of the pelvic girdle. Later, weakness involves muscles of the shoulder girdle. Eventually peripheral muscles are affected. *Facioscapulohumeral dystrophy* occurs in both sexes. Muscle weakness, which may be delayed in onset to any time between the ages five and fifty, is usually mild. Facial and shoulder muscles are involved first; later, as the disease progresses, pelvic muscles are also affected.

Myotonic dystrophy is characterized by dystrophy and by myotonia, an impairment of muscular relaxation. Muscle involvement includes the hands and anterior tibial muscles, the facial muscles, the neck flexors and the muscles of the eyelids. Hip and shoulder girdle muscles are usually spared. Weakness is associated with progressive atrophy. The most common symptom related to myotonia is an inability to rapidly open the clenched fist. Delayed muscle relaxation can be demonstrated by striking involved muscles, such as the thenar eminence, with a reflex hammer; slow muscle relaxation is readily noted. Other manifestations of the disease include cataracts, frontal baldness, testicular atrophy and mental deterioration. The disease is inherited as an autosomal dominant. Mild elevations of serum muscle enzymes may be seen. Electromyography reveals a characteristic continuous firing of muscle fibers, commonly described as a "dive-bomber" pattern.

Muscle weakness may be a major clinical symptom of endocrine disorders. *Thyrotoxicosis* is a primary example of this type of disorder. Weakness is prominent in the proximal musculature, but diffuse weakness develops in severe disease. Serum muscle enzymes, interestingly, are usually normal. Muscle weakness is also noted in patients with *hypothyroidism,* even though gross evidence of myxedema may not be present. Myalgia may be minimal and weakness the predominant manifestation. In contrast to thyrotoxic myopathy, serum muscle enzymes are often elevated. Neuromuscular findings characterized by weakness and atrophy of muscles, particularly of the lower extremities, have been described in patients with primary[27,28] and secondary[29] *hyperparathyroidism.* In most of these patients, clinical electromyographic and histopathologic findings are consistent with neurogenic atrophy as the cause of symptoms.[28] Findings consistent with myopathic disease have, however, been described.[27] Patients with *hypercortisonism* due to Cushing's syndrome may exhibit variable degrees of muscle weakness in severe cases. Similarly, patients receiving corticosteroid preparations in the therapy of various disorders may develop a toxic *steroid myopathy.* In these patients, proximal muscles of the lower extremities are involved early. Involvement of proximal upper extremity, distal and trunk muscles ensues as the disorder progresses. Urinary excretion of creatine is increased but serum muscle enzyme levels are characteristically normal. Although myalgia may occur, pain is usually minimal. Weakness of involved muscles is the prominent clinical manifestation. Symptoms respond to reduction in steroid dose. Myopathy has also been described with *acromegaly.*[30] Weakness begins insidiously and progresses slowly. The weakness is mild in degree and proximal in distribution, sparing the axial and cranial muscles. Serum enzymes are usually normal but may be slightly elevated. Muscle biopsy studies generally show little in the way of abnormalities except for rare scattered muscle fiber degeneration and increased central migration of nuclei. Myopathy improves slowly after hypophysectomy.

Metabolic disorders may be associated with muscle weakness. Patients with diabetes mellitus may develop a syndrome of muscle weakness termed *diabetic amyotrophy.* Symptoms are usually slow in onset and most pronounced in the proximal aspect of the lower extremities. The pathogenesis of the disorder is uncertain; it may reflect changes primarily of muscle origin, but anterior horn cell degeneration has also been suspected. Symptoms may improve with control of the diabetes, but progressive changes often ensue despite good diabetic management. Several myopathic syndromes have been described in patients with *chronic alcoholism.*[31] One such disorder simulates McArdle's syndrome in that muscle weakness is associated with an inability to metabolize glycogen. Symptoms are usually associated with acute bouts of alcoholism and generally resolve rapidly as alcoholic intake stops. A second syndrome is characterized by chronic muscle weakness that may improve as alcoholic intake ceases, although it may persist despite abstinence from alcohol. The clinical picture simulates polymyositis in that proximal muscles of the extremities are involved most frequently and most severely. *Chronic hypokalemia* is associated with variable degrees of muscle weakness. In other patients, sudden falls in serum potassium are associated with the syndrome *hypokalemic familial periodic paralysis.* Although most often idiopathic, this latter syndrome may be associated with thyrotoxicosis. Symptoms are characterized by acute attacks of diffuse weakness or flaccid paralysis. Weakness may last for hours or days. Lower limbs are usually involved first, followed by involvement of the upper extremities, trunk and face. Speech and swallowing may be affected. Death in an attack is rare. Laboratory studies demonstrate a fall in serum potassium coincident with paralysis. Occasionally, however, familial periodic paralysis is seen in association with normal or high levels of serum potassium.

Muscle weakness has long been recognized in patients with *osteomalacia.*[32] Findings are predominantly proximal in distribution; weakness may be asymmetrical. Muscle wasting is variable, and tendon reflexes are generally normal. This cause of muscle weakness should be suspected in patients with gastrointestinal malabsorption states, or in patients with vitamin D resistance, including chronic renal failure. The pathogenesis of the disorder is unclear. Weakness rarely correlates with serum calcium levels, and the response to phosphate restoration is inconsistent. Alterations in muscle function related to lack of or resistance to vitamin D may be at fault.

Muscle weakness may be associated with *amyloidosis,* particularly of the primary type. Weakness progresses slowly as deposition of amyloid in muscle becomes more severe and diffuse. Granulomatous involvement of muscle occurs in many patients with *sarcoidosis.* Despite this finding, clinical symptoms of weakness are uncommon. Nevertheless, some patients develop severe progressive weakness and muscle atrophy. The clinical features resemble chronic polymyositis or one of the dystrophies. Noncaseating granulomas are seen on muscle biopsy.

Muscle weakness may result from a number of rare congenital disorders such as central core disease, myotubular disease, nemaline myopathy, mitochondrial disease[33] and fingerprint body myopathy.[34] These disorders are generally manifest at or shortly after birth. Muscles are hypotonic and walking is delayed. The diseases usually progress slowly, if at all. Diagnosis depends on use of histochemical, light and electron microscopic techniques. These entities should be considered in the differential diagnosis of myopathic disorders not otherwise consistent with the more common entities.

DIAGNOSTIC STUDIES

Obviously, many of the foregoing muscle diseases overlap with respect to clinical symptomatology. Differential diagnosis depends on a clear delineation of subtleties of clinical presentation. A detailed history and physical examination to define age of onset, initial areas of muscle involvement, pattern and pace of disease progression and presence or absence of pain are important clues to diagnosis. Associated systemic findings characteristic of the basic disorder or evidence of associated disease states must also be sought. The following studies are valuable in the diagnosis and management of disorders of muscle.

A detailed manual muscle examination to determine distribution and severity of muscle weakness should be performed as early in the disease as possible; such information is helpful in differential diagnosis. In addition, accurately recorded serial findings can be compared to determine disease progression and response to therapy. Determinations of the ability to rise from a chair with or without the use of hands, the ability to rise from the floor to a standing position, the ability to walk a constant distance and the ability to climb stairs are particularly valuable. These functions should be timed with a stopwatch in order to compare measurements as the patient is observed during the course of disease.

Complete blood count, erythrocyte sedimentation rate, and tests for serum rheumatoid factor and antinuclear antibody are helpful in delineating the presence of associated connective tissue diseases and in differentiating inflammatory from noninflammatory myopathies.

Enzymes released into serum from degenerating muscle cells are important in diagnosis and management. Elevated levels support the presence of a primary myopathic disorder, because they are increased only occasionally and to mild degree in patients with neurogenic atrophy. In addition, these enzyme levels are valuable in following disease progression and response to therapy. The enzyme determinations used most commonly in studies of muscle diseases are serum creatine phosphokinase (CPK), serum glutamic oxaloacetic transaminase (SGOT), and aldolase (see Chapter 2).

As noted, elevated serum enzyme levels support a diagnosis of primary myopathy. However, serum enzyme levels are frequently normal in the presence of significant muscle pathology. Accordingly, normal values for these enzymes do not necessarily exclude primary muscle disease. Elevations of serum enzyme levels are usually proportional to the severity of muscle degeneration or necrosis. High levels are seen in all patients with progressive muscular dystrophy of the Duchenne type until late in the disease. Elevations are common in limb-girdle dystrophy. In facioscapulohumeral dystrophy, enzyme abnormalities are less frequent and only modest in degree. At least one or more of the enzymes are elevated in 80 to 90% of patients with polymyositis. Enzyme levels are frequently elevated in alcoholic and myxedematous myopathies, but are characteristically normal in thyrotoxic and steroid myopathies.

Quantitative determinations of the ratio of creatine to creatinine excreted in the urine are valuable in diagnosis and followup of patients with primary muscle disease (see Chapter 2). Because the degree of creatinuria parallels muscle damage, urinary determinations of creatine-creatinine ratio are valuable not only in diagnosis but also in following disease progression and response to therapy. Elevations in the creatine-creatinine ratio also result from other causes of muscle dysfunction, such as disuse or neurogenic atrophy of muscle.

The electromyogram (EMG) is particularly helpful in distinguishing primary myopathic from neurogenic causes of muscle weakness (see Chapter 2). However, although electromyography and nerve conduction velocity studies will help to differentiate myopathic from neuropathic disorders, they will not differentiate specific disease entities *within* each of these categories.

Muscle biopsy helps to differentiate muscle disorders of neurogenic cause from those of primary myopathic origin; in addition, specific primary myopathies can often be distinguished. Atrophy of groups of muscle fibers innervated by single motor units appears in muscle weakness due to lower motor neuron disease. In polymyositis, several pathologic findings may be noted (Fig. 9-5). Degenerative changes of fibers are common. Central

Figure 9-5. Muscle biopsy, polymyositis. Note fiber degeneration, variation in fiber size and shape, and inflammatory cells. (Hematoxylin and eosin) (Courtesy, Dr. A. Mackenzie)

migration of sarcolemmal nuclei occurs. Regeneration is characterized by basophilic staining. Severe cases show fiber necrosis. Variation in muscle fiber size and shape is common. Inflammatory reaction may be prominent and involves interstitial connective tissues, vascular and perivascular structures. Fibrosis occurs as the disease progresses. Perifascicular atrophy at the perimeter of the muscle bundle is particularly characteristic. Many of these findings may be noted to various degrees in patients with different forms of muscular dystrophy and, in many cases, biopsy study will not differentiate these entities from polymyositis. However, a striking inflammatory reaction strongly indicates polymyositis. In trichinosis, necrotizing vasculitis, amyloidosis and sarcoid, evidence of Trichinella spiralis larvae, vascular inflammation, positive stains for amyloid, and noncaseating granulomas respectively on muscle biopsy provides specific diagnosis.

Special histochemical stains on biopsy material provide additional information. Specific involvement of Type I or Type II fibers, or both, can be determined. Some myopathies are more likely to involve the slowly-contracting Type I fibers, which depend primarily on oxidative mechanisms for energy, while other diseases primarily involve the fast-contracting Type II fibers, which depend on glycogen utilization for energy release. Enzyme analyses and histochemical and biochemical studies are required to demonstrate glycogen and lipid abnormalities in patients with hereditary disorders of glycogen and lipid metabolism. Electron microscopic studies are necessary to diagnose some of the other less common myopathies.

To be most informative, muscle biopsy requires the appropriate selection of involved muscles. Prior manual muscle testing or electromyography should be performed in order to determine which muscles are involved. If the disease is acute and recent in onset, biopsy of the weakest muscle is most likely to yield positive findings. In chronic disease, biopsy of a very weak muscle may demonstrate only end-stage, nonspecific characteristics; in these cases, a moderately weak muscle should be selected.

Miscellaneous additional studies are indicated when specific disorders are suspected. Appropriate diagnostic studies to detect possible neoplasms should be performed in patients over 40 years of age who have dermatomyositis or polymyositis. Temporal artery biopsy with arteriography should be considered in patients with polymyalgia rheumatica syndrome. Studies for malignancy may be indicated in patients with this syndrome if there is no clinical or biopsy evidence of temporal arteritis.

Additional laboratory studies are helpful in excluding metabolic abnormalities as the cause of the patient's disorder. These should include serum thyroxine determination, glucose tolerance test, serum potassium, and serum calcium, phosphorus and alkaline phosphatase studies. Rectal biopsy for amyloid study is valuable if amyloidosis is suspected.

THERAPY

In most cases of muscle disease, the diagnosis can be pursued with appropriate deliberation with no undue hazard from delay. Symptoms related to inflammation with associated pain are often relieved by a conservative program that utilizes full doses of aspirin, other analgesics, rest and heat. Physical therapy is important, even early in the course of muscle disease, to maintain muscle tone and to retard or prevent deterioration of muscle strength.

The therapeutic response to primary fibrositis is frequently frustrating both to the patient and the physician. Reassurance regarding the absence of serious underlying disease and the overall benign nature of the syndrome is an important part of the therapeutic program. Close attention should be paid to chronic tension factors and other psychiatric problems when these are evident. Activities such as swimming or tennis directed toward overall physical fitness may be helpful when tolerated. Specific physical therapy utilizing stretching mobilizing exercises and heat or ice packs is useful. Injection of local trigger areas of spasm and pain with a combination of long-acting steroids and 1% lidocaine is effective in providing variable periods of symptomatic relief. This therapy is safe in limited administration; several courses may be required. Narcotics should be assiduously avoided. Full doses of aspirin or other nonsteroidal anti-inflammatory agents are helpful in a limited number of patients with this disorder. Tranquilizing drugs which have associated muscle relaxant properties such as meprobamate or diazepam are useful adjuncts. Sleep disturbance and overall symptoms may be helped by the nighttime administration of amitriptyline, 25 to 100 mg in one dose taken at bedtime. Biofeedback relaxation has helped some patients. Maintenance of employment should be encouraged.

Specific treatment of other diseases varies with the diagnosis. Unfortunately, many patients suffer from disorders for which little specific treatment is available. Adrenocorticosteroids, such as prednisone, are effective in the treatment of polymyositis and polymyalgia rheumatica (see Chapter 19). Corticosteroid therapy may be used as a diagnostic test to differentiate polymyositis from one of the dystrophies, because a positive therapeutic response supports a diagnosis of polymyositis. Steroids are also therapeutically valuable in patients with necrotizing vasculitis and trichinosis. The weakness associated with hyperthyroidism responds to appropriate therapy to diminish overactive thyroid function; the weakness of hypothyroidism responds to thyroid replacement. Diabetic amyotrophy may improve if good control of the diabetes is attainable. Abstinence from alcohol is indicated in the presence of alcoholic myopathy, although unfortunately the disease may persist in some cases despite cessation of alcohol intake. Hypokalemic myopathy usually responds well to potassium replacement. Acute attacks of familial periodic paralysis are precipitated by high sugar intake, which results in rapid utilization of potassium and subsequent lowering of serum potassium levels. A diet high in protein and limited in carbohydrates is often therapeutic. Management of muscle weakness associated with osteomalacia is directed to the underlying primary disorder. Vitamin D replacement may be effective in patients with vitamin D deficiency or resistance states.

CASE HISTORIES

History 9-1. Primary Fibrositis

B.L., a 38-year-old white female was first seen for evaluation in January, 1972. She had been in apparently good health until approximately six months prior, at which time she noted insidious onset of aching and stiffness involving the posterior cervical, upper dorsal and shoulder girdle regions. Symptoms were aggravated by tension situations. Continuous low-grade aching was punctuated by episodes of pain of increased intensity. Symptoms were worse in cool, damp weather. Musculoskeletal pain was frequently associated with severe blinding headaches similar to migraine headaches from which she had suffered 15 years earlier. There were no complaints of joint swelling, tenderness or limitation. System review was negative for Raynaud's phenomenon, alopecia, sun sensitivity, skin rash, pleurisy, dry eyes or mouth, dysphagia or drug allergy. Past medical history was unremarkable, although family and social history was significant. The patient's mother had died suddenly of myocardial infarction three months prior to onset of the patient's illness; several months later, her mother-in-law died of acute leukemia. In addition to this already severe emotional trauma, the patient was seriously concerned about her daughter when she learned that children of mothers who had received high doses of stilbestrol during pregnancy (as did the patient) had an increased incidence of carcinoma of the cervix.

Physical examination in this pleasant but obviously tense woman was normal except for tenderness and spasm of the upper trapezius and posterior cervical muscles. Deep pressure over areas of maximal spasm and tenderness triggered increased pain, similar in quality to that experienced by the patient during symptomatic flares. No muscle weakness was noted. Temporal arteries were nontender with normal pulsations. Musculoskeletal examination was otherwise negative. Laboratory examinations, which included urinalysis, hematocrit, white blood cell count and differential, erythrocyte sedimentation rate, serologic test for syphilis, serum protein electrophoresis, serum uric acid, protein bound iodine, serum calcium, phosphorus and alkaline phosphatase, serum cholesterol and lipid studies, serum glutamic oxaloacetic transaminase, creatine phosphokinase, serum rheumatoid factor and antinuclear antibody studies were normal or negative, as were roentgenograms of the chest and cervical spine. A presumptive diagnosis of primary fibrositis was made on the basis of her clinical history and physical examination and negative laboratory findings.

The patient was treated with aspirin, 640 mg QID, diazepam, 5 mg TID, and propoxyphene hydrochloride, 65 mg TID PRN for pain. Periodic injections with steroid and lidocaine were made locally into trigger sites of pain and spasm. Physical therapy, which included hot packs and cervical traction, was extremely helpful in further relieving symptoms. Extensive discussions were carried out regarding the nature of her problem and the important role that emotional factors might play in etiology. With reassurance and better understanding of the illness, the patient was able to tolerate her symptoms with much less distress. No other disease states became apparent over a prolonged period of observation. Her symptoms were relatively mild except during periods of extreme emotional stress, at which time exacerbations usually responded to an intensified physical therapy program.

Discussion: At the time this patient was first seen, a diagnosis of primary fibrositis could be made on a presumptive basis only. Similar symptoms are frequently seen in association with systemic disorders, such as one of the connective tissue diseases, temporal (cranial) arteritis, polymyalgia rheumatica, subacute thyroiditis and hypothyroidism. The diagnosis became more secure after observation over a period of time. Appropriate initial and periodic clinical and laboratory evaluations were indicated to exclude more serious disorders. Although many cases of primary fibrositis are associated with emotional factors, psychologic relationships are not always so overt as in this case.

History 9-2. Idiopathic Polymyalgia Rheumatica

J.G., a 75-year-old white male, was seen for evaluation in July, 1973. He was well until November, 1972, at which time he noted pain and stiffness of the shoulders, buttocks and hips. Symptoms were constant, and increased in intensity with activity. Morning stiffness lasted for three or four hours daily. Fever was absent but the patient had noted anorexia and a weight loss of eight pounds during the previous eight months. System review was otherwise negative. In particular, there were no complaints of headaches, dysphagia or joint symptoms. Past medical history was noncontributory. Physical examination revealed slight limitation of motion of the shoulders and severe pain when he attempted to raise his arms above his head. Hip examination was normal except for pain at extreme ranges of motion. Muscle strength was normal and no other abnormalities were noted. Complete physical examination was otherwise unremarkable.

The hematocrit was 36%, the white blood cell count was 8100/mm³ with a normal differential, and the erythrocyte sedimentation rate was 82 mm/hour (Wintrobe). Serum antinuclear antibody and rheumatoid factor studies were negative as were LE cell examinations. Stool examination for occult blood was negative. Serum muscle enzyme determinations were normal. Twenty-four-hour urinary creatine-creatinine ratios were 6% and 8% on two separate evaluations. Serum protein electrophoresis showed 22% gamma globulin with a reversal of the albumin-globulin ratio. Roentgenograms of the chest, upper gastrointestinal tract and colon, and intravenous pyelogram were normal. Sigmoidoscopic examination was unremarkable. Biopsy of the right temporal artery revealed no inflammatory changes. Clinical impression was polymyalgia rheumatica.

The patient was given prednisone, 10 mg TID; significant symptomatic improvement was noted in 48 to 72 hours. The dose of prednisone was gradually decreased as symptoms improved and the erythrocyte sedimentation rate fell to high normal levels. Symptoms were eventually controlled with prednisone, 5 mg daily. The patient was closely observed over a period of three years with clinical evaluations, and monthly determinations of the erythrocyte sedimentation rate. Prednisone was slowly discontinued with the patient eventually remaining symptom-free without therapy.

Discussion: The clinical findings were consistent with a diagnosis of idiopathic polymyalgia rheumatica. Symptoms are usually severe in the areas of the shoulder and hip girdle muscles. Although muscle weakness is absent, pain may limit muscle function. Since this syndrome is frequently associated with temporal (cranial) arteritis and, at times with neoplasm, careful studies to exclude both entities should be carried out. Clinical response of symptoms to steroid therapy is usually dramatic and supports the diagnosis. The clinical course of the syndrome is usually self-limited with resolution of disease-related abnormalities in most patients over a period of several years.

History 9-3.   Temporal (Cranial) Arteritis with Polymyalgia Rheumatica

B.R., an 82-year-old white female, was first seen for evaluation in July, 1973. She was in good general health until six months prior, at which time she noted a flu-like syndrome characterized by anorexia, malaise and low-grade fever. Shortly thereafter, she developed muscle aching that was particularly severe in the shoulder and hip girdle areas. Weight loss of 15 pounds was noted. The patient had no history of eye symptoms and no muscle weakness. She complained of temporal and occipital headaches. System review was otherwise noncontributory and past medical history was unremarkable. On physical examination blood pressure was 120/70 mm Hg, pulse 72 per minute, and temperature 37° C. Both temporal arteries were thickened and tender to palpation. Eye examination was normal. There was full range of motion of all joints with no tenderness or swelling. Muscles were nontender and had normal strength. A clinical diagnosis of temporal (cranial) arteritis with polymyalgia rheumatica was made and the patient hospitalized for further studies.

Hematocrit was 31%, white blood cell count was 6400/mm^3 with a normal differential, reticulocyte count was 1.1%, platelet count was 225,000/mm^3, erythrocyte sedimentation rate was 55 mm/hour (Wintrobe), and urinalysis was normal. Serum electrolytes, calcium, phosphorus and alkaline phosphatase, fasting blood sugar and liver function studies were normal or negative. Serum protein electrophoresis revealed slight elevation of alpha-2 globulin. Chest roentgenogram was negative, and electrocardiogram was normal. Sigmoidoscopy and roentgenograms of the upper and lower gastrointestinal tract were normal. Erythrocytes appeared normal on smear, and red cell indices revealed normochromic, normocytic results. Stools were negative for occult blood. Serum iron content and total iron binding capacity were normal; saturation was 37%. Bone marrow examination was within normal limits. Arteriography and biopsy of the left temporal artery were performed on November 13, 1973. The arteriogram revealed focal areas of vessel narrowing. Histopathologic examination showed extensive infiltration of all layers of the artery with lymphocytes and polymorphonuclear cells. The internal elastic membrane was well preserved and giant cells were not identified. Therapy consisted of prednisone, 20 mg QID, antacids, and a no-salt-added diet. Within 24 hours the patient had notable relief of pain and tenderness in the area of the temporal vessels and loss of muscle stiffness and pain.

Discussion: This patient's history was characteristic of temporal (cranial) arteritis with polymyalgia rheumatica. Response to steroid therapy was dramatic. The patient was discharged to the care of her physician with the recommendation to continue high dose steroid therapy until the erythrocyte sedimentation rate had returned to essentially normal values. At that time, gradual reduction in dose was to be carried out and the patient maintained on the lowest dose possible that would keep her free of symptoms with a normal sedimentation rate. Treatment for a period of years is usually required. Although the temporal arteritis that was clinically apparent in this patient with polymyalgia rheumatica provided a reasonable explanation for her anemia, a neoplasm evaluation was considered necessary for completion of her workup.

History 9-4. Dermatomyositis

D.K., a two-year-old black male, was in good health until age 21 months, at which time his mother noted that the child appeared "lazy." He was less active than usual and refused to walk stairs, complaining that he was too tired. Weakness became more overt and the patient had difficulty walking, rising from a chair, or rising from the floor to a sitting or standing position. He walked with a waddling gait. He had no history of difficulty in chewing or swallowing nor changes in speech or articulation. System review was otherwise completely negative. Past medical history was noncontributory. The patient was hospitalized approximately six weeks after the onset of symptoms. Physical examination revealed moderate erythema over the knuckles of the proximal interphalangeal (PIP) joints of the hands. No muscle fasciculations were noted. The child was unable to lift his neck off the bed and there was moderate weakness of shoulder and hip girdle muscles. Neurologic examination was normal.

Urinalysis, white blood cell count and differential, serologic test for syphilis, and erythrocyte sedimentation rate were normal or negative. Serum electrolytes were normal. Serum glutamic oxaloacetic transaminase was 11 Henry units (normal, 9 to 25 units), and creatine phosphokinase was 1200 IU/ml (normal, less than 150 IU/ml). Twenty-four-hour urinary creatine–creatinine ratio determinations were 54% and 48% on two successive days. Serum protein electrophoresis and protein bound iodine were normal.

Chest roentgenogram and electrocardiogram were normal. Barium swallow revealed no abnormalities of esophageal function. Electromyographic study showed multiple polyphasic potentials consistent with primary myopathic disease. Spinal fluid studies revealed normal pressure, no cells, protein 10 mg/100 ml, sugar 41 mg/100 ml. Biopsy of the right vastus lateralis muscle was performed. Histopathologic examination revealed extensive variability of muscle fiber size, degenerative vacuolation, and regenerative changes. Moderate numbers of inflammatory cells were seen throughout the specimen. An occasional vessel was slightly thickened and hyalinized. No perivascular infiltrates were seen. No changes specific for one of the congenital myopathies were noted on electron microscopic study.

A diagnosis of childhood dermatomyositis was made and the patient was placed on prednisone, 15 mg TID. Antacids were added as a prophylactic measure. Progressive improvement in strength was noted. Serum muscle enzyme determinations returned to normal levels over a period of two months. Urinary creatine–creatinine ratios similarly improved. Prednisone therapy was gradually reduced and symptoms were well controlled on a dose of 5 mg daily. Following this, the patient was successfully converted to an alternate day program in which prednisone, 10 mg, was administered every other day only. This latter schedule was utilized in the hope of lessening growth retardation and other complications of steroid therapy. Attempts to further reduce his steroid dosage were associated with slow onset of increased weakness.

Discussion: This patient had a history consistent with childhood dermatomyositis. Initial diagnostic considerations included infectious polyneuritis and other forms of primary myopathic disease. Laboratory and pathologic studies and the response to steroid therapy were consistent with a diagnosis of dermatomyositis.

History 9-5. Amyotrophic Lateral Sclerosis

W.J., a 70-year-old white male, was in good health until approximately six months prior to consultation. At that time he noted a change in his usual strong voice, which became high-pitched and nasal. In addition, he had difficulty swallowing and regurgitated food through the nose. He developed weakness in climbing stairs and, later, weakness in his upper extremities. There was no history of diplopia nor difficulty in chewing. On physical examination there was notable atrophy of interosseous muscles. Extensor and flexor muscles of the wrists were weak, and diffuse atrophy of the muscles of the shoulder and hip girdles was noted. The patient spoke with a nasal voice. Sensory examination was normal except for a slight decrease in vibratory sensation of both feet. Bilateral positive Babinski reflexes were elicited. Deep tendon reflexes of the left arm were increased. No clonus was present. Eye examination was normal and there was no weakness of extraocular muscles. Diffuse fasciculations were noted in the muscles of the upper extremities, trunk, abdominal wall, and thighs.

Chest x-ray and upper gastrointestinal series were normal. Roentgenograms of the skull and cervical spine were within normal limits. Electrocardiogram was normal. Other laboratory studies revealed normal hematocrit and white blood cell count and differential. Urinalysis revealed slight albuminuria. Serum uric acid was 6.2 mg/100 ml. Serum calcium, phosphorus and alkaline phosphatase studies, serum protein electrophoresis, and serum electrolytes were normal. Protein bound iodine was 6.3 μg%. Fasting blood sugar was normal. Twenty-four-hour urinary creatine–creatinine ratios were 25 and 20% on two different occasions. Serum muscle enzyme determinations were normal. Electromyographic study revealed large spikes consistent with denervation atrophy. A diagnosis of amyotrophic lateral sclerosis was made.

Discussion: The findings of diffuse weakness, muscle atrophy, muscle fasciculations and involvement of the corticospinal tracts were characteristic of the diagnosis of amyotrophic lateral sclerosis. Abnormal sensory changes are not seen. The disease is usually gradual in onset and relentless in progression. Fasciculations are characteristic of neurogenic atrophy and differentiated the symptoms in this patient from those seen in primary myopathy. Abnormal creatinuria occurs in muscle disorders related both to primary myopathy and neurogenic atrophy. The clinical picture as described in this patient should not be readily confused with primary myopathic disease.

History 9-6. Thyrotoxic Myopathy

N.A., a 43-year-old black female, was first seen in consultation in the hospital in January, 1974. She had been in good health until several months prior when she noted onset of fatigue and generalized weakness. She had difficulty climbing stairs, needed help getting up from her bed, and had to use her hands to get up from a chair. Despite increased appetite and food intake, she had lost 13 pounds in the previous two months. System review revealed palpitations of the heart, increased sweating, and heat intolerance. Diarrhea alternated with constipation. She had a choking feeling in the anterior neck area. No aching was noted in the joints or muscles. There was no family history of muscle disease, and the patient gave no history of rash, sun sensitivity, Raynaud's phenomenon, dryness of the eyes or mouth, pleurisy, alopecia or drug allergy. Past medical history was noncontributory.

On physical examination, blood pressure was 120/70 mm Hg, pulse rate was regular at 100 beats per minute, and temperature was 37° C. The skin was smooth and moist and hair texture was fine. A slight tremor of the hands was noted. No lid lag or exophthalmos was seen. The thyroid was diffusely enlarged to approximately three times normal size and a bruit was heard over the gland. Lungs were clear to examination. Cardiac examination revealed a Grade II/VI systolic murmur, best heard at the apex. Deep tendon reflexes were symmetric but generally increased. Neurologic examination was otherwise within normal limits. Muscle evaluation revealed mild to moderate weakness of the muscles of the hip and shoulder girdles and neck flexors.

Hematocrit was 31%, white blood cell count was 4200/mm³ with a normal differential, platelet count was 350,000/mm³, and erythrocyte sedimentation rate was 52 mm/hour (Wintrobe). Urinalysis showed trace albumin. Serum electrolytes, fasting blood sugar, protein electrophoresis and routine serologic test for syphilis were normal or negative. Serum iron content, iron binding capacity and iron saturation were 65 μg/100 ml, 300 μg/100 ml and 22% respectively. Serum studies for rheumatoid factor and antinuclear antibody were negative. Serum creatine phosphokinase was 30 IU/ml (normal, less than 150 IU/ml). Serum glutamic oxaloacetic transaminase was normal. Twenty-four-hour urinary creatine-creatinine ratio determination was 32%. Serum protein bound iodine was 14.4 μg/100 ml. Total serum thyroxine was "over 16 μg/100 ml." T-3 sponge resin uptake and 24-hour I¹³¹ uptake studies were significantly elevated. Serum calcium was 10.9 mg/100 ml and 12.1 mg/100 ml on two separate occasions. Serum phosphorus was 6 mg/100 ml. Serum creatinine was 0.5 mg/100 ml and creatinine clearance was 92 ml/min. Chest roentgenogram was normal.

Endocrine consultation was requested. A diagnosis of classic Grave's disease with associated thyrotoxic myopathy was made. The increased calcium was considered a manifestation of thyrotoxicosis. The patient was placed on therapy with propranolol, 10 mg QID, and referred for I¹³¹ therapy. Although other causes of muscle weakness and hypercalcemia were not completely excluded, it was elected to observe the patient following I¹³¹ therapy and to perform further diagnostic studies if muscle weakness and laboratory evidence of hypercalcemia did not resolve.

Discussion: This patient had classic clinical findings of hyperthyroidism. Muscle weakness was severe and was a major initial complaint. The distribution of muscle weakness was characteristic of thyrotoxic myopathy but was also consistent with other primary myopathies such as polymyositis. Clinical observation after discharge revealed progressive improvement in muscle strength and a fall in serum calcium to normal values.

REFERENCES

1. Kraft, G. H., Johnson, E. W. and La Ban, M. M.: The fibrositis syndrome. Arch Phys Med and Rehab 49:155, 1968.
2. Smythe, H. A.: Fibrositis as a disorder of pain modulation. Clinics in Rheumatic Diseases 5:823, 1979.
3. Moldofsky, H. et al.: Musculoskeletal symptoms and non-REM sleep disturbance in patients with fibrositis syndrome and healthy subjects. Psychosomatic Med 37:341, 1975.
4. Healey, L. A., Parker, F. and Wilske, K. R.: Polymyalgia rheumatica and giant cell arteritis. Arthritis Rheum 14:138, 1971.
5. Papaionnou, C. C. et al.: Circulating immune complexes in giant cell arteritis and polymyalgia rheumatica. Arthritis Rheum 23:1021, 1980.
6. Jones, J. G. and Hazelman, B. L.: Prognosis and management of polymyalgia rheumatica. Ann Rheum Dis 40:1, 1981.
7. Hamilton, C. R., Shelly, W. M. and Tumulty, P. A.: Giant cell arteritis including temporal arteritis and polymyalgia rheumatica. Medicine 50:1, 1971.
8. Hunder, G. G., et al.: Daily and alternate-day corticosteroid regimens in treatment of giant cell arteritis: comparison in a prospective study. Ann Intern Med 82:613, 1975.
9. Healey, L. A. and Wilske, K. R.: Manifestations of giant cell arteritis. Med Clin N Amer 61:261, 1977.
10. Blankenhorn, M. A., Zeek, P. and Knowles, H. C.: Periarteritis nodosa and other forms of necrotizing angiitis: a clinical pathological correlation. Trans Assoc Am Physicians 66:156, 1953.

11. Churg, J. and Strauss, L.: Allergic granulomatosis, allergic angiitis, and periarteritis nodosa. Am J Path 27:277, 1951.
12. Gocke, D. J. et al.: Association between polyarteritis and Australia antigen. Lancet 2:1149, 1970.
13. Baker, A. L. et al.: Polyarteritis associated with Australia antigen-positive hepatitis. Gastroenterology 62:105, 1972.
14. Fye, K. H. et al.: Immune complexes in hepatitis B antigen-associated periarteritis nodosa. Am J Med 62:783, 1977.
15. Fauci, A. S., Haynes, B. F. and Katz, P.: The spectrum of vasculitis—clinical, pathologic, immunologic and therapeutic considerations. Ann Intern Med 89: 660, 1978.
16. Citron, B. P. et al.: Necrotizing angiitis associated with drug abuse. N Eng J Med 283:1003, 1970.
17. Bron, K., Stratt, C. and Shapero, A.: The diagnostic value of angiographic observations in polyarteritis nodosa. Arch Int Med 116:450, 1965.
18. Travero, R. L., et al.: Polyarteritis nodosa: a clinical and angiographic analysis of 17 cases. Sem Arth Rheum 8:184, 1979.
19. Leonhardt, E. T. G. and Kullenberg, K. P. G.: Bilateral atrial myxomas with multiple arterial aneurysms—a syndrome mimicking polyarteritis nodosa. Am J Med 62:792, 1977.
20. Barnes, B. E.: Dermatomyositis and malignancy. Ann Intern Med 84:68, 1976.
21. Carpenter, S. et al.: Inclusion body myositis: a distinct variety of idiopathic inflammatory myopathy. Neurology 28:8, 1978.
22. Bank, W. J. et al.: A disorder of muscle lipid metabolism and myoglobinuria—absence of carnitine palmityl transferase. N Eng J Med 292:443, 1975.
23. Agamanolis, D. P. et al.: Muscle phosphofructokinase deficiency: two cases with unusual polysaccharide accumulation and immunologically active enzyme protein. Muscle and Nerve 3:456, 1980.
24. Bosch, E. P. and Munsat, T. L.: Metabolic myopathies. Med Clin N Amer 63: 759, 1980.
25. Chapoy, P. R. et al.: Systemic carnitine deficiency—a treatable inherited lipid-storage disease presenting as Reye's syndrome. N Eng J Med 303:1389, 1980.
26. Rooke, E. D. et al.: Myasthenia and malignant intrathoracic tumors. Med Clin N Am 44:977, 1960.
27. Frame, B. et al.: Myopathy in primary hyperparathyroidism. Ann Intern Med 68:1022, 1968.
28. Patten, B. M. et al.: Neuromuscular disease in primary hyperparathyroidism. Ann Intern Med 80:182, 1974.
29. Mallette, L. E., Patten, B. M. and Engel, W. K.: Neuromuscular disease in secondary hyperparathyroidism. Ann Intern Med 82:474, 1975.
30. Pickett, J. B. E. et al.: Neuromuscular complications of acromegaly. Neurology 25:638, 1975.
31. Perkoff, G. T.: Alcoholic myopathy. Ann Rev Med 22:125, 1971.
32. Schott, G. D. and Wills, M. R.: Muscle weakness in osteomalacia. Lancet, March 20, 1976, p 626.
33. Pearson, C. M. et al.: Skeletal muscle: basic and clinical aspects and illustrative new diseases. Ann Int Med 67:614, 1967.
34. Engel, E. G., Angelini, C. and Gomez, M. R.: Fingerprint body myopathy. A newly recognized congenital muscle disease. Mayo Clin Proc 47:377, 1972.

CHAPTER 10

SKIN RASH AND ARTHRITIS

Joint symptoms are the common thread connecting the various rheumatic disorders. Since these joint manifestations frequently resemble one another, close attention to ancillary associated findings such as skin lesions is important in diagnosis. Careful observation and characterization of these cutaneous manifestations can often lead to the correct rheumatologic diagnosis.

DIFFERENTIAL DIAGNOSIS

Diseases to be considered:

Systemic lupus erythematosus
Dermatomyositis
Scleroderma
Eosinophilic fasciitis
Psoriasis
Reiter's syndrome
Behçet's syndrome
Stevens-Johnson syndrome
Erythema nodosum
Vasculitis
Cryoglobulinemia
Rheumatic fever
Rheumatoid arthritis

Juvenile rheumatoid arthritis
Rubella arthritis
Gonococcal arthritis
Subacute bacterial endocarditis
Ulcerative colitis and regional
  enteritis
Hepatitis-associated arthritis
Lyme arthritis
Arthritis with pancreatic disease
Lipoid dermatoarthritis (multicentric reticulohistiocytosis)
Arthritis with acne
Sweet's syndrome

Cutaneous lesions are common in *systemic lupus erythematosus* (SLE) at all stages of the disease. These lesions may be the initial symptoms, with joint symptoms following later. In other cases skin lesions occur concomitantly with or follow other manifestations of the disease. The classic lesion is the macular erythematous butterfly rash of the face in which involvement of malar areas is bridged by a lesion across the skin of the nose (Fig. 6-1). Other areas of frequent involvement are the neck, upper chest,

Figure 10-1.   Rash, systemic lupus erythematosus. Involvement between knuckles is prominent, although extension over knuckles is also seen.

Figure 10-2.   Rash, dermatomyositis. Lesions over the extensor surfaces of the knuckles are characteristic. (Courtesy, the Arthritis Foundation)

Figure 10-3. Rash, discoid lupus erythematosus. Chronic le-
sions reveal atrophy and
scarring. (Courtesy, Dr.
B. Michel)

and the extremities. The lesions tend to be symmetric. The rash may be transient, lasting only a few days, or may be chronic. Chronic lesions are characterized by erythematous plaques with scaling and follicular plugging; the skin often becomes atrophic and scarred. Other characteristic components of the rash are erythematous lesions in the paronychial areas of the fingers, and lesions scattered over the palms associated with palmar erythema. Lesions of the hands in SLE characteristically involve the dorsal skin *between* the knuckles (Fig. 10-1) rather than at the knuckles. This differentiates them from the skin lesions of dermatomyositis, which characteristically involve extensor surfaces over the knuckles (Fig. 10-2). The skin lesions of SLE and dermatomyositis may overlap in form and location, however, and be difficult to differentiate.

The rash of chronic discoid lupus is similar to chronic lesions of systemic lupus erythematosus (Fig. 10-3). The dermatitis is usually focal and often confined to the face, neck and scalp. In some patients, discoid lupus is present in disseminated form, with numerous discrete lesions occurring in many locations.

Skin rash is a prominent component of *dermatomyositis*. The characteristic rash consists of a symmetric dusky erythematous lesion in the periorbital region, associated with periorbital edema (Fig 9-3). Their unusual violaceous color has given rise to the term "heliotrope eyelids." The facial rash may be more diffuse, involving a butterfly distribution on the face as in systemic or discoid lupus, and extending to the forehead, neck and upper thorax and back. Lesions on the extremities characteristically affect extensor areas such as elbows and knees, and malleoli at the ankles. These lesions, similar to those seen in the face and neck area, consist of dusky red patches that are slightly elevated and sometimes slightly scaly. Hyperemia occurs about the base of the fingernails. The areas of skin involvement may become somewhat atrophic with time. Less common skin features include cutaneous changes that simulate those of scleroderma, with thickening of the skin of the hands and arms and evidence of hyperpigmentation or vitiligo. A distinctive cutaneous lesion has been described involving the hands of patients with connective tissue diseases associated with inflammatory myopathy.[1] The rash consists of a non-pruritic, hyperkeratotic eruption accompanied by scaling, fissuring, and hyperpigmentation, suggestive of the calloused hands of a manual laborer. Mixed connective tissue disease, dermatomyositis, or systemic lupus erythematosus were present in patients described. Bilateral symmetrical proximal muscle weakness and inflammatory myopathy on muscle biopsy were consistent findings. Although not specific for dermatomyositis, awareness of this cutaneous lesion as a manifestation of underlying myositis may be helpful in the evaluation of patients with early undifferentiated connective tissue disease.

Skin rash is the classic and most characteristic change seen in patients with *scleroderma*. Early, changes are characterized by painless edema of the hands, fingers, feet and legs. This swelling, which lasts for variable periods of time, is gradually replaced by chronic thickening and tightening of the skin. The term acrosclerosis is often used to describe the form of the disease in which lesions are localized to the hands and feet. In other patients, cutaneous lesions are diffuse and involve not only peripheral areas of the extremities but the trunk as well. Following the initial phase of cutaneous edema, the skin becomes less pliant and somewhat shiny (Fig. 10-4). A hardening of the tissues leads to loss of normal skin folds; a

Figure 10-4.   Scleroderma.   Cutaneous involvement leads to tightening of the skin. Small healed ulcerations are seen at the proximal interphalangeal joints.

Figure 10-5. Scleroderma. Note the characteristic "pinched facies" and telangiectases. (Courtesy, Dr. A. Mackenzie)

Figure 10-6. Scleroderma. Telangiectases of the tongue are seen as dark red areas.

characteristic "pinched facies" is noted (Fig. 10-5.) Generalized hyperpigmentation of the skin and areas of patchy vitiligo are common. Telangiectases are frequently noted on the fingers, face (Fig. 10-5), lips and tongue (Fig. 10-6) as the disease becomes chronic. Ulceration (Fig. 10-4) and infection of the fingers and bony eminences and subcutaneous calcification are noted. The clinical combination of calcinosis, Raynaud's phenomenon, esophageal dysfunction, sclerodactyly and telangiectasis in scleroderma has been given the term CREST syndrome, after the initials of the five associated manifestations.[2] These symptoms probably reflect degenerative changes that have been allowed to develop in patients with more benign scleroderma of longer duration rather than a specific disorder.

Distinctive in vivo capillary abnormalities have been described in skin at the edge of the nail-fold in patients with scleroderma. Characteristic abnormalities include large dilated capillary loops, with loss of capillaries from adjacent areas leading to marked avascularity[3-5] (Fig. 10-7). These changes, seen in over 80% of patients with scleroderma, also occur in mixed connective tissue disease, dermatomyositis and prescleroderma Raynaud's disease. Patients who have only Raynaud's phenomenon, but in whom these characteristic capillary abnormalities are seen, appear to be at higher risk for development of connective tissue disease in the future. Capillary abnormalities can be demonstrated in vivo utilizing widefield microscopy. Screening observations may be performed at the bedside using a regular ophthalmoscope set at +20 to +40 diopters, after immersion oil has been placed on the nail-fold skin. Capillary microscopy has been proposed as a simple practical procedure useful in early recognition of scleroderma and related diseases.

Eosinophilic fasciitis is characterized by a scleroderma-like thickening of the skin of the extremities, with less frequent involvement of the trunk.[6-9] Onset tends to be rapid and joint contractures are common. Disease onset not infrequently follows unusual physical exertion. Peripheral blood eosinophilia is characteristic. In contrast to scleroderma, Raynaud's phenomenon and telangiectasia are relatively uncommon. Extracutaneous manifestations, initially thought infrequent include synovitis, pulmonary function abnormalities, and hematologic disorders such as aplastic anemia and thrombocytopenic purpura. In addition to eosinophilia, hypergammaglobulinemia and elevated erythrocyte sedimentation rate are noted. Rheumatoid factor and antinuclear antibodies are only infrequently positive.

Specimens for biopsy study should include skin, subcutaneous tissue, fascia, and muscle. Characteristic findings reveal collagen hypertrophy of subdermal fascia, associated with a marked cellular infiltrate within the fascia, composed usually of lymphocytes, plasma cells, histiocytes and, at times, eosinophils. Muscle inflammation is often prominent. Although tissue eosinophilia is common, its absence in a number of cases has led to the suggestion that the entity be called diffuse fasciitis with eosinophilia.

Figure 10-7.   (A) Normal capillary nail-fold pattern. (B) Capillary nail-fold pattern in patient
with scleroderma. Note large dilated capillary loops and loss of capillaries from
adjacent areas. (Reprinted from Clinics in Rheumatic Diseases 5:81, 1979 with kind
permission of W. B. Saunders Co. and H. R. Maricq, M.D.)

In contrast to scleroderma, the majority of patients with eosinophilic fasciitis respond to prednisone therapy, although prolonged use of this agent to suppress disease manifestations may be required. It has been suggested that other therapeutic agents such as hydroxychloroquine or potassium para-aminobenzoate may be of benefit.[8] The prognosis of patients with this disease is still uncertain. Spontaneous improvement has been described. On the other hand, relapse has been noted after a prolonged period of disease remission. Although eosinophilic fasciitis bears a close resemblance to scleroderma, clinical and laboratory differences suggest that it may be a major variant of scleroderma, or may represent a distinct disorder.

There is an increased frequency of arthritis of various forms in patients with *psoriasis*[10] (see Chapter 7). In any form of psoriatic arthritis, joint symptoms may be acute or insidious, and few or many joints may be involved. Spondylitis involving the spine and sacroiliac joints is common. In most cases, psoriasis precedes the onset of arthritis; in others, psoriasis and arthritis begin concomitantly. In a few patients, arthritis precedes psoriatic lesions by one or more years. Nail and skin lesions are identical to those seen in psoriatic patients without arthritis; they are often minimal and overlooked. Nail changes in women may be missed if nail polish is worn at the time of examination. Nail lesions are characterized by discoloration, pitting, thickening and onycholysis. Skin lesions are characterized by erythematous scaling plaques, located most frequently on extensor areas such as the elbows and knees. Involvement of the scalp and intergluteal areas is common. In addition, any region of the skin may be affected.

Involvement of the skin and mucous membranes in *Reiter's syndrome* is so frequent that a tetrad of symptoms consisting of arthritis, urethritis, conjunctivitis and mucocutaneous lesions is often used to clinically define the syndrome.[11] Lesions of the penis are especially common. They are characterized by superficial ulcerations, especially around the urethral meatus (Fig. 10-8). Coalescence of lesions on the glans penis gives rise to a characteristic circular lesion called balanitis circinata. Mucous membrane ulcers are seen frequently in the mouth, with involvement of the buccal mucosa, tongue and gums. The lesions are often small and painless but may be irritating and painful in some patients. Papular and pustular lesions are common on the palms of the hands and soles of the feet. They may be small and discrete at onset, but frequently become confluent and covered by a thick keratotic crust that eventually peels with no evidence of scar formation. The diffuse keratotic lesions of the soles have been termed keratodermia blennorrhagica (Fig. 6-2). Hyperkeratosis may occur around the finger and toe nails. The lesions of Reiter's syndrome may be almost identical in appearance to those seen in pustular psoriasis and, indeed, impossible to differentiate. In some patients, there appears to be an actual overlap between psoriatic arthritis and Reiter's syndrome, with various features of both diseases being present at the same or different times. The

Figure 10-8. Mucocutaneous lesions of the penis in a patient with Reiter's syndrome. (Courtesy, Dr. C. Denko)

skin and joint lesions of Reiter's syndrome are usually self-limiting and resolve after several weeks or months. Of pathogenic and diagnostic interest is the recent observation that histocompatibility antigen, HLA-B27, is present in 80% or more of patients with Reiter's syndrome, whether or not spondylitis is present.[12,13]

Behçet's syndrome is characterized by a basic triad of lesions that includes mucocutaneous ulcers of the oral and genital tracts and recurrent iritis. Arthritis is common. Oral ulcerative mucous membrane lesions resemble aphthous stomatitis (Fig. 7-8). Ulcerative lesions of the penis are common and usually painful. In women, similar ulcerations may be seen on the vulva and in the vagina. They are characteristically painfree and easily overlooked. Pyoderma gangrenosum and lesions that resemble erythema nodosum are common.

Stevens-Johnson syndrome may be regarded as a variant of erythema multiforme. Characteristically, patients have high fever and severe stomatitis characterized by ulcerative lesions of the oral mucous membranes. Similar lesions may appear on the genitalia. A bullous erythematous skin eruption may occur elsewhere on the body. Symptoms in joints and muscles may be present but are usually a minor manifestation of the disease. Transient arthralgia is the most frequent associated musculoskeletal finding. The presence of bullous vesicular lesions and stomatitis is usually required to make the diagnosis.

The syndrome of *erythema nodosum* is characterized by painful subcutaneous nodules. Hilar adenopathy, fever and arthritis are frequent associated findings (see Chapter 6). The syndrome is more frequent in females. Characteristic skin lesions consist of cutaneous and subcutaneous inflammatory nodules that appear in crops. Lesions are red, tender and painful. Their color may change as the lesion ages, becoming somewhat violaceous in hue. Lesions usually heal completely without scarring. In most cases, lesions are confined to the legs below the knees and involve the anterior tibial areas (Fig. 6-3). In some patients, however, the lesions are more widespread and involve the upper extremities as well. Joint symptoms usually occur concomitantly with skin findings, but they may precede or follow cutaneous manifestations. Joint symptoms may be limited to arthralgia, but swelling and synovial effusion are common. Although knees and ankles are most frequently involved, other joints may be affected. Erythema nodosum may occur as a primary disease, or secondary to other disorders, which should be diagnostically excluded (see Chapter 6).

Skin lesions are a prominent component of various forms of *vasculitis,* such as polyarteritis nodosa, allergic angiitis and Henoch-Schönlein purpura. The lesions are extremely pleomorphic and many forms may be seen simultaneously. Purpuric eruptions are very common (Fig. 10-9). Other forms include nodular lesions, vesicular or bullous eruptions, urticaria, livedo reticularis and gangrene. Small necrotic lesions that involve the paronychial or subungual areas (Fig. 10-10) are common and are similar to the splinter hemorrhages seen in subacute bacterial endocarditis.

Other somewhat specific forms of vasculitis have been described. *Hypocomplementemic vasculitis* is characterized clinically by recurrent urticarial skin eruptions.[14] Fever, and joint and abdominal pain are commonly asso-

Figure 10-9.   Necrotizing vasculitis. Typical purpuric lesions of skin.

Figure 10-10. Necrotizing vasculitis. Paronychial and subungual lesions
secondary to ischemia. (Courtesy, Dr. A. Mackenzie)

ciated. Urinalysis may reveal hematuria, proteinuria and casts due to kidney involvement. Hypocomplementemia parallels disease activity. Urticarial
venulitis likely represents the same disorder.[15,16]

Cutaneous vasculitis is a common concomitant of the clinical picture in
patients with *mixed cryoglobulinemia.*[17,18] Palpable purpura usually involves the lower extremities. Polyarthralgias, lymphadenopathy, hepatosplenomegaly, and glomerulonephritis are often present. Serum cryoglobulins, rheumatoid factor and hypocomplementemia are seen. This syndrome
occurs as a secondary manifestation of other connective tissue diseases
such as rheumatoid arthritis, Sjögren's syndrome or systemic lupus erythematosus, or may be essential (idiopathic) in origin. Hepatitis antigen
(Hb_sAg) or its antibody is seen in many of these patients, suggesting a
relationship of this virus to disease pathogenesis.[17]

Subcutaneous nodules and erythema marginatum are the characteristic
skin lesions of *rheumatic fever.* Subcutaneous nodules vary in size from a
few millimeters to one or two centimeters and appear most frequently over
bony surfaces such as the olecranon areas and at the wrists and malleoli.
Although these nodules are similar in appearance to those seen in patients
with rheumatoid arthritis, certain differences are notable: the nodules in
rheumatic fever appear more commonly at the point of the olecranon process, rather than in the subolecranon area characteristic of rheumatoid
arthritis. In addition, the nodules in rheumatic fever tend to last for a
shorter period of time; the duration rarely exceeds more than three or four
weeks.

Erythema marginatum is characterized by nonpruritic macular pink lesions that tend to be evanescent. The trunk and limbs are affected most
often; the face is never involved. The lesion extends peripherally while the
skin in the center gradually returns to normal. Lesions that are continuous
and form a ring are called erythema annulare; they probably represent a
form of erythema marginatum. Lesions may appear and disappear over a
matter of hours. They change shape rapidly and are often more evident
following a hot bath or shower. Both the subcutaneous nodules and erythema marginatum lesions are considered major manifestations in diagnosis.

Although joint manifestations are the hallmark of *rheumatoid arthritis,* extra-articular lesions are common and can be helpful in diagnosis. Rheumatoid nodules, characterized by firm subcutaneous nodular lesions, are a significant diagnostic finding. Although located most frequently in subcutaneous areas, they often involve deeper connective tissue structures such as periosteum and tendon sheaths, as well as tendons themselves. They tend to appear in areas subjected to repeated trauma, such as the subolecranon areas of the elbow (Fig. 1-3), the ischial tuberosities, the Achilles tendons, and the scapular areas of the back. Involvement of hands and feet is common in severe cases. These lesions must be differentiated from gouty tophi, sebaceous cysts, xanthoma tuberosum, granuloma annulare, amyloid deposits and the subcutaneous nodules of rheumatic fever.

Other cutaneous manifestations associated with rheumatoid arthritis are seen when necrotizing vasculitis is a complicating manifestation of the disease. The lesions are similar to those described in the preceding section on vasculitis. Particularly frequent are purpuric lesions of the skin and infarctive lesions of the fingernail beds. The purpuric lesions should be distinguished from ecchymotic or purpuric lesions that occur spontaneously or follow mild trauma in rheumatoid arthritis patients on prolonged steroid therapy. Secondary skin ulcers are common.

A characteristic erythematous rash occurs in approximately 30% of patients with *juvenile rheumatoid arthritis* (JRA). The rash consists of macular and maculopapular lesions that are usually discrete but are sometimes confluent (Fig. 10-11). They are distributed mainly on the limbs and trunk, but are also seen on the face, palms and soles. As with erythema marginatum, the rash of juvenile rheumatoid arthritis tends to be evanescent. It frequently appears primarily in the evening or concomitantly with high fever spikes. Heat or irritation intensify the rash. Pruritus occurs but is uncommon. In contrast to the frequent finding of subcutaneous nodules in adult rheumatoid arthritis, subcutaneous nodules are uncommon in children, especially at the youngest age levels. A similar rash associated with high spiking fevers and arthritis that begins in adulthood (adult onset Still's disease) has been described with increased frequency.[19]

Rubella infection is characterized by a diffuse maculopapular rash, fever, and suboccipital lymphadenopathy. Acute polyarthralgia or polyarthritis commonly occurs in adolescents or young adults.[20] Joint symptoms usually occur in association with the rash, but may precede or follow it. Small joints of the hands are affected most commonly, but large joints may also be involved. Joint manifestations are usually self-limited.

A distinctive skin rash is seen in patients with *gonococcal arthritis.*[21] The lesions represent either septic metastatic foci with infectious angiitis, or a systemic hypersensitivity reaction. Small erythematous macules, vesicles and pustules are common (Fig. 10-12). As the lesions progress, central

Figure 10-11.   Rash, juvenile rheumatoid arthritis. Diffuse macular and maculopapular lesions are seen. (Courtesy, the Arthritis Foundation)

Figure 10-12.   Pustular necrotic lesion of leg in patient with acute gonococcal arthritis. (Courtesy, Dr. F. Bishko)

necrosis occurs. Bullous lesions are occasionally seen. Skin lesions in all stages of development may be present simultaneously.

Subacute bacterial endocarditis is associated with musculoskeletal symptoms in approximately 30% of patients.[22] Arthralgias and myalgias, particularly in the low back area, may be prominent. Arthritis is usually pauci-articular, involving proximal large joints. This diagnosis should be considered in patients with undiagnosed arthritis, fever and leukocytosis.

Skin lesions and arthritis are seen in patients with *ulcerative colitis* and *regional enteritis.* Erythema nodosum is present in approximately 5% of patients with ulcerative colitis and somewhat less often in patients with regional enteritis. Oral ulcerations are common. Pyoderma gangrenosum, associated with ulcerative colitis, is seen most frequently on the lower extremities. Early lesions appear as pustules that later coalesce and ulcerate. The lesions are frequently multiple and may become quite extensive. They are slow to heal and scarring is common. New lesions may appear at sites of trauma.

Skin rash is a common concomitant of the *arthritis associated with hepatitis.*[23] Although urticarial pruritic lesions are seen most frequently, erythematous maculopapular lesions, petechiae, and tender erythematous nodules have been described. Large joints are involved most commonly in the associated arthritis. Low serum complement levels and a positive test for hepatitis B antigen (HB_sAg) are characteristic laboratory findings.

Lyme arthritis, named after the small community in Connecticut where it was first described, is characterized by intermittent attacks of arthritis primarily affecting large joints.[24] Asymmetric, pauci-articular joint involvement is most common. Cutaneous manifestations are related to the bite of a tick involved in disease transmission. The skin lesion, known as erythema chronicum migrans, begins as a small red macule or papule which expands to form a large outer ring with central clearing. Arthritis, when it occurs, develops within weeks to months after the cutaneous lesion. Other manifestations of the disorder include fever, chills, central nervous system abnormalities such as meningitis and cranial nerve palsies, and myocardial conduction defects. Circulating immune complexes may be of pathogenic importance in the development of multisystem organ involvement.[25]

Cutaneous nodular panniculitis and arthritis are seen in association with *pancreatitis or pancreatic neoplasms.*[26] Joint and skin manifestations may precede evidence of pancreatic disease. Subcutaneous nodules at times resemble erythema nodosum. Cutaneous and joint manifestations appear related to release of pancreatic enzymes. Periarticular fat necrosis and intramedullary lytic defects of bone are seen.

Lipoid dermatoarthritis (multicentric reticulohistiocytosis) is an uncommon disorder characterized by cutaneous nodules and severe, often mutilating, polyarthritis.[27] In most cases arthritis precedes the skin rash, but the two may occur simultaneously. Skin lesions consist of firm brownish-yellow papular nodules, seen most commonly on the face, hands, scalp, neck and chest. Small raised lesions, similar to coral beads in appearance, appear around the nail folds. Lesions tend to vary in size and usually disappear without a trace. Mucosal papules occur on the lips, tongue and buccal mucosa. The associated polyarthritis is usually symmetric and often simulates rheumatoid arthritis. Some patients suffer from severe arthritis mutilans. Roentgenograms of involved joints show extensive destructive changes with loss of cartilage and absorption of subchondral bone. Biopsy study of lesions reveals multinucleated giant cells and histiocytes with a ground-glass appearance.

An asymmetric, self-limited, nondeforming peripheral arthritis has been described in association with *acne conglobata and acne fulminans.*[28,29] A similarity between the arthritic manifestations associated with these cutaneous disorders and "reactive arthritis," such as seen in Reiter's disease has been suggested. Spondylitis is occasionally observed. *Sweet's syndrome* (acute febrile neutrophilic dermatosis) is characterized by fever, raised tender plaques on the skin, and leukocytosis.[30] Joint symptoms occur in up to 25% of patients; manifestations, although acute, are usually self-limited. Biopsy study of the cutaneous lesion reveals neutrophilic infiltration of the dermis.

DIAGNOSTIC STUDIES

Close attention to history and physical examination is important in the initial differential diagnosis of disease characterized by skin rash and arthritis. Appropriate laboratory studies are then directed toward the most highly suspected diagnoses. Skin biopsy can be performed with little hazard and discomfort utilizing a punch biopsy technique under local anesthesia. Pathologic findings on routine histologic study are often sufficiently characteristic to allow accurate diagnosis. Special immunofluorescent studies of biopsy tissue are often helpful when a diagnosis of chronic discoid lupus or systemic lupus erythematosus is being considered (see Chapter 2). Immunofluorescent localization of gamma globulin at the epidermal-dermal junction is seen in 85 to 95% of cases of discoid or systemic lupus erythematosus (SLE) in biopsy specimens from involved skin. Similar findings are noted in normal uninvolved skin in up to 80% of patients with SLE but are absent in studies of normal skin of patients with chronic discoid lupus.

THERAPY

Treatment of the cutaneous manifestations varies with the specific diagnosis. The lesions of discoid and systemic lupus erythematosus are usually aided by direct application of local steroid creams or by intralesional injections of corticosteroids. Enclosing the areas of treatment with an occlusive covering augments the therapeutic response to local steroid creams. More severe lesions require the use of systemic agents such as hydroxy-chloroquine (Plaquenil), or quinacrine hydrochloride (Atabrine), and oral or parenteral steroids. Sun screen lotions diminish aggravation of the rash by sun exposure. The rash of dermatomyositis may respond to systemic steroids utilized in treatment of the muscular component of the disease, in addition to local steroid creams. Antimalarial agents are helpful in some patients. Management of cutaneous changes in scleroderma requires trial with a variety of agents (see Chapter 19). Eosinophilic fasciitis is characterized by a generally good response to corticosteroid therapy. Psoriasis responds to various regimens including coal tar ointments and ultraviolet light, or local steroid creams or ointments. Intractable cases may require more potent agents, such as methotrexate, 6-mercaptopurine, azathioprine or hydroxyurea. All of these agents except methotrexate are still investigational for use in this disease. PUVA (oral methoxypsoralens followed by ultra-violet radiation) is effective in many patients. The cutaneous lesions of Reiter's syndrome usually respond to local steroid therapy. Oral lesions benefit from applications of triamcinolone (Kenalog) in Orobase. Tetra-cycline suspension used three or four times a day as a mouthwash is effective in reducing secondary infection. Pain is often lessened by use of Viscous Xylocaine. Genital ulcerations similarly respond to local steroids. Severe diffuse lesions may require systemic steroids. Management of Stevens-Johnson syndrome usually requires high-dose steroids, such as prednisone, 15 mg QID, by mouth. Offending allergenic drugs implicated in etiology should be discontinued. The lesions of Behçet's syndrome that involve the mouth or genitalia are treated similarly to lesions in Reiter's syndrome. Systemic steroids or immunosuppressive agents[31] are worthy of trial in severe cases.

The nodular lesions of erythema nodosum require little specific therapy if the disease is mild. Full doses of aspirin reduce inflammation and relieve pain. Local steroids combined with plastic wrap occlusion may be beneficial. Severe cases may require systemic steroids for relief of joint and cutaneous manifestations. The skin lesions of necrotizing vasculitis require high-dose systemic steroids for management; 60 to 100 mg of prednisone daily are not unusual. Use of topical steroids with occlusion may also be beneficial. In patients with generalized systemic vasculitic involvement, immunosuppressive therapy in addition to corticosteroids has been recommended.[32,33] Plasmapheresis to remove cryoproteins, steroid therapy and use of cytotoxic drugs deserve consideration in management of cryoglobulinemic syndromes. When secondary in etiology, treatment should also be directed to the underlying disorder. The cutaneous lesions of rheumatic fever spontaneously disappear and do not require specific attention. Subcutaneous nodules in patients with rheumatoid arthritis are often asymptomatic, in which case no specific therapy is required. Large lesions in pressure-sensitive areas may benefit from local steroid injection therapy. Large persistent nodules require surgical removal. Recurrences are lessened by avoiding pressure over previously involved areas. No specific therapy is indicated for the rash of juvenile rheumatoid arthritis. Antipruritic lotions or oral antihistamines are helpful if pruritus is bothersome. Gonococcal skin lesions respond readily to penicillin therapy used in management of the basic gonococcal infection.

Musculoskeletal symptoms associated with subacute bacterial endocarditis respond to appropriate treatment of the offending organism. Pyoderma gangrenosum may be benefited by local therapy such as gentian violet applications and steroid injections. More severe lesions require consideration of systemic corticosteroid therapy and, at times, immunosuppressive agents. Appropriate management of related underlying disorders such as ulcerative colitis is helpful. Erythema chronicum migrans, seen in patients with Lyme disease, resolves faster in patients given penicillin or tetracycline.[34] Preliminary study suggests that penicillin therapy may prevent or attenuate subsequent arthritis; neurologic and cardiac abnormalities are unaffected.[34] These findings remain to be confirmed. In patients with subcutaneous panniculitis and arthritis related to pancreatic disease, treatment should be directed at the underlying disorder. Anti-inflammatory medications may be helpful. Although no one agent has been shown of consistent benefit in the treatment of the arthritis or cutaneous lesions of lipoid dermatoarthritis, prednisone and immunosuppressive agents have been described as possibly beneficial.[35]

CASE HISTORIES

History 10-1. Dermatomyositis

C.H., a 15-year-old white female, had a history of weakness of the pelvic and shoulder girdle muscles beginning nine months earlier. This symptom was associated with periorbital edema and the presence of slightly scaly violaceous macular lesions over the extensor surface of both elbows and knees and the malleoli of the ankles. Muscle weakness progressed in severity over the ensuing months. Shortly prior to consultation the patient observed pallor and paresthesia of the fingers on exposure to cold. There was no history of dysphagia, sun sensitivity, pleurisy, dry eyes or mouth, frequent canker sores, arthralgia or arthritis. System review was otherwise negative, and past history was unremarkable. Family history for muscle disorders was negative.

On physical examination, the cutaneous lesions were readily visible. No thickening of the skin was observed. Moderate weakness of the hip and shoulder girdle muscles and the cervical and abdominal flexors was demonstrated. Muscles were nontender. The remainder of the examination was normal.

Hematocrit was 38%, white blood cell count was 6200/mm³ with a normal differential, and erythrocyte sedimentation rate was 18 mm/hour (Wintrobe). Routine serologic test for syphilis was negative; serum protein electrophoresis was normal. Urinalysis revealed trace protein. Serum glutamic oxaloacetic transaminase and alkaline phosphatase were normal. Studies for serum rheumatoid factor and antinuclear antibody were negative. Serum creatine phosphokinase (CPK) was 1500 IU/ml (normal, up to 150 IU/ml). Twenty-four-hour urinary creatine-creatinine ratio determinations were 34% and 39% on two successive days. Electromyographic study of involved muscles demonstrated small numbers of polyphasic potentials. Right deltoid muscle biopsy was performed. Examination of the specimen revealed variation in fiber size, increased amounts of connective tissue, and mononuclear inflammatory infiltrates. A diagnosis of dermatomyositis was made and the patient was placed on prednisone, 15 mg QID.

Excellent response with improvement in muscle strength was noted over a period of six weeks. Repeat serum CPK was 70 units. Urinary creatine-creatinine ratios were 16% and 21%. Slow reduction of prednisone dosage was instituted and the patient monitored closely by periodic manual muscle evaluation, serum CPK and urinary creatine-creatinine ratio studies. Muscle symptoms were eventually well-controlled on a maintenance dose of prednisone, 2.5 mg TID. Cutaneous lesions improved but did not disappear despite additional therapy utilizing local steroid creams.

Discussion: The clinical diagnosis related to muscle weakness in this patient was simplified by the presence of cutaneous lesions characteristic of dermatomyositis. Periorbital edema with a violaceous rash of the eyelids (heliotrope eyelids) is a typical finding, as is the presence of the rash over extensor surfaces such as the knuckles, elbows, and knees. Cutaneous lesions improved but did not completely resolve with steroid therapy, despite excellent response of muscle weakness.

History 10-2. Psoriatic Arthritis

S.B., a 42-year-old white male dentist, was first seen in consultation in January, 1972. Approximately one year prior he noted arthralgias of the proximal interphalangeal (PIP) joints of the hands, wrists, elbows, and knees. Six months later he developed persistent swelling of the metatarsophalangeal (MTP) joints of the feet, both knees, and the right wrist. Morning stiffness was minimal. In November, 1971, he had onset of scaly erythematous pruritic patches on the extensor surfaces of both elbows and over the right scalp. There was no history of pleurisy, colitis, back pain, sciatica, iritis, or urethritis. Physical examination revealed scaly erythematous lesions over both olecranon areas and the right scalp. There was swelling of the IP joint of the left thumb, the right second and third PIP and DIP joints, the left knee, and the second, third and fourth MTP joints of the right foot. In addition, the interphalangeal joints of the left third and fourth toes showed a sausage-like fusiform swelling. Several fingernails exhibited pitting and thickening with whitish discoloration.

Urinalysis, white blood cell count and differential, hematocrit and serologic test for syphilis were normal or negative. Erythrocyte sedimentation was 18 mm/hour (Wintrobe). Serum studies for rheumatoid factor and antinuclear antibody were negative. Serum uric acid was 5.4 mg/100 ml. Roentgenograms of the hands showed several small erosions of periarticular bone in the second and third PIP joints of the right hand. A diagnosis of psoriatic arthritis was made.

The patient was treated with aspirin, 640 mg QID, physical therapy, and transverse metatarsal pads for the shoes. Psoriatic cutaneous lesions responded well to local use of steroid creams. Joint symptoms were well controlled for several months on this conservative program. Indomethacin, 25 mg TID, was substituted for salicylates when a moderately severe episode of the arthritis did not respond to increased doses of aspirin. Swelling and pain were well controlled, and the patient was able to carry on his dental activities without major difficulty.

Discussion: The involvement of distal interphalangeal joints of the hands and sausage-like fusiform swelling of the interphalangeal joints of the toes were characteristic manifestations of psoriatic arthritis in this patient. As may occasionally occur, joint symptoms preceded onset of psoriatic skin lesions.

History 10-3. Reiter's Syndrome

R.B., a 32-year-old white male, was admitted to hospital on January 19, 1972. His illness began two weeks prior, at which time he noted pain and burning on urination and a white urethral discharge. The right eye appeared red. Pain and swelling of the right knee and left ankle developed one week later. During hospitalization, the right heel became painful and tender, and inflammation of the right eye increased. In addition, several scaly maculopapular lesions were noted on the plantar surfaces of both feet and a scaly erythematous lesion appeared in the area of the penile meatus. There was an erythematous aphthous lesion of the tongue. Further history revealed extramarital sexual contact seven days prior to onset of his acute illness. Physical examination showed acute swelling and inflammation of the right knee and left ankle, and mucocutaneous lesions on the feet, penis and tongue.

The hematocrit was 42%, and the white blood cell count was 5700/mm^3 with a normal differential. Erythrocyte sedimentation rate was 33 mm/hour (Wintrobe). Urine contained 1+ albumin with a few white cells per high power field. Smear and culture of the urethra and urine culture were negative. Study of fluid aspirated from the right knee revealed 7000 white cells/mm^3, 45% of which were polymorphonuclear cells. Synovial fluid glucose was 80 mg/100 ml when blood glucose was 100 mg/100 ml. No crystals were seen. Synovial fluid culture was negative. Serum studies for rheumatoid factor and antinuclear antibody were negative. Creatinine clearance was normal. Serum protein electrophoresis revealed slight elevation of alpha-2 globulin. Roentgenograms of the chest and involved joints were normal except for soft tissue swelling of the right knee. Ophthalmologic examination revealed conjunctivitis and mild uveitis. A diagnosis of Reiter's syndrome was made.

Tetracycline, 500 mg QID, was begun for his genitourinary symptoms, with resolution of complaints after a period of five to six days. Attempts to control his relatively severe arthritic symptoms with full doses of aspirin, indomethacin and, later, phenylbutazone were unsuccessful. The patient was placed on prednisone, 10 mg QID, for treatment of uveitis and joint symptoms. In addition, steroid eye drops were used locally. Triamcinolone in Orabase was prescribed for his oral lesion. The patient responded well to the above program and prednisone dosage was gradually reduced as joint and eye symptoms improved. Clinical symptoms resolved completely after four months and all therapy was discontinued. The patient did well for approximately one and a half years, at which time he had recurrence of iritis in the right eye. This was treated successfully with oral and local steroids and was not associated with recurrence of joint, genitourinary or mucocutaneous lesions.

Discussion: The patient presented with a classic tetrad of symptoms of Reiter's syndrome, including arthritis, conjunctivitis and iritis, urethritis, and mucocutaneous lesions of the skin, mouth and genitalia. Although all components of the tetrad were present simultaneously in this patient, it is not uncommon for various facets of the syndrome to occur independently of one another at separate times during the clinical course of this disease. Joint symptoms in many patients with this syndrome will respond satisfactorily to conservative therapy with salicylates or other non-steroidal anti-inflammatory agents, but some patients require short courses of steroids to control severe articular manifestations. Steroids used both systemically and locally are valuable for treatment of iritis. Genitourinary symptoms may respond to a short course of tetracycline therapy.

History 10-4. Behçet's Syndrome

A.H., a 15-year-old black male, was first seen for evaluation in December, 1973. He was well until approximately four weeks prior, when he noted onset of fever, malaise, myalgia and polyarthralgia. Several days later he developed swelling, tenderness and limitation of motion of the right ankle. Shortly afterwards, pain was noted in both shoulders and he developed swelling and pain in the right knee. The patient was treated with buffered aspirin, 640 mg QID, with some relief of muscle and joint pain. Three weeks prior to admission he developed painful subcutaneous nodules over the anterior aspect of the right leg and the dorsal aspect of the right forearm. Furuncle-like lesions were noted over the right side of his forehead. Temperature elevations up to 38.5° C daily were recorded. There was no history of eye symptoms, pleurisy, Raynaud's phenomenon, sun sensitivity, dry eyes or dry mouth, dysuria or drug allergy. Several days prior to admission, the patient developed painful oral ulcers and a painless ulcer on the scrotum. He was admitted to hospital by his pediatrician for evaluation and rheumatologic consultation. Further system review was negative, and past medical history was noncontributory.

Physical examination revealed normal blood pressure, pulse and respiration. Intermittent daily temperature elevations to 38.5° C were noted. Furuncle formation was seen over the right side of his forehead. Multiple oral ulcerations were present in the buccal mucosa and at the inferior aspect of the tongue. Small lymph nodes were palpable in each axillary area. Cardiorespiratory examination was normal. Abdominal examination revealed no enlargement of the liver or spleen. Examination of the extremities revealed slight swelling and tenderness of the right knee, and more extensive swelling, tenderness and limitation of motion of the right ankle. Tender, erythematous, warm discrete nodules, measuring 2 × 3 cm, appeared over the anterior aspect of the right leg and the dorsal aspect of the right forearm. A small ulcer of the scrotum was observed. The remainder of the musculoskeletal examination and muscle evaluation was normal.

The hematocrit was 41%, white blood cell count was 10,000/mm³ with a normal differential, and the platelet count was 342,000 per mm³. The erythrocyte sedimentation rate was 12 mm/hour (Wintrobe). The serum uric acid was 6 mg/100 ml, serum calcium was 10.7 mg/100 ml and serum phosphorus was 4.4 mg/100 ml. Serum protein electrophoresis, creatinine, and muscle enzymes were normal. Serologic test for syphilis was negative. Serum studies for rheumatoid factor and antinuclear antibody were negative, as were blood studies for LE cells. Throat culture revealed normal flora. Culture of the furuncle from the right forehead revealed Staphylococcus albus. Blood and urine cultures were negative. Upper gastrointestinal series, barium enema and chest x-rays were normal. Roentgenograms of both knees and ankles were unremarkable. Sigmoidoscopic examination to 25 cm revealed slightly edematous mucosa at 20 cm. No ulcers were seen. Ophthalmologic examination was normal. PPD and fungus skin tests were negative. A diagnosis of probable Behçet's syndrome was made.

Aspirin was increased to 960 mg QID. Oral ulcerations were treated with tetracycline suspension used as a mouthwash, Viscous Xylocaine, and triamcinolone in Orobase. It was advised that prednisone, 20 to 30 mg daily, be started if the patient failed to respond to a conservative program of therapy. Joint symptoms, myalgia, malaise and fever responded after four days of conservative therapy, however, and the patient was discharged to the care of his pediatrician.

Discussion: The symptoms in this patient, which included orogenital ulcerations, pyoderma, erythema nodosum-like lesions, arthritis and fever were consistent with a diagnosis of Behçet's syndrome. Although the classic syndrome includes conjunctivitis or iritis, components of the basic triad of symptoms may occur at separate times. Other diagnostic considerations included Reiter's syndrome and ulcerative colitis. Absence of symptoms involving the eye and genitourinary tract militated against a diagnosis of Reiter's syndrome. No evidence of ulcerative colitis was noted on radiologic or sigmoidoscopic study.

History 10-5. Erythema Nodosum

C.T., a 26-year-old white female, was seen in consultation in March, 1969. She was well until approximately one month prior, when she noted aching in the knees, hips and shoulders associated with mild morning stiffness. Two weeks later, she developed increased aching in numerous peripheral joints and objective swelling of the ankles and knees. Red, painful, tender nodules were noted in both anterior tibial areas. Nodule formation occurred in crops at intervals of several days. Treatment with aspirin, 640 mg QID, provided mild relief. She gave no past history of arthritis or rheumatic fever. Recent history was negative for upper respiratory infection or sore throat. On system review the patient denied pleurisy, Raynaud's phenomenon, sun sensitivity, dry eyes or mouth, iritis, canker sores, diarrhea or drug allergy. There was no known exposure to tuberculosis and the patient had not traveled outside the midwest for several years. The patient gave no history of prior drug ingestion; in particular, no intake of bromides, iodides, sulfonamides or contraceptive pills was noted.

Physical examination revealed blood pressure 100/64 mm Hg. Cutaneous examination showed a number of discrete, warm, erythematous nodules on the anterior aspects of both tibial areas. Individual lesions were characterized by a central area of induration. Lesions varied from 1 to 1½ cm in diameter. Cardiorespiratory examination revealed a Grade I/VI apical systolic murmur. Liver and spleen were not palpably enlarged. Musculoskeletal examination showed swelling of both wrists and both ankles with mild limitation of motion.

Hematocrit was 38%, and white blood cell count was 7700/mm³ with 8% eosinophils on differential white count. Erythrocyte sedimentation rate was 27 mm/hour (Wintrobe). Urinalysis was normal. Serum calcium was 9.4 mg/100 ml. Routine serologic test for syphilis and C-reactive protein studies were negative. Antistreptolysin-O titer was less than 100 Todd units. Heterophile antibody titer was 1:28. Serum studies for rheumatoid factor and antinuclear antibody were negative, and LE cells were not seen. Throat culture revealed normal flora. PA and lateral roentgenograms of the chest showed bilateral hilar adenopathy. Electrocardiogram was normal. Skin test with intermediate PPD was negative. A diagnosis of erythema nodosum was made.

The patient was continued on aspirin, 960 mg QID. When seen in followup one month later the cutaneous lesions had almost completely resolved. Joint swelling was absent and only mild polyarthralgia remained. Repeat chest x-ray at that time was completely normal. The patient went on to complete clearing of symptoms over a period of several more weeks and had no recurrence of a similar syndrome during prolonged followup.

Discussion: The findings of tender, erythematous nodular skin lesions over the anterior tibial areas, arthritis, and hilar adenopathy were consistent with a diagnosis of erythema nodosum. History, physical examination and laboratory studies did not reveal the presence of any underlying disease with which erythema nodosum is commonly associated. Lesions responded to a conservative program of management.

Prolonged observation for the presence of primary disease states that are associated with erythema nodosum is important, because the underlying disorder may not become evident for some time. A diagnosis of primary idiopathic erythema nodosum can be made safely only after a reasonable period of followup.

History 10-6. Henoch-Schönlein (Anaphylactoid) Purpura

G.G., a 10-year-old white male, was admitted to hospital for evaluation in April, 1973. He was well until one week prior, at which time he noted onset of fatigue, fever, red spots on the skin about the ankles, and pain in both elbows and knees. The night prior to admission he developed nausea and epigastric pain and vomited clear gastric fluid. Physical examination revealed many discrete purpuric cutaneous lesions, 3 mm to 2 cm in size, over the lower extremities and buttocks. Lesions did not blanch with pressure. Cardiorespiratory examination was normal. There was generalized abdominal tenderness and the spleen was palpable 1 cm below the costal margin. Joint examination was normal except for tenderness of the elbows and knees to palpation.

The urine contained 10 to 20 red blood cells per high power field. Hematocrit was 38%, white blood cell count was 11,500/mm^3 and differential white cell count was normal. Erythrocyte sedimentation rate was 26 mm/hour (Wintrobe). Prothrombin time, partial thromboplastin time, platelet count, bleeding time and coagulation time were normal. Throat culture revealed normal throat flora, and antistreptolysin-O titer was negative. Studies for serum rheumatoid factor, antinuclear antibody, complement and serum protein electrophoresis were normal or negative. Serologic test for syphilis was negative. Stool guaiac studies were strongly positive. Creatinine clearance was 104 ml/minute. Electrocardiogram and roentgenograms of the chest and abdomen revealed no abnormal findings.

Re-examination on the second day of hospitalization demonstrated definite swelling of the right wrist and the presence of fresh blood in the stool. Purpuric cutaneous lesions became larger and more widespread and the patient continued to pass grossly bloody stools. Prednisone was begun in a dose of 10 mg BID by mouth. After four days, skin lesions notably diminished, there was no abdominal tenderness or gross gastrointestinal bleeding, and joint examination was normal. Urinalysis revealed no abnormalities. The patient was discharged with plans to slowly decrease steroid therapy while under clinical observation. Clinical manifestations continued to improve and steroids were discontinued after three weeks.

Discussion: The clinical findings of purpura, abdominal pain and gastrointestinal bleeding, hematuria and joint symptoms were typical of those seen in patients with Henoch-Schönlein (anaphylactoid) purpura. Prognosis is generally good unless chronic renal disease intervenes. Other forms of necrotizing vasculitis that might produce similar clinical manifestations must be excluded if symptoms are atypical.

History 10-7. Gonococcal Arthritis

P.D., a 19-year-old black male, was first seen in consultation in December, 1972. He had been in good health until four days prior to admission, at which time he noted pain in the right wrist with use. Pain increased in intensity, with severe symptoms at rest. Pain was followed by swelling of the right wrist and the dorsum of the right hand. Two days prior to admission, the patient developed fever and chills. There was no history of sun sensitivity, Raynaud's phenomenon, morning stiffness, skin rash, diarrhea, urethritis or pleurisy. The patient denied past history of venereal disease and recent sexual intercourse. System review was otherwise normal and past medical history was unremarkable.

Physical examination revealed temperature of 38° C. No lymphadenopathy was present. Examination of the heart and lungs revealed no abnormal findings. The abdomen was soft and the liver and spleen were not palpably enlarged. Several acute papulovesicular lesions with erythematous borders were observed. Joint examination revealed acute inflammation of the right wrist and hand with notable erythema, increased heat and tenderness. Movement of the fingers produced pain in the region of the dorsum of the right hand and the wrist. No other abnormal joint findings were observed.

Hematocrit was 42%, the erythrocyte sedimentation rate was 30 mm/hour (Wintrobe), and white blood cell count was 9000/mm³ with 88% neutrophils. Urinalysis, liver function studies, electrocardiogram and chest roentgenogram were normal. Roentgenograms of the right wrist and hand revealed only soft tissue swelling. A few drops of purulent-looking material were removed by arthrocentesis from the right wrist. Gram stain revealed a moderate number of polymorphonuclear cells but no bacteria. Culture was positive for Neisseria gonorrhoeae. Blood, urethral, and throat cultures were negative. A diagnosis of acute gonococcal arthritis and tenosynovitis was made.

The patient was treated with aqueous crystalline penicillin, 6 million units daily in divided doses, by intravenous route. Swelling of the right hand and wrist and fever subsided notably over a two-day period. He was discharged five days after admission to continue oral penicillin for a total of 14 days of therapy.

Discussion: Gonococcal arthritis may appear in several different clinical forms. Acute migratory polyarthralgia or polyarthritis may precede localization of infection to one or two joints. Systemic findings such as fever and chills and cutaneous lesions are common associated symptoms. In some patients, preceding polyarticular disease may be absent and the infection appears as an acute monoarthritis. In this patient, joint symptoms were limited to the right wrist and dorsum of the right hand. The right hand symptoms were consistent with acute tenosynovitis, a common manifestation of gonococcal infection. Cutaneous lesions were characteristic of those seen in gonococcal infection and strongly suggested the correct diagnosis even before bacterial confirmation. Although a history of recent sexual exposure can frequently be elicited, the diagnosis cannot be excluded in the absence of such information.

History 10-8.   Eosinophilic fasciitis

C. H., a 29-year-old white male was admitted with a six-month history of knee aching associated with morning stiffness, which developed shortly after a week of strenuous physical activity related to painting a living room. Two months later, after baling hay, he developed aching in his wrists and hands with arthralgias spreading to multiple other joints. The patient denied facial rash, hair loss, Raynaud's phenomenon or photosensitivity, and there was no history of asthma or other allergies.

On physical examination blood pressure was 140/90 and pulse 80. There was mild thickening of the skin over the forearms and hands. On joint examination, there was mild swelling of the right second, third, and fourth proximal interphalangeal joints; the left second, fourth, and fifth proximal interphalangeal joints; and both wrists and elbows, with moderate limitation of full extension of the latter. Both knees were slightly swollen, and could not be fully extended. There was a palpable rubbing sensation when the right knee was flexed. The rest of the examination was within normal limits.

Laboratory data included a hematocrit of 44%, with a white blood cell count of 8,300 cells/mm³. Platelet count was within normal limits. Examination of multiple peripheral blood films showed 8 to 18% eosinophils, with total eosinophil counts varying between 1,500 and 1,800. The erythrocyte sedimentation rate (Wintrobe) varied from 23 to 27 mm/hour. There was a slightly elevated A.M. serum cortisol of 23.2 μg/dl (upper limit of normal, 20 μg/dl). Serum protein electrophoresis showed an elevated gamma globulin of 1.5 g/100 ml with a normal albumin of 4.1 g/100 ml, and normal alpha-one, alpha-two, and beta fractions. Serum protein immunoelectrophoresis showed an IgG of 1,490 mg/100 ml (149% of normal), IgA of 52.5 mg/100 ml (23% of normal) and IgM of 84 mg/100 ml (80% of normal). There was a normal serum creatine phosphokinase (42 units/liter), and a normal 24 hour urine creatine to creatinine ratio of less than 1%. Trichinosis titers (complement fixation) were negative. Serologic evaluation included a negative latex fixation, weakly positive ANA (1:10, homogeneous pattern), negative anti-DNA (Crithidia luciliae method), negative antibody to extractable nuclear antigen (hemagglutination technique), negative hepatitis associated antigen, negative indirect Coombs test, and a nonreactive VDRL. EKG showed minor aberrant intraventricular conduction. Chest radiographs, periodontal films, esophagram, and upper gastrointestinal series were within normal limits. However, findings on barium enema suggested wide-mouthed diverticula, and radiographs of the hands showed slight narrowing of the proximal interphalangeal joint of the left fifth finger. Pulmonary function studies were interpreted as consistent with a mild reversible obstructive defect.

A full thickness biopsy of skin, subcutis, fascia and muscle was taken from the clinically involved right forearm. Direct immunofluorescent studies of skin were negative. Microscopic examination showed fibroinflammatory changes involving the fascia, skeletal muscle, subcutis and dermis. Lymphocytes and histiocytes were predominant, with occasional plasma cells. Eosinophils were rare and were seen only in the muscle. Examination of a bone marrow biopsy revealed a moderately increased number of eosinophil precursors and mature eosinophils.

The patient was started on aspirin 6 to 8 tablets/day, and prednisone 20 mg b.i.d. Over the next six weeks, he showed decreasing stiffness in his feet and shoulders, and decreasing swelling in his hands and wrists. Over the next 14 months, the daily prednisone dose was slowly decreased as the patient continued to show improvement. Skin thickening over the forearms and hands had resolved, and only slight edema of the hands could be detected. Range of motion of hand and wrist joints was normal. Sedimentation rate remained under 10 mm/hour. On alternate day steroids, 10 mg p.o. q.o.d., the patient developed shoulder stiffness, hand edema, a sedimentation rate of 18 mm/hour, and reappearance of eosinophils up to 8%. Hydroxychloroquine, 200 mg b.i.d., was added to his regimen. When seen in follow-up, stiffness and aching had improved. Physical examination revealed minimal hand swelling and slight limitation of extension of both elbows. Sedimentation rate was 8 mm/hr and eosinophils were 6% of the white cell differential. Slow reduction in his prednisone dose was recommended and his hydroxychloroquine intake was reduced to 200 mg every other day.

Discussion: This patient had characteristic clinical and laboratory findings of eosinophilic fasciitis. Onset of symptoms following strenuous physical activity has been noted in other reported cases. Joint swelling, mild pulmonary dysfunction, and wide-mouth diverticula on barium enema study represented extracutaneous manifestations of the eosinophilic fasciitis spectrum. Inflammation was noted in muscle and subcutaneous fascia. Response to steroid therapy was good but the patient required prolonged prednisone therapy to control symptoms and abnormal laboratory parameters. Although the addition of hydroxychloroquine was associated with symptomatic improvement, the role of this agent in the treatment of this disorder requires further definition.

REFERENCES

1. Stahl, N. I., Klippel, J. H. and Decker, J. L.: A cutaneous lesion associated with myositis. Ann Intern Med 91:577, 1979.
2. Velayos, E. E. et al.: The "CREST" syndrome: comparison with systemic sclerosis (scleroderma). Arch Int Med 139:1240, 1979.

3. Maricq, H. R. and LeRoy, E. C.: Patterns of finger capillary abnormalities in connective tissue disease by "wide-field" microscopy. Arthritis Rheum 16:619, 1973.
4. Maricq, H. R., Spencer-Greene, G. and LeRoy, E. C.: Skin capillary abnormalities as indicators of organ involvement in scleroderma (systemic sclerosis), Raynaud's syndrome, and dermatomyositis. Am J Med 61:862, 1976.
5. Maricq, H. R. et al.: Diagnostic potential of in vivo capillary microscopy in scleroderma and related disorders. Arthritis Rheum 23:183, 1980.
6. Shulman, L. E.: Diffuse fasciitis with hypergammaglobulinemia and eosinophilia: a new syndrome. Trans Assoc Am Physicians 88:70, 1975.
7. Moore, T. L. and Zuckner, J.: Eosinophilic fasciitis. Semin Arth Rheum 19:228, 1980.
8. Kent, L. T., Cramer, S. F. and Moskowitz, R. W.: Eosinophilic fasciitis: clinical, laboratory and micrsocopic considerations. Arthritis Rheum 24:677, 1981.
9. Michett, C. J., Doyle, J. A. and Ginsburg, W. W.: Eosinophilic fasciitis. Report of 15 cases. Mayo Clinic Proc 56:27, 1981.
10. Moll, J. M. H. and Wright, V.: Psoriatic arthritis. Semin Arthritis Rheum 3:55, 1973.
11. Ford, D. K.: Reiter's syndrome. Bull Rheum Dis 20:588, 1970.
12. Morris, R. et al.: HLA-W27—a clue to the diagnosis and pathogenesis of Reiter's syndrome. N Eng J Med 290:554, 1974.
13. Fox, R. et al.: The chronicity of symptoms and disability in Reiter's syndrome: an analysis of 131 consecutive patients. Ann Intern Med 91:190, 1979.
14. McDuffie, F. C. et al.: Hypocomplementemia with cutaneous vasculitis and arthritis: possible immune complex syndrome. Mayo Clinic Proc 48:340, 1973.
15. Soter, N. A., Austen, K. F. and Gigli, I.: Urticaria and arthralgias as manifestations of necrotizing angitis (vasculitis). J Invest Dermat 63:485, 1974.
16. Soter, N. A.: Chronic urticaria as a manifestation of necrotizing venulitis. N Eng J Med 296:1440, 1977.
17. Meltzer, M. et al.: Cryoglobulinemia—a clinical and laboratory study. II. Cryoglobulins with rheumatoid factor activity. Am J Med 40:837, 1966.
18. Levo, Y. et al.: Association between hepatitis B virus and essential mixed cryoglobulinemia. N Eng J Med 296:1501, 1977.
19. Gupta, R. C. and Mills, D. M.: Still's disease in an adult: a link between juvenile and adult rheumatoid arthritis. Am J Med Sci 269:137, 1975.
20. Yanez, J. E. et al.: Rubella arthritis. Ann Int Med 64:772, 1966.
21. Keiser, H. L. et al.: Clinical forms of gonococcal arthritis. N Eng J Med 274:234, 1968.
22. Churchill, M. A., Geraci, J. E. and Hunder G. G.: Musculoskeletal manifestations of bacterial endocarditis. Ann Int Med 87:754, 1977.
23. McCarty, D. J. and Ormiste, V.: Arthritis and HB Ag positive hepatitis. Arch Int Med 132:264, 1973.
24. Steere, A. C. et al.: Erythema chronicum migrans and Lyme arthritis. Ann Int Med 86:685, 1977.
25. Steere, A. C. et al.: Lyme arthritis—correlation of serum and cryoglobulin IgM with activity, and serum IgG with remission. Arthritis Rheum 22:471, 1979.
26. Tannenbaum, H., Anderson, L. G. and Schur, P. H.: Association of polyarthritis, subcutaneous nodules and pancreatic disease. J Rheum 2:15, 1975.
27. Barrow, M. V. and Holubar, K.: Multicentric reticulohistiocytosis. Medicine 48:287, 1969.
28. Lane, J. M., Lyden, J. J. and Spiegel, R. J.: Acne arthralgia. J Bone Joint Surg 58A:673, 1976.
29. Goldschmidt, H., Leyden, J. J. and Stein, K. H.: Acne fulminans. Arch Dermat 113:444, 1977.
30. Krauser, R. E. and Schumacher, H. R.: The arthritis of Sweet's syndrome. Arthritis Rheum 18:35, 1975.
31. Buckley, G. E. III and Gills, J. P. Jr.: Cyclophosphamide therapy of Behçet's disease. J Allerg 43:273, 1969.

32. Fauci, A. S., Doppman, J. L. and Wolff, S. M.: Cyclophosphamide-induced remission in advanced polyarteritis nodosa. Am J Med 64:890, 1978.
33. Lieb, E. S., Restivo, C. and Paulus, H. E.: Immunosuppressive and corticosteroid therapy of polyarteritis nodosa. Am J Med 67:941, 1979.
34. Steere, A. C. et al.: Antibiotic therapy in Lyme disease. Ann Int Med 93:1, 1980.
35. Hanauer, L. B.: Reticulohistiocytosis. Remission after cyclophosphamide therapy. Arthritis Rheum 15:636, 1972.

CHAPTER 11

GASTROINTESTINAL SYMPTOMS AND ARTHRITIS

Patients with arthritis may suffer from diseases characterized by gastrointestinal abnormalities. In some patients, the arthritis and gastrointestinal symptoms occur concomitantly, or the arthritis follows gastrointestinal manifestations. In others, the arthritis may occur first, in which case the relationship between the two sites of involvement becomes obvious only with observation over a period of time.

DIFFERENTIAL DIAGNOSIS

Diseases to be considered:

Ulcerative colitis, regional enteritis
Whipple's disease
Reiter's syndrome
Yersinia arthritis
Behçet's syndrome
Hypertrophic osteoarthropathy
Scleroderma
Necrotizing vasculitis
Carcinoma of the bowel
Amyloidosis
Tuberculosis
Gastrointestinal shunts
Miscellaneous gastrointestinal disorders

Arthritis often accompanies *chronic ulcerative colitis*[1,2] or *regional enteritis.*[2,3] Although the arthritic features of these disorders are similar, different patterns of peripheral joint involvement occur. In classic cases, peripheral joint symptoms parallel gastrointestinal symptoms with respect to remissions and exacerbations. Large and small joints are involved. Arthritis may be limited to one or a few joints or involve numerous articulations. Migratory spread is common. Some patients complain of arthralgia with little or no objective swelling or tenderness. Rheumatoid factor tests are characteristically negative. Prognosis is usually good with regard to permanent joint disability.

In some patients, joint symptoms may more closely simulate rheumatoid arthritis; attacks are prolonged and lack an association with exacerbations and remissions of bowel disease. In other patients with inflammatory bowel disease, joint symptoms may be a reflection of associated disorders, including erythema nodosum and hypertrophic osteoarthropathy. Systemic manifestations of inflammatory bowel disease such as pyoderma gangrenosum, oral ulcerations, uveitis, and hepatic abnormalities are common associated findings.

Spondylitis that resembles ankylosing spondylitis occurs with increased frequency in patients with ulcerative colitis and regional enteritis. Evidence supports the interpretation that the spondylitis seen in these patients is an independent associated finding rather than a systemic manifestation of the bowel disease. For example, spondylitis often antedates bowel symptoms and there is little clinical correlation between the spondylitis and bowel disease. Effective treatment of the bowel is usually unassociated with relief of back symptoms. Interestingly, HLA-B27 histocompatibility antigen has been found in approximately 75% of patients with spondylitis and inflammatory bowel disease.[4,5] This increased frequency parallels the increased association of this antigen in patients with ankylosing spondylitis. No such increase is seen in patients with colitis or enteritis in the absence of spondylitis.

Whipple's disease is characterized by abdominal pain, diarrhea, fever, cutaneous hyperpigmentation, peripheral lymphadenopathy and arthritis[6,7] (see Chapter 8). In addition, there is a tendency to hypotension and pleural reactions. Peripheral joint manifestations are similar to those described for patients with colitis and regional enteritis. Joint complaints often precede symptoms of diarrhea; symptoms of arthritis and diarrhea usually do not occur simultaneously. The arthritis is usually episodic with a migratory pattern. Joint symptoms last for one to several days and long remissions are frequent. Chronic residual arthritis is rare. Large joints such as the knees and ankles are involved most frequently; fingers, wrists, elbows and other joints are also affected. Back symptoms may be present and findings of spondylitis have been described.[6,7] Rheumatoid factor studies are negative.

Diagnosis of Whipple's disease depends on demonstrating PAS-positive inclusion bodies in macrophages of small intestinal mucosa or mesenteric nodes. Biopsy of the jejunum by a peroral approach is utilized to obtain tissue for study. Electron microscopic studies demonstrate rod-shaped organisms infiltrating the lamina propria of the intestinal mucosa. Although these rod-shaped structures are probably related to disease etiology, experimental transmission of disease to animals has not been successfully accomplished. Initial treatment with penicillin and streptomycin for 10 to 14 days, followed by tetracycline for 10 to 12 months, has given favorable results in most cases.

Reiter's syndrome is associated with arthritis, urethritis, conjunctivitis and mucocutaneous ulcerative lesions. In addition, patients occasionally have involvement of the gastrointestinal tract. Diarrhea is usually mild and short in duration; in some cases, however, it is severe, bloody and prolonged. A relationship between Reiter's syndrome and Shigella flexneri infections during episodes of epidemic dysentery has been described.

Arthritis is most frequently seen in large joints, but toes and fingers may be involved. As in patients with ulcerative colitis and regional enteritis, spondylitis with involvement of sacroiliac joints and the spine is a common sequela of the disease. Close evaluation of roentgenographic spinal changes is helpful in differentiating the spondylitis of Reiter's syndrome from that seen in ulcerative colitis and ankylosing spondylitis. In Reiter's syndrome, paravertebral spurs (syndesmophytes) are more rounded and thicker than those seen in ankylosing spondylitis. Unilateral syndesmophytes are common in Reiter's syndrome.

A seronegative reactive arthritis similar if not identical to that observed in Reiter's syndrome occurs with *Yersinia enterocolitica* infection.[8,9] Acute infection with this organism usually presents as diarrhea. Subacute pauciarticular synovitis involving large and small joints is common; sacro-iliitis has been described. Additional manifestations include conjunctivitis, urethritis, myocarditis and erythema nodosum. HLA-B27 antigen is found in approximately three-quarters of the patients with arthritis.

Behçet's syndrome is a multisystem disorder characterized by a triad of recurrent oral and genital ulcerations and relapsing iritis. In addition, lesions occur in the gastrointestinal tract that may be severe and resemble the pathologic changes of ulcerative colitis. In most patients, arthralgia is more frequent than true arthritis. Large joints such as knees, ankles, wrists and elbows are involved most frequently. Fortunately, chronic permanent changes and joint disability rarely develop.

Hypertrophic osteoarthropathy is characterized by clubbing of the fingers and toes, periostitis of the ends of long bones and arthritis. Although usually seen secondary to infectious or neoplastic diseases of the lungs and pleura (see Chapter 12), this syndrome also occurs in association with gastrointestinal disorders such as ulcerative colitis, regional enteritis, intestinal tuberculosis, spruc, and carcinoma of the colon.

Joint and gastrointestinal symptoms are common concomitant findings in *scleroderma*. In most patients joint symptoms are characterized by pain with little or no swelling; other patients, however, show mild to severe degrees of joint disability. Involvement of skeletal muscle results in weakness

Figure 11-1.   Dental roentgenograms, scleroderma. Widening of the periodontal membrane due to collagen deposition is contrasted with normal findings. (Courtesy Dr. A. Mackenzie)

which, when severe, simulates polymyositis. Lesions of the gastrointestinal tract may be present from the mouth to the anus. Roentgenograms of the teeth show widening of the periodontal membrane (Fig. 11-1). Esophageal dysfunction with symptoms of dysphagia and esophagitis is common; on roentgenographic examination, peristaltic activity may be diminished or totally absent (Fig. 11-2). Hiatal hernia is frequent as reflux of gastric juices leads to stricture and secondary herniation. Involvement of the small bowel causes bloating, cramps, vomiting, episodic diarrhea and constipation. Malabsorption syndrome results from severe involvement of the small bowel.[10] Roentgenologic examination reveals dilatation of the second and third portions of the duodenum (Fig. 11-3). Roentgenographic examination of the small intestine demonstrates irregular flocculation of barium, areas of dilata-

Figure 11-2.   Roentgenogram of esophagus, scleroderma, showing generalized dilatation. Fluoroscopic study revealed loss of peristaltic activity. (Courtesy, Dr. A. Mackenzie)

Figure 11-3. Roentgenogram of stomach and small bowel, scleroderma. Note widely dilated duodenum. (Courtesy, Dr. A. Mackenzie)

Figure 11-4. Roentgenogram of large intestine, scleroderma. Note numerous wide-mouthed diverticula. (Courtesy, Dr. A. Mackenzie)

tion, hypersegmentation and evidence of hypomotility. Pneumatosis cystoides intestinalis may be seen in the form of radiolucent cysts or streaks of gas within the walls of the small bowel. When rupture of one of these cysts leads to pneumoperitoneum, the symptoms are highly suggestive of a perforated viscus. The disproportion between radiologic findings and benign clinical symptoms is the clue to diagnosis. Atrophy of the muscularis of the large intestine produces characteristic wide-mouthed diverticula (Fig. 11-4).

Gastrointestinal symptoms may be a major clinical feature in patients with various forms of *necrotizing vasculitis*. Abdominal pain is often accompanied by nausea, vomiting, diarrhea or bloody stools. The latter result from ischemic involvement of the bowel. Acute inflammation of various abdominal viscera, such as the appendix, intestine, stomach, gallbladder or pancreas, causes acute abdominal pain and sometimes rupture of the involved viscus. Mesenteric arteritis leads to thrombosis and bowel infarction; the clinical picture may superficially resemble ulcerative colitis. Henoch-Schönlein purpura is a specific vasculitic syndrome characterized by arthralgia or arthritis, cutaneous macules, papules and purpura, renal disease and gastrointestinal symptoms. Crampy abdominal pain and gastrointestinal hemorrhage are common. Intussusception may be a complicating factor.

Carcinoma of the bowel, as with carcinomas elsewhere, may be associated with peripheral arthritis that simulates rheumatoid arthritis.[11] Joint symptoms may appear when the neoplasm is occult and the true diagnosis becomes evident only after prolonged observation. The association of arthritis and malignancy should always be considered as a diagnostic possibility when arthritis begins in older persons. Large joints are characteristically involved but small joints may also be affected. Joint symptoms may recede following resection or other forms of treatment of the carcinoma. Recurrence of joint symptoms should suggest the possibility of recurrence of the neoplasm.

Arthritis may be a manifestation of either primary or secondary *amyloidosis*. Actual joint swelling may be noted. Cutaneous deposits of amyloid form subcutaneous nodules that simulate those seen in rheumatoid arthritis. Amyloidosis is frequently accompanied by gastrointestinal symptoms, including gastrointestinal bleeding. Infiltration of the esophagus or small bowel may lead to obstruction. Malabsorption syndrome results from infiltration of the small bowel. The diagnosis of amyloid may be made safely by study of tissue obtained by biopsy of the rectum, gingiva, or subcutaneous abdominal fat.[12]

An uncommon cause of arthritis and gastrointestinal symptoms is *tuberculosis*. These patients are usually severely ill and other findings to support the diagnosis are usually obvious.

An unusual form of arthritis is that seen in association with gastrointestinal *shunts occurring after jejunocolostomy or jejunoileostomy*.[13–17] Musculoskeletal complaints consist of arthralgias, myalgias, and arthritis involving both large and small joints. Tendinitis may be seen. Although arthritis is usually transitory and unassociated with permanent joint deformities, frequent recurrences or persistence of symptoms may require reconstitution of the bowel. Urticarial, pustular and nodular cutaneous vasculitic lesions have been described, and Raynaud's phenomenon may be associated.[17] Studies suggest that immune complexes are involved in the pathogenesis of the arthritis and other manifestations of this disorder such as cutaneous vasculitis, pleural effusions and impaired renal function.[15–17] Immune complexes containing immunoglobulin, complement components and antibodies to gram negative organisms such as *E. coli* and *B. fragilis* may result from antibody stimulation in response to intestinal absorption of bacterial antigens.[15–17]

Peptic or gastric ulceration is common in patients with various diseases of connective tissue. Their frequency is increased by use of various therapeutic agents that are highly irritating to the gastrointestinal tract. Indomethacin, commonly used in the treatment of inflammatory arthritides, may cause ulcerative lesions of the bowel. It is contraindicated in the presence of ulcerative colitis, regional enteritis and diverticulitis.

DIAGNOSTIC STUDIES

In addition to general diagnostic studies, specific examinations directed to the bowel are required. Sigmoidoscopic examination and barium enema are indicated if ulcerative colitis is suspected. Small bowel roentgenograms are utilized in patients with symptoms consistent with regional enteritis. The diagnosis of Whipple's disease is based on demonstration of specific pathologic findings in small bowel specimens obtained by peroral biopsy as previously described. Roentgenologic findings in patients with gastrointestinal symptoms due to Reiter's syndrome may be nonspecific or absent. The diagnosis usually rests on the overall clinical presentation. Ulcerative bowel lesions on radiologic study of patients with Behçet's syndrome are usually difficult to differentiate from ulcerative colitis. Indeed, the two diseases may be clinically indistinguishable. Sigmoidoscopic and vaginal examination to demonstrate ulcerative lesions characteristic of Behçet's syndrome are diagnostically helpful.

Studies in patients with hypertrophic osteoarthropathy should be directed toward diseases to which it is a secondary manifestation; chest roentgenograms are mandatory. Tuberculin skin testing, chest roentgenogram, and cultures of sputum and urine are indicated in patients with symptoms suggestive of intestinal tuberculosis.

Scleroderma is usually obvious on clinical examination, but visceral changes may occur with minimal or no skin changes. Roentgenograms often reveal characteristic changes at various levels of the bowel, as previously described. Radiologic changes in vasculitis of the bowel are nonspecific and resemble changes seen in other types of bowel ischemia. Dilatation and irritability of the bowel may be seen in association with edema and thickening of the bowel wall. Muscle biopsy is usually indicated for diagnosis. Arteriography of mesenteric, hepatic or renal vessels may demonstrate characteristic areas of thrombosis and aneurysm formation.

Carcinoma requires careful radiologic and sigmoidoscopic evaluation for diagnosis. Amyloidosis can be diagnosed in many cases by specific amyloid stains of tissue obtained at biopsy. A history of a gastrointestinal bypass shunt procedure provides the clue necessary for consideration of this disorder as the cause of articular symptoms.

THERAPY

The management of arthritis associated with the foregoing disorders includes nonspecific measures directed toward symptomatic relief and specific measures directed to the underlying disorders. Nonspecific therapeutic programs such as rest, heat, exercise and mild anti-inflammatory and analgesic agents can often be instituted safely prior to completion of studies without obscuring the diagnosis. Full doses of aspirin, such as 640 to 960 mg four times daily, are effective in relieving painful joint manifestations to some degree. Aspirin should be used with caution, if at all, in patients whose underlying disease state may be aggravated by its use, such as patients with peptic ulcer disease. Special forms of salicylates, such as enteric-coated aspirin, can be utilized more safely in such cases. Other nonsteroidal inflammatory agents may be utilized if salicylate therapy is unsuccessful or not well tolerated. These agents are contraindicated in the presence of peptic ulcer disease and should be used with caution in patients with ulcerative disease of the small or large bowel. Analgesic agents including acetaminophen, 320 to 640 mg QID, propoxyphene hydrochloride, 65 mg QID, or ethoheptazine citrate (Zactane), 75 mg QID, may be substituted or added without fear of causing significant gastric irritation. Systemic corticosteroid therapy should not be instituted for symptomatic relief, but should be limited to those specifically diagnosed conditions in which it has a definite and safe therapeutic effect. However, local steroid injections into the joint can be safely considered as a nonspecific approach to overall management.

The arthritis of ulcerative colitis or regional enteritis often responds to measures directed at control of the disease. Therapeutic agents include salicylazosulfapyridine (Azulfidine), systemic corticosteroids and, at times, immunosuppressive agents such as azathioprine. Colectomy or small bowel resection should be considered only for treatment of bowel disease unresponsive to conservative measures, and not as a therapeutic approach for the arthritis per se. The symptoms of Whipple's disease, including the arthritis, usually respond favorably to antibiotic therapy. Initially, procaine penicillin G, 1.2 million units, and streptomycin, 1 gm daily, are given for a period of 10 to 14 days. This is followed by tetracycline, 250 mg QID, which is continued for at least 10 to 12 months.

The arthritis of Reiter's syndrome, if mild, may respond to high doses of salicylates. In many cases, a better response of the arthritis is noted with use of the newer nonsteroidal anti-inflammatory agents. More severe cases with intractable symptoms may require consideration of therapy with corticosteroids or immunosuppressive agents.[18] Patients with Behçet's syndrome are handled in similar fashion with respect to joint manifestations. Severe cases with diffuse systemic symptoms warrant consideration of high-dose steroids or immunosuppressive agents[19] for control.

Treatment of the arthritis of hypertrophic osteoarthropathy involves non-specific anti-inflammatory agents or corticosteroids for symptomatic relief. Prolonged or complete relief depends on the ability to effectively treat and remove those factors to which the syndrome is often secondary. Therapy of musculoskeletal symptoms in scleroderma is usually a minor part of overall management. Although joint symptoms may be severe, they are more often mild and respond to the simpler anti-inflammatory agents. Various forms of therapy are effective for gastrointestinal symptoms, depending upon the area of bowel involved. Dysphagia is improved by use of bethanechol (Urecholine), 5 to 10 mg TID, chewed 30 minutes before meals. Metoclopramide, a procaine amide derivative, stimulates motility of the gastrointestinal tract including the esophagus. Its use in scleroderma esophageal disease remains investigational.[20] Antacids are helpful in relief of esophagitis. Malabsorption symptoms sometimes respond to periodic or continuous administration of tetracycline. A diet utilizing short-chain fatty acids may also provide some symptomatic relief. Bowel softeners or mild laxatives, such as dioctyl sodium sulfosuccinate (Colace) or bisacodyl (Dulcolax), relieve severe constipation.

Bowel manifestations of vasculitis reflect the basic underlying vascular pathology seen elsewhere and may respond to corticosteroid therapy. Unfortunately, steroid therapy may represent a two-edged sword, in that rapid healing may result in ischemic occlusion of mesenteric and other vessels. Nevertheless, steroid therapy is usually indicated because uncontrolled vasculitis will usually lead to even more serious pathologic manifestations. Recent studies suggest that immunosuppressive agents should be added to the therapeutic regimen in patients in whom vasculitic manifestations are severe.[21,22]

Joint symptoms related to carcinoma of the bowel are relieved to variable extent by nonspecific anti inflammatory agents. Successful removal of the neoplasm is sometimes associated with rapid and complete relief of articular symptoms. Incomplete relief or recurrence of joint symptoms suggests incomplete removal or recurrence of the tumor. Tuberculosis of the joints and bowel is managed by the usual antitubercular regimens. Multiple drug therapy using various combinations of isoniazid, ethambutol and rifampin are usually indicated. Treatment should be continued for a minimum of one year to 18 months, and in certain cases even longer, before the patient is considered permanently cured.

Amyloid disease is difficult to treat; no consistently effective specific therapy has been found. The recent suggestion that prolonged colchicine treatment may be beneficial is of interest but requires further confirmation.[23] Arthritic manifestations associated with gastrointestinal shunts are aided by various anti-inflammatory agents such as high-dose salicylates and the newer nonsteroidal anti-inflammatory agents; corticosteroid therapy is necessary in severe cases. Treatment of the blind loop with antibiotics, and sphincteroplasty to prevent reflux into the blind loop is helpful in some cases.[17] Restoration of normal bowel anatomy may be required if symptoms are severe and persistent despite more conservative measures.

CASE HISTORIES

History 11-1. Chronic Ulcerative Colitis with Arthritis

J.B., a 49-year-old white female, was first seen in January, 1974. She gave a history of having been well until approximately two years prior, when she noted onset of fever, abdominal cramps and bloody diarrhea. Gastrointestinal studies revealed changes consistent with chronic nonspecific ulcerative colitis. At that time, the patient was placed on therapy with prednisone and salicylazosulfapyridine (Azulfidine). Remission of symptoms occurred after approximately one month. All medications were discontinued several months later when the patient continued to be completely asymptomatic. She did well until September, 1973, when symptoms of colitis recurred; this was controlled with prednisone, 5 mg BID. A mild exacerbation of symptoms was noted in December, 1973. At that time the patient developed acute onset of pain and swelling in both ankles. Symptoms were worse in the morning and did not respond to aspirin, 960 mg QID, added to her usual dose of prednisone. There were no ancillary symptoms of connective tissue disease such as pleurisy, alopecia, sun sensitivity, drug allergy, Raynaud's phenomenon, dry eyes or mouth, or frequent canker sores in the mouth. On physical examination no abnormal findings were noted except for moderate swelling, increased heat and tenderness of both ankles.

Laboratory studies revealed negative serum rheumatoid factor and antinuclear antibody studies and a normal serum uric acid. Hematocrit, white blood cell count and differential were normal. Erythrocyte sedimentation rate was 29 mm/hour (Wintrobe). Roentgenograms of both ankles were normal. Studies of synovial fluid aspirated from the left ankle revealed a white cell count of 8300/mm^3 with 42% mononuclear cells. No crystals were seen. Smears and cultures for routine organisms, tuberculosis and fungi were negative. A presumptive diagnosis of arthritis related to ulcerative colitis was made. The patient responded well to local injections of steroid with lidocaine into both ankles. She was maintained in a relatively comfortable state on a program of aspirin, 960 mg QID, added to her daily dose of prednisone, 5 mg BID.

Discussion: Although a diagnosis of arthritis associated with ulcerative colitis was only presumptive in this patient with joint symptoms of recent origin, the clinical findings were consistent with the diagnosis. No evidence of articular disease of other etiology was present on clinical or laboratory study. Onset of joint symptoms at a time of exacerbation of her colitis was supportive of the diagnosis. Further observation substantiated the initial clinical impression.

History 11-2. Regional Enteritis with Arthritis

G.W., a 15-year-old white male, was in good health until age 13, at which time he developed anorexia, vomiting, weight loss and fever. Diagnostic studies were consistent with regional enteritis and the patient was begun on prednisone therapy, 15 mg daily. Six months later, he had a severe episode of gastrointestinal symptoms associated with a painless effusion of the left knee. Swelling improved following joint aspiration and injection of intra-articular steroids. Prednisone was increased to 10 mg BID for a short period of time, and reduced later to a maintenance dose of 5 mg BID. Subsequently, the patient had intermittent swelling of the left knee which was treated with periodic injections of local steroids. The patient was referred for rheumatologic evaluation when swelling of the right knee was noted. There was no history of morning stiffness, pleurisy, Raynaud's phenomenon, dysphagia, sun sensitivity, iritis, urethritis, psoriasis or other skin rash. Bowel symptoms were quiescent and other aspects of the system review were negative.

Physical examination revealed a slightly pallid, well-developed young man. Abdominal examination was within normal limits. Musculoskeletal examination revealed moderate swelling and increased warmth of the right knee and minimal swelling of the left knee. No limitation of knee motion was noted. Examination of other joints was negative.

Hematocrit was 40%, white blood cell count was 9700/mm^3 with a normal differential, erythrocyte sedimentation rate was 10 mm/hour (Wintrobe) and urinalysis was normal. Serum glutamic oxaloacetic transaminase, serologic test for syphilis, serum studies for antinuclear antibody and rheumatoid factor, and LE cell studies were normal or negative. Slight elevation of gamma globulin was seen on serum protein electrophoresis study. Analysis of synovial fluid removed from the right knee revealed a mildly inflammatory fluid that was negative on culture for routine organisms, tuberculosis and fungi. Chest roentgenogram was normal. Roentgenograms of the knees showed a small suprapatellar effusion in the right knee. Barium enema revealed a normal mucosal pattern of the colon. Small bowel roentgenograms showed narrowing and mucosal irregularities consistent with regional enteritis. The right knee was treated with an intra-articular injection of steroid and lidocaine. The patient was continued on prednisone, 10 mg daily, in addition to aspirin, 640 mg QID. A physical therapy program was instituted.

Discussion: The clinical and laboratory findings in this case are consistent with a diagnosis of arthritis related to regional enteritis. No evidence of other forms of arthritis was noted. The patient did satisfactorily on a program of rest, physical therapy, and salicylates added to his maintenance prednisone. Joint symptoms were relatively mild and not disabling.

History 11-3. Arthritis Associated with Gastrointestinal Shunt

I.H., a 46-year-old black female, was in good health until 1945 when, at age 26, she underwent uterine myomectomy, right salpingo-oophorectomy and coincidental appendectomy for treatment of chronic pelvic inflammatory disease. Six years later, she had surgical lysis of adhesions for treatment of intestinal obstruction. Panhysterectomy was performed later that same year for management of menometrorrhagia. Over the ensuing 11 years, abdominal surgery was performed on four more occasions for treatment of recurrent intestinal obstruction due to adhesions. Surgical management included lysis of adhesions, multiple small bowel resections and, in 1962, performance of a jejunocolostomy.

In 1963 the patient developed severe diarrhea, with 10 to 25 bowel movements a day. Stools were characterized as frothy and foul-smelling and were noted to float in the toilet bowl. Diagnostic studies revealed marked malabsorption with associated metabolic changes. The patient's clinical problems were later complicated by the development of hypercalcemia in 1969. Diagnostic studies suggested a diagnosis of hyperparathyroidism. Exploration of the parathyroid glands revealed a large parathyroid adenoma. Parathyroidectomy was performed.

The patient was first evaluated by the rheumatology service in February, 1972, when she was admitted to hospital with complaints of pain and swelling of the right knee and right ankle since May, 1971. Persistent swelling had been treated with intermittent injections of intra-articular steroids, aspirin, and analgesic medications. System review revealed diarrhea, with five to six stools daily. There was no history of Raynaud's phenomenon, hair loss, pleurisy, skin rash, psoriasis, dry mouth or eyes, sun sensitivity or drug allergy. On physical examination blood pressure was 150/90 mm Hg. Moderate swelling of the right knee and right ankle were noted. The patient had been on no medications other than buffered aspirin, 960 mg four times a day, and diphenoxylate hydrochloride with atropine sulfate (Lomotil) as needed for diarrhea.

Hematocrit was 37%, white blood cell count was 4200/mm^3 with a normal differential count, and erythrocyte sedimentation rate was 25 mm/hour (Wintrobe). Urinalysis, serum electrolytes, serum calcium, phosphorus and alkaline phosphatase, serum muscle enzymes and uric acid determinations were normal. Routine serologic test for syphilis was negative. Serum studies for rheumatoid factor and antinuclear antibody were negative, as were LE cell determinations. Serum protein electrophoresis was normal. Chest roentgenogram was unremarkable. Roentgenographic examination of the knees revealed bilateral calcification of menisci consistent with pseudogout. No calcifications of the ankles were noted. During hospitalization, the patient developed swelling of the right wrist. Roentgenograms of both wrists were normal; no calcium deposits were seen. Synovial fluid was aspirated from the right knee for study. The fluid was mildly inflammatory; no crystals wree observed. Histopathologic study of synovial tissue removed at closed biopsy of the right knee revealed inflammatory granulation tissue and mild infiltration of mononuclear cells. No granulomas or calcium deposits were present. A diagnosis of arthritis secondary to jejunocolostomy was made.

The patient was placed on prednisone, 2.5 mg TID, in addition to buffered aspirin, 640 mg QID. Psyllium hydrophilic mucilloid (Metamucil) 4 ml TID, and dicyclomine hydrochloride (Bentyl), 20 mg TID, were used in treatment of diarrhea. The patient was followed regularly after discharge. Joint symptoms were limited to chronic swelling of the right ankle, right knee and right wrist with periodic acute exacerbations. No evidence to suggest a different diagnosis as a cause of her symptoms was seen. Repeated studies of synovial fluid were consistently negative for the presence of crystals. Symptoms were only poorly controlled with prednisone, 2.5 mg QID, aspirin 960 to 1280 mg QID, and periodic injections of intra-articular steroids. Chlorambucil therapy, 2 mg BID, was initiated when persistent symptoms became disabling. Subsequently, the patient had fewer acute exacerbations and moderately good reduction in chronic synovial swelling. Improvement persisted and prednisone dosage was reduced to 2.5 mg BID. Chlorambucil therapy was subsequently discontinued without exacerbation of symptoms.

Discussion: This patient presented an interesting diagnostic challenge with respect to her rheumatologic symptoms. No evidence to support a diagnosis of one of the more common causes of chronic arthritis was seen. Although chondrocalcinosis (pseudogout syndrome) may cause chronic polyarthritis, absence of crystals in the synovial fluid and the absence of calcium deposits on synovial biopsy suggest that her symptoms were due to some other disorder. The association of hyperparathyroidism and chondrocalcinosis was of interest. The patient's joint findings were consistent with arthritis described in patients with jejunocolostomy and malabsorption syndrome. This clinical syndrome has been described in a number of patients in whom jejunocolostomy or jejunoileostomy was performed as a short-circuiting procedure for control of obesity.

REFERENCES

1. Wright, V and Watkinson, G.: The arthritis of ulcerative colitis. Br Med J 2: 670, 1965.
2. Palumbo, P. J. et al.: Musculoskeletal manifestations of inflammatory bowel disease. Mayo Clin Proc 48:411, 1973.
3. Soren, A.: Joint affections in regional ileitis. Arch Int Med 117:78, 1966.
4. Morris, R. I. et al.: HL-A-W27—a useful discriminator in the arthropathies of inflammatory bowel disease. N Eng J Med 290:1117, 1974.
5. Mallas, E. G. et al.: Histocompatibility antigen in inflammatory bowel disease. Gut 17:906, 1976.
6. Kelly, J. J. and Weisiger, B. B.: The arthritis of Whipple's disease. Arthritis Rheum 6:615, 1963.
7. LeVine, M. E. and Dobbins, W. O.: Joint changes in Whipple's disease. Semin Arthritis Rheum 3:79, 1973.
8. Arvastson, B., Damgaard, K. and Winblad, S.: Clinical symptoms of infections with Yersinia enterocolitica. Scand J Inf Dis 3:37, 1971.
9. Laitinen, O., Leiresalo, M. and Skylv, G.: Relation between HLA-B27 and clinical features in patients with Yersinia arthritis. Arthritis Rheum 20:1121, 1977.
10. Kahn, I. J., Jeffries, G. H. and Sleisinger, M. H.: Malabsorption in intestinal scleroderma. Correction by antibiotics. N Eng J Med 274:1339, 1966.
11. Calabro, J. J.: Cancer and arthritis. Arthritis Rheum 10:553, 1967.
12. Westermark, P. and Stenkvist, B.: A new method for the diagnosis of systemic amyloidosis. Arch Int Med 132:522, 1973.
13. Shagrin, J. W., Frame, B. and Duncan, H.: Polyarthritis in obese patients with intestinal bypass. Ann Int Med 75:377, 1971.
14. Wands, J. R. et al.: Arthritis associated with intestinal bypass procedure for morbid obesity. N Eng J Med 294:121, 1976.
15. Rose, E., Espinoza, L. R. and Osterland, C. K.: Intestinal bypass arthritis: association with circulating immune complexes. J Rheumatol 4:129, 1977.
16. Ginsberg, J. et al.: Musculoskeletal symptoms after jejunoileal shunt surgery for intractable obesity. Clinical and immunologic studies. Am J Med 67:443, 1979.
17. Stein, H. B. et al.: The intestinal bypass arthritis-dermatitis syndrome. Arthritis Rheum 24:684, 1981.
18. Farber, G. A., Forshener, J. G. and O'Quinn, S. E.: Reiter's syndrome treatment with methotrexate. JAMA 200:171, 1967.
19. Buckley, G. E. III and Gills, J. P. Jr.: Cyclophosphamide therapy of Behçet's disease. J Allerg 43:273, 1969.
20. Ramirez-Mata, M., Ibanez, G. and Alarcon-Segovia, D.: Stimulatory effect of metoclopramide on the esophagus and lower esophageal sphincter of patients with progressive systemic sclerosis. Arthritis Rheum 20:30, 1977.
21. Fauci, A. S., Doppman, J. L. and Wolff, S. M.: Cyclophosphamide-induced remission in advanced polyarteritis nodosa. Am J Med 64:890, 1978.
22. Leib, E. S., Restivo, C. and Paulus, H. E.: Immunosuppressive and corticosteroid therapy of polyarteritis nodosa. Am J Med 67:941, 1979.
23. Ravid, M., Robson, M. and Kedar (Keizman), I.: Prolonged colchicine treatment in four patients with amyloidosis. Ann Int Med 87:568, 1977.

CHAPTER 12

PULMONARY-ARTICULAR SYNDROMES

Pulmonary disease is commonly seen in association with various forms of arthritis. In some patients, the pulmonary lesions represent systemic extra-articular manifestations of the primary rheumatologic disorder. In others, the pulmonary lesions are primary and articular manifestations secondary.

DIFFERENTIAL DIAGNOSIS

Diseases to be considered:

Rheumatoid arthritis   Sarcoidosis
Systemic lupus erythematosus   Erythema nodosum
Polymyositis-dermatomyositis   Hypertrophic osteoarthropathy
Necrotizing vasculitis   Tuberculosis; fungal infection
Rheumatic fever   Lung carcinoma
Scleroderma

Pulmonary manifestations are common in association with many of the systemic connective tissue diseases. Although the lung changes in these disorders may be similar, they are frequently specific enough to be useful clues in differential diagnosis.

Lesions involving the lung and pleura are common in patients with *rheumatoid arthritis*.[1] They occur more frequently in males and sometimes precede the actual onset of arthritis. The form of involvement varies. Rheumatoid nodules, similar to those seen in subcutaneous areas of the skin, develop within the pleura or within the lung parenchyma (Fig. 12-1). They are more likely to be seen when serum rheumatoid factor is present in high titer. The nodules may persist for some time without change or they may disappear spontaneously. Other nodules slowly enlarge, with considerable progression in size. Nodules may be single or multiple; differ-

Figure 12-1. Chest roentgenogram in patient with rheumatoid arthritis. A solitary nodule (arrow) had the pathologic characteristics of a typical rheumatoid nodule when studied following thoracotomy. (Courtesy, Dr. M. Pazirandeh)

entiation of these discrete shadows from primary or metastatic carcinoma on x-ray may be impossible. Cavitation occurs but is not common. In addition to discrete nodules, rheumatoid lung disease is characterized by diffuse interstitial fibrosis. Progression is associated with dyspnea, cough, sputum and occasionally clubbing of the fingers. Early, roentgenologic examination reveals soft fluffy patches of fine reticular mottling, most prominent at the lung bases. With disease progression, the fibrosis becomes more dramatic: a honeycombing picture, with cyst formation and fibrosis characterizes the end-stage disease (Fig. 12-2). Pleural disease is also common in the form of asymptomatic pleural effusion or pleural thickening on roentgenogram.[2] The fluid is exudative with increased protein and cells. Characteristically, the glucose content of the pleural fluid is reduced[3]; this finding, however, is

Figure 12-2. Chest roentgenogram, rheumatoid arthritis. Diffuse interstitial fibrosis with honeycomb appearance. (Courtesy, Dr. M. Pazirandeh)

variable. Examination of the fluid for rheumatoid factor frequently yields positive results and helps to confirm the diagnosis. Pleural fluid complement levels may be reduced.[4] Empyema has been described; decreased resistance to infection related to corticosteroid administration may play a role in this complication.[5] Management of empyema in these patients is similar to that of patients without rheumatoid disease.

An interesting type of rheumatoid lung disease is that associated with pneumoconiosis, the so-called *Caplan's syndrome*. Pulmonary lesions result from the interplay of silicosis and rheumatoid arthritis, both of which are present in these patients. Radiologic examination of the lung reveals well-defined nodular lesions usually greater than 1 cm in diameter. Cavitation is common and nodules are usually diffuse. Characteristic fibrotic and nodular changes of pneumoconiosis appear in the background. A similar syndrome has been described for rheumatoid arthritis and lung disease associated with agents other than silica, such as asbestos and abrasives.

Pulmonary symptoms are extremely common in patients with *systemic lupus erythematosus* (SLE)[6] as a result of pleural involvement, pneumonitis or congestive heart failure. Pleuritic pain and associated pleural effusions are frequent. Basilar plate-like atelectasis is a notable finding. Pleural effusions associated with congestive heart failure may be difficult to differentiate from similar changes induced by inflammatory pleuritis. A low pleural fluid complement indicates an inflammatory origin.[4] The combination of pleural disease and plate-like atelectasis on roentgenogram is a common finding in patients with SLE. Because secondary infection is not uncommon in patients with SLE, infectious pneumonitis due to bacteria or fungi should always be considered in the differential diagnosis of pulmonary lesions.

Diffuse pulmonary fibrosis may develop in patients with *dermatomyositis* or *polymyositis* (Fig. 12-3). The symptoms may be difficult or impossible to differentiate from those seen in rheumatoid arthritis or other entities

Figure 12-3. Diffuse pulmonary fibrosis in a patient with dermatomyositis. Similar lesions are seen in rheumatoid arthritis and scleroderma. (Courtesy, Dr. M. Pazirandeh)

causing pulmonary fibrosis. Pulmonary neoplasms should be routinely excluded, because of the increased overall association of malignancy with dermatomyositis in persons over age 40.

Necrotizing vasculitis is associated with pulmonary manifestations. Roentgenologic study reveals a patchy nonspecific pneumonitis that resembles that seen in a number of diverse infectious or inflammatory pulmonary disorders. Involvement is often progressive. In some cases, new areas of the lung become involved while lesions in formerly involved areas spontaneously regress.

Pulmonary artery involvement is rare in periarteritis nodosa but is commonly seen in allergic angiitis, in which case thrombosis with infarction may develop. Wegener's granulomatosis is characterized by systemic necrotizing vasculitis, granulomatous inflammation of the upper respiratory tract, vasculitic and granulomatous disease of the lungs, and necrotizing glomerulonephritis. Pulmonary involvement is characterized by discrete nodules or diffuse widespread pneumonitis.[7] Cavitation is not uncommon. In some patients with a forme-fruste of the disease, pulmonary lesions alone may be seen for variably long periods of time.[8] Organ system involvement in Wegener's granulomatosis includes in addition necrotizing otitis media, necrotizing glomerulonephritis, mononeuritis multiplex, and polyarthralgias or polyarthritis.

Wegener's granulomatosis may be difficult to differentiate from a more recently described form of vasculitis, lymphomatoid granulomatosis, in which the inflammatory reaction is composed of lymphocytoid and plasmacytoid cells.[9] Cutaneous, pulmonary, cerebral and renal involvement are common in the latter disorder as well. Benign lymphocytic angiitis with granulomatosis, felt by some to represent a separate disease entity, likely represents an early stage of lymphomatoid granulomatosis.[10]

The syndrome of *"rheumatic fever pneumonitis"* is open to question. Patients with rheumatic fever and rheumatic heart disease frequently develop congestive heart failure; the associated pulmonary and pleural changes may simulate nonspecific inflammation or infection.

Pulmonary involvement occurs in many patients with *scleroderma*. The most common lesion is interstitial pulmonary fibrosis. This may be accompanied clinically by dyspnea on exertion, chronic cough with little or no sputum, and bouts of pleuritic chest pain. Many patients, however, are asymptomatic for prolonged periods of time. Roentgenologic evaluation reveals a reticular pattern of linear and nodular densities, usually most pronounced in the lower two-thirds of the lung fields. Honeycombing, the result of cystic lesions, is common in advanced cases and is similar to that seen in rheumatoid arthritis.

Laboratory studies reveal low pulmonary diffusion capacity and a restrictive ventilatory deficit. Bronchograms of the lungs show a characteristic bronchiectatic pattern. Electron microscopic examination of lung tissue

Figure 12-4. Clubbing of fingers in a patient with hypertrophic osteoarthropathy. (Courtesy, Dr. A. Mackenzie)

occasionally reveals a notable thickening of the basement membrane of alveolar lining cells. Alveolar or bronchiolar cell carcinoma occurs with some increased frequency in patients with scleroderma. These lesions may result from the chronic intense stimulation of bronchiolar epithelial cells that accompanies the fibrosis.

A diagnosis of *sarcoidosis* should be strongly considered when joint symptoms occur in association with pulmonary symptoms. Sarcoid arthropathy is characterized by diffuse polyarthralgia, monoarthritis or polyarthritis. Chronic joint inflammation simulates that seen in rheumatoid arthritis. Pulmonary lesions include hilar adenopathy, diffuse parenchymal nodular granulomatous lesions, restrictive lung disease with fibrosis, and secondary cor pulmonale. Increased isotope uptake on pulmonary [67]gallium scan[11] and elevated serum levels of angiotensin-converting enzyme[12,13] are helpful in diagnosis.

Erythema nodosum (see Chapter 6) is characterized by tender painful subcutaneous nodules occurring most commonly on the anterior aspects of the legs. Hilar adenopathy is common on roentgenologic examination. Cutaneous lesions are often associated with an acute or subacute polyarthritis that lasts for weeks or several months.

The syndrome of *hypertrophic osteoarthropathy* is characterized by clubbing of the fingers (Fig. 12-4) and toes, periostitis of the ends of long bones, synovial swelling of joints, and sometimes gynecomastia. Large joints, such as the wrists, knees and ankles, are involved most frequently. The syndrome may be idiopathic but frequently occurs secondary to some other disorder, such as neoplasm, subacute bacterial endocarditis, cirrhosis, and chronic diarrheal disorders. An association with bronchogenic carcinoma and pleural mesotheliomas is particularly common. Although in the past this syndrome was commonly seen secondary to pulmonary infections such as empyema, lung abscess, and bronchiectasis, this relationship is now infrequent due to the availability of more successful antibiotic therapy for the underlying infections. Rarely, osteoarthropathy may be associated with pulmonary tuberculosis or pneumoconiosis.

Chronic infectious arthritis may be associated with pulmonary infection with *tuberculosis, atypical mycobacteria, or fungal organisms*. Articular lesions are usually limited to one or a few joints.

Chronic joint findings characterized by pain, swelling, and objective evidence of synovitis may be associated with *carcinoma*. Although seen with neoplasms originating in almost any site, tumors of the lungs and the genitourinary and gastrointestinal tracts are frequent associated lesions. Joint manifestations often simulate rheumatoid arthritis, but subcutaneous nodules are not characteristically seen. Studies for serum rheumatoid factor are usually negative; when present, rheumatoid factor may diminish or disappear when the tumor is effectively removed. Positive tests for antinuclear antibodies have been described,[14] complicating disease differentiation from other connective tissue disorders. This diagnosis should always be entertained when joint disease has its onset in older persons.

Pulmonary lesions and joint symptoms may rarely be associated with other disorders, such as Reiter's syndrome, Behçet's syndrome and ulcerative colitis. These causes should be considered when the more common disorders affecting the two systems have been excluded.

DIAGNOSTIC STUDIES

Detailed history and physical examination will usually limit the diagnostic entities to be considered to a reasonable number. Routine laboratory studies should include a complete blood count, erythrocyte sedimentation rate, urinalysis, studies for rheumatoid and antinuclear factors, and serum protein electrophoresis. Serial roentgenologic examinations of the chest may prove invaluable in defining the problem at hand. Pleural fluid, when present, should be removed for analysis and studied for total and differential white cell count, protein, glucose, complement, cytology, and culture for routine organisms, tuberculosis and fungi. A low pleural fluid glucose strongly suggests a diagnosis of rheumatoid arthritis. Low pleural complement is seen in rheumatoid arthritis and systemic lupus erythematosus. Rheumatoid factor may be present in fluid from rheumatoid patients. Fluid from patients with systemic lupus erythematosus may reveal LE cells on appropriate cytologic study.

Skin tests for tuberculosis and fungi should be performed when these diseases are suspected. Fungus skin tests should be delayed, however, until sera have been drawn for complement-fixation studies. In some cases, open or closed biopsy of the lung or pleura is necessary for diagnosis.

THERAPY

Management of the arthritis associated with pulmonary disease can be divided into nonspecific symptomatic measures and specific measures directed at the basic disease process. Symptomatic measures include rest, heat and mild anti-inflammatory and analgesic agents. In patients with one of the systemic connective tissue diseases, specific measures of value can be added when the diagnosis has been confirmed (see Chapter 19). Acute sarcoid arthritis may respond to full therapeutic doses of colchicine as used in attacks of acute gout.[15] The chronic polyarthralgia or polyarthritis of sarcoid may benefit from daily use of salicylates, or other non-steroidal anti-inflammatory agents. Corticosteroid therapy may be indicated in severe cases. Antimalarial agents, such as hydroxychloroquine (Plaquenil), 200 mg BID, are helpful in selected instances. The dose can be reduced to once daily after three or four months if a response has been obtained. Baseline and periodic eye examinations for antimalarial toxicity are essential.

Oral salicylates or other non-steroidal anti-inflammatory agents benefit patients with arthritis related to erythema nodosum if symptoms are mild; severe cases require steroid therapy. Underlying causes of erythema nodosum should be removed or treated if possible. Articular symptoms of hypertrophic osteoarthropathy respond to non-steroidal anti-inflammatory agents; steroid therapy may be necessary if joint symptoms are severe. Removal of any underlying causes is usually essential for complete remission of symptoms. Tuberculous or fungal infections of the joints are treated with the same agents used in treatment of these diseases in other locations. Long-term therapy is indicated. Joint symptoms associated with carcinoma may benefit to some degree from nonspecific anti-inflammatory agents. Complete or significant remission depends on the ability to adequately treat the tumor.

Therapy of the pulmonary manifestations of these disorders varies with the diagnosis. The treatment of the pulmonary lesions of rheumatoid arthritis is often difficult. Lung manifestations may respond to antimalarial agents, gold, D-penicillamine or steroids used in management of the basic rheumatoid process. In many cases, however, lung changes persist despite improvement in joints. Pleural effusions may clear spontaneously. Persistent effusions should be aspirated in order to prevent pleural thickening and loss of lung volume. Treatment with intrapleural administration of nitrogen mustard or radioactive colloidal gold is sometimes successful. Surgical decortication may be indicated if ventilatory restriction is severe. Moderate to high doses of steroids may prevent progression of pulmonary fibrosis; this therapy should be considered in patients with deteriorating pulmonary function. The pulmonary manifestations of systemic lupus erythematosus usually respond to systemic steroid therapy; the lesions are usually short-lived and reasonably well-controlled with this agent. The progressive pulmonary fibrosis seen in dermatomyositis does not lend itself to any specific therapeutic agent. Treatment with steroids is worth a try when progressive deterioration in pulmonary function ensues.

CASE HISTORIES

History 12-1.   Rheumatoid Arthritis with Pulmonary Manifestations

I.K., a 64-year-old white male, was first seen in September, 1970, with a history of rheumatoid arthritis of ten years' duration. Physical examination revealed classic joint deformities of rheumatoid arthritis and subcutaneous rheumatoid nodules. Serum latex fixation test for rheumatoid factor was positive in a titer of 1:1280; antinuclear antibody was absent. The patient was continued on his prior therapeutic program of aspirin, 960 mg QID, hydroxychloroquine, 200 mg daily, and prednisone, 2.5 mg TID. Symptoms improved only slightly and Myochrysine therapy was substituted for hydroxychloroquine. In March, 1971, the patient complained of sticking pains in the left lower chest unassociated with cough, expectoration of sputum, or hemoptysis. Chest roentgenogram revealed a left pleural effusion and the patient was admitted for study. Repeat chest roentgenogram after aspiration of pleural fluid showed no parenchymal lung disease. Pleural fluid cell count, differential and protein studies were consistent with a mild exudate. Blood sugar and pleural fluid sugar determinations done simultaneously with the patient in a fasting state were 96 mg/100 ml and 16 mg/100 ml respectively. Serum CH^{50} complement was 90 units; pleural fluid complement was 42 units. Pleural fluid cultures for tuberculosis and fungi were negative, and cytologic examination revealed no abnormalities. Intermediate PPD, histoplasmin and coccidioidin skin tests were negative. Pulmonary consultation was requested.

Clinical findings were considered consistent with a diagnosis of rheumatoid pleural effusion and further studies such as pleural biopsy were deemed unnecessary. The patient's medical regimen was continued unchanged and he was discharged to be followed with periodic chest roentgenograms and clinical observation. Periodic followup chest roentgenograms showed no recurrence of pleural effusion nor other pulmonary abnormalities. Joint symptoms slowly improved.

Discussion: The development of pleural effusion in a patient with rheumatoid arthritis requires exclusion of other causes such as tuberculous or fungal infection or neoplasm. The presence of a reduced pleural fluid glucose, characteristically seen in rheumatoid pleural effusion, was strong evidence that the pulmonary symptoms in this patient were related to his basic rheumatologic disorder. A fall in pleural fluid complement levels has been reported in pleural effusion secondary to rheumatoid arthritis or systemic lupus erythematosus. No special management other than aspiration of the pleural fluid and maintenance of his primary treatment program for rheumatoid arthritis was necessary in this patient. Pulmonary manifestations of rheumatoid arthritis are not uncommon, particularly in patients with high serum rheumatoid factor and subcutaneous nodules, both of which were noted in this patient.

History 12-2.   Necrotizing Vasculitis with Vasculitic Pneumonitis

J.R., a 60-year old white male, was first seen in April, 1972, when he was referred to hospital for evaluation of fever and arthritis. The patient gave a history of rheumatoid arthritis of five years' duration for which he had been treated with aspirin, 960 mg QID, and prednisone, 5 mg BID. Ten days prior to admission he noted increased stiffness in his joints, high fever and shaking chills. Physical examination in hospital revealed multiple rheumatoid arthritis deformities with active synovitis. Numerous small purpuric lesions were diffusely scattered over both lower extremities. Neurologic examination showed decreased sensory response to pinprick in the distal aspects of both lower extremities. Initial diagnostic considerations included acute exacerbation of rheumatoid arthritis, pyogenic or granulomatous infection, and vasculitis.

Hematocrit was 48%, white blood cell count was 16,500/mm³ with a normal differential, and blood urea nitrogen was 27 mg/100 ml. Erythrocyte sedimentation rate was 42 mm/hour (Wintrobe). Urinalysis demonstrated trace albumin and occasional white cells, red cells and hyaline casts. Serum rheumatoid factor was positive in a titer of 1:1280. Serum study for antinuclear antibody was negative. No LE cells were seen. Creatinine clearance was 89 ml/min. Cultures of the pharynx, blood and urine were negative. Chest roentgenogram was within normal limits.

On the third day of hospitalization, the patient developed sudden onset of numbness and weakness of dorsiflexion of the right foot. Peripheral pulses were normal. Biopsy of the right gastrocnemius muscle was performed the following morning. Histopathologic examination revealed diffuse inflammatory infiltrates of lymphocytes and polymorphonuclear cells throughout all coats of numerous small and medium-sized arteries. Fibrinoid necrosis of some vessel walls was evident. Prednisone was increased to 15 mg QID with excellent response of clinical symptoms over a period of 48 hours. Intermittent high fever receded and the patient had notable improvement in muscle aching. The right foot-drop improved over a period of several weeks, during which good position was maintained with physical therapy exercises and a foot-drop splint. The patient was discharged on prednisone, 15 mg BID, one month after admission. Isoniazid, 300 mg daily and pyridoxine, 50 mg daily, were added while awaiting culture results. Symptoms of vasculitis and rheumatoid arthritis were in good control.

The patient was readmitted to hospital ten days after discharge for evaluation of acute right sided chest pain and fever. He gave no history of cough, dyspnea or hemoptysis. His therapeutic program had not been altered. Physical examination revealed dry rales at the right lung base. Chest roentgenogram showed patchy infiltrates in the right first and second interspace. Chest films taken at intervals of one to two days revealed enlargement and consolidation of the right lung lesions; infiltrates were seen in the left lower lobe as well. Pertinent laboratory studies revealed negative blood cultures, normal throat culture, and absence of acid-fast and fungus organisms on examination of sputum smears. Serum cold agglutination study was positive in a titer of 1:128. Pulmonary consultation was requested.

Differential diagnosis lay chiefly between rapidly progressive necrotizing vasculitis of the lungs versus pneumonia due to a pyogenic organism. Pulmonary mycosis, tuberculosis, atypical pneumonia or Pneumocystis carinii infection seemed less likely causes of the pulmonary findings. Repeat sputum culture showed small numbers of gram-positive diplococci. Intravenous oxacillin and gentamicin were added to his therapeutic program. Despite several days of high dose antibiotic therapy, the lung lesions progressed rapidly. Prednisone was increased to 20 mg QID, and tetracycline, 2 g daily, was added. The patient had an excellent response to this program over 48 hours. Antibiotic therapy was discontinued after several days, and prednisone therapy alone was maintained. Progressive clinical improvement was associated with clearing of pulmonary infiltrates on roentgenogram. The patient was discharged on a program of gradually decreasing doses of prednisone. He did well over a prolonged period of observation, but required a maintenance dose of prednisone, 5 mg BID, to control vasculitis symptoms.

Discussion: This patient with biopsy evidence of necrotizing vasculitis developed a severe progressive pneumonitis. Numerous diagnostic possibilities had to be considered and excluded. The clinical course and response to steroid therapy were consistent with pulmonary lesions due to necrotizing vasculitis.

History 12-3. Hypertrophic Osteoarthropathy

J.H., a 56-year-old white male, was first seen for evaluation in December, 1972. He had been in good health until two months prior when he developed pain and swelling of both knees and wrists. Swelling and disability were relieved only slightly by aspirin, 640 mg QID. The patient had no other complaints except for a seven-pound weight loss over the preceding two months. System review was completely negative and past medical history was noncontributory. On physical examination both knees and wrists were tender, warm and swollen. In addition, moderate clubbing of the fingers and toes was present.

Hematocrit was 35%, white blood cell count was 7200/mm³ with a normal differential, urinalysis was normal, and erythrocyte sedimentation rate was 38 mm/hour (Wintrobe). Serum rheumatoid factor and antinuclear antibody tests were negative. Chest roentgenogram revealed a mass lesion in the right middle lobe. Tuberculin and fungus skin tests were negative. Cytologic examination of induced sputum samples was normal. Roentgenograms of the wrists and knees revealed periosteal new bone formation at the distal aspects of the radial and femoral bones. A clinical diagnosis of bronchogenic carcinoma with pulmonary hypertrophic osteoarthropathy was made.

Exploratory thoracotomy was performed. Pathologic studies revealed bronchogenic carcinoma and a right pneumonectomy was performed. The patient had mild remission of musculoskeletal symptoms postoperatively. Residual joint symptoms were controlled with aspirin, 640 mg QID, and indomethacin, 25 mg TID. The patient returned to his referring physician for followup.

Discussion: This patient appeared with arthritis consistent with that seen in many of the connective tissue diseases. The presence of clubbing suggested a clinical diagnosis of hypertrophic osteoarthropathy. Roentgenographic studies of involved joints revealed abnormalities characteristic of this syndrome. Variable degrees of symptomatic remissions may be seen following tumor resection.

REFERENCES

1. Walker, W. C. and Wright, V.: Pulmonary lesions and rheumatoid arthritis. Medicine 47:501, 1968.
2. Lillington, G. A., Carr, D. T. and Mayne, J. G.: Rheumatoid pleurisy with effusion. Arch Int Med 128:764, 1971.
3. Carr, D. T. and Mayne, J. G.: Pleurisy with effusion in rheumatoid arthritis, with reference to the low concentration of glucose in pleural fluid. Am Rev Resp Dis 85:345, 1962.
4. Hunder, G. G., McDuffie, F. C. and Hepper, N. G. G.: Pleural fluid complement in systemic lupus erythematosus and rheumatoid arthritis. Ann Int Med 76:357, 1972.
5. Jones, F. L. and Blodgett, R. C.: Empyema in rheumatoid pleuropulmonary disease. Ann Int Med 74:665, 1971.
6. Eisenberg, H. et al.: Diffuse interstitial lung disease in systemic lupus erythematosus. Ann Int Med 79:37, 1973.
7. Israel, H. L. and Patchefsky, A. S.: Wegener's granulomatosis of lungs: diagnosis and treatment. Ann Int Med 74:881, 1971.

8. Carrington, C. B. and Liebow, A. A.: Limited forms of angiitis and granulomatosis of Wegener's type. Am J Med 41:497, 1966.
9. Liebow, A. A., Carrington, C. R. B. and Friedman, P. J.: Lymphomatoid granulomatosis. Human Pathol 3:457, 1972.
10. Israel, H. L., Patchefsky, A. S. and Saladana, M. J.: Wegener's granulomatosis, lymphomatoid granulomatosis, and benign lymphocytic angiitis and granulomatosis of the lung. Recognition and treatment. Ann Int Med 87:691, 1977.
11. Siemsen, J. K., Grebe, S. F. and Waxman, A. D.: The use of gallium[67] in pulmonary disorders. Sem Nucl Med 8:235, 1978.
12. Lieberman, J. et al.: Serum angiotensin-converting enzyme for diagnosis and therapeutic evaluation of sarcoidosis. Amer Rev Resp Dis 120:329, 1979.
13. DeRemee, R. A. and Rohrbach, M. S.: Serum angiotensin-converting enzyme activity in evaluating the clinical course of sarcoidosis. Ann Int Med 92:361, 1980.
14. Husian, M. N., Neff, J., Derby, E. et al.: Antinuclear antibodies: clinical significance of titers and fluorescence patterns. Amer J Clin Pathol 61:59, 1974.
15. Kaplan, H.: Further experience with colchicine in the treatment of sarcoid arthritis. N Eng J Med 268:761, 1963.

CHAPTER 13

VASCULAR ABNORMALITIES AND CONNECTIVE TISSUE DISEASE

Vascular symptoms may be the initial complaint in patients with systemic connective tissue disease. In some patients, the vascular manifestations precede articular symptoms by several or many years. In others, the vascular changes occur concomitant with or subsequent to articular symptoms. An awareness of the important inter-relationship of vascular changes and connective tissue disease is helpful in diagnosis.

RAYNAUD'S PHENOMENON AND RAYNAUD'S DISEASE

Clinical Features

Although several vascular diseases are associated with systemic connective tissue disorders, the most common abnormality is *Raynaud's phenomenon*.[1,2] This entity is characterized by color changes in the skin that occur either spontaneously or in response to certain precipitating factors such as cold. Color changes occur most frequently in the hands, but the toes, nose, and ears may sometimes be involved. In the typical sequence, the skin first becomes white because of arteriolar spasm and subsequent diminished blood supply. Cyanosis follows, caused by stagnation of blood in capillaries and venules. As warming and reactive vasodilation ensue, the skin becomes red. Thus, the classic color sequence is white to blue to red. In many patients, this sequence is not present, and various combinations of color change are seen. Tingling and paresthesia are common accompanying symptoms and may occur in the absence of definitive color changes. Severe recurrent Raynaud's phenomenon may produce chronic vasomotor instability with a persistent blue mottling of the skin on which the typical color changes are intermittently superimposed. Although the exact cause of Raynaud's phenomenon is still unknown, an abnormal local increase in the viscosity of blood in response to a fall in temperature has

Figure 13-1. Cyanosis and trophic ulceration of the fingertip in a patient with long-standing Raynaud's disease. (Courtesy, Dr. A. Mackenzie)

been described.[3] Among the connective tissue diseases, Raynaud's phenomenon occurs most frequently in patients with systemic lupus erythematosus and scleroderma. Rheumatoid arthritis, dermatomyositis, and necrotizing vasculitis are less common causes.

Raynaud's phenomenon should be differentiated from *Raynaud's disease*. The latter is an idiopathic primary disorder with color changes identical to those seen in patients with Raynaud's phenomenon; however, evidence of an underlying disorder is persistently absent. Over a period of time, vascular insufficiency may produce trophic changes such as ulceration of the fingertips (Fig. 13-1). A diagnosis of Raynaud's disease should be made with caution when symptoms are recent in onset, because secondary Raynaud's phenomenon may be present for long periods of time prior to the appearance of other symptoms of connective tissue disease. The presence of Raynaud's changes for over two years in the absence of any underlying disorder supports a diagnosis of idiopathic Raynaud's disease. Unfortunately, some patients manifest Raynaud's changes for years before connective tissue disease becomes apparent. Constant reappraisal of the significance of the patient's vascular symptoms is usually indicated.

As previously noted (see Chapter 10), widefield capillary microscopy of cutaneous vessels may be of diagnostic help in the diagnosis of scleroderma and related disorders such as mixed connective tissue disease and dermatomyositis.[4-6] Characteristic changes seen in patients with scleroderma include large dilated capillary loops near the edge of nail-folds, with adjacent dropout of capillary loops leading to avascular changes. Similar abnormalities are seen at times in patients with Raynaud's phenomenon and no obvious connective tissue disease. Such patients appear to be at higher risk for development of connective tissue disease in the future than are patients with Raynaud's symptoms whose vascular patterns are normal.

Differential Diagnosis

Besides occurring in association with connective tissue diseases, Raynaud's phenomenon may occur secondary to other disorders. The following are non-connective tissue diseases that must be considered as possible underlying disorders in the differential diagnosis of Raynaud's phenomenon.

Patients with *disorders of the cervical spine, such as cervical disk herniation or thoracic outlet compression syndromes,* may develop Raynaud's phenomenon secondary to vascular instability induced in the involved extremity. *Carpal tunnel compression* may produce similar vascular abnormalities.

Patients may develop Raynaud's phenomenon as a result of *chronic trauma,* as occurs in pneumatic hammer workers or in industrial occupations that require repetitive pounding motions of the hands. Raynaud's phenomenon is associated with diseases of large vessels, such as *atherosclerosis obliterans* and *Buerger's disease (thromboangiitis obliterans).* Peripheral pulses are usually diminished.

Raynaud's phenomenon is seen in patients with various *hematologic disorders* such as polycythemia vera. Patients with multiple myeloma, hypergammaglobulinemia of Waldenström, lymphoma, chronic leukemia or idiopathic cryoglobulinemia may have Raynaud's phenomenon. The vascular changes may result from the presence of blood cryoglobulins, cryofibrinogens or cold agglutinins or from hyperviscosity changes.

Intoxication with heavy metals, such as arsenic, or poisoning with ergot derivatives may produce Raynaud's phenomenon. Induction of Raynaud's phenomenon in patients receiving β-adrenergic blockers such as propranolol has been described.[7] A careful history and studies for suspected toxic agents are essential in diagnosis.

Laboratory Diagnosis

A full laboratory evaluation should include a complete blood count, erythrocyte sedimentation rate, serologic test for syphilis (for false-positive serology), serum studies for rheumatoid and antinuclear factors, serum cold agglutinins and cryoglobulins, plasma cryofibrinogen, and serum protein electrophoresis. Chest roentgenograms may demonstrate an associated underlying disorder. Cervical spine roentgenograms including PA, lateral and oblique views are helpful in excluding etiologic factors emanating from this area. Barium swallow often demonstrates abnormal function in patients with scleroderma. This finding is not diagnostic, however, because similar dysfunction may be noted in patients with idiopathic Raynaud's disease. Other laboratory studies, such as serum immunoelectrophoresis, serum complement, blood lipids and sugar, are indicated when suggested by clinical findings. Special diagnostic procedures such as bone marrow aspiration, muscle or lymph node biopsy, and arteriography may be required.

Management

Raynaud's disease and Raynaud's phenomenon often respond to various symptomatic measures. Patients should be cautioned to avoid exposure to cold. Light cotton gloves are useful for this purpose and should be worn during routine household activities. Warm outer clothing should be utilized as well, because symptoms result from cold exposure to the body in general. Patients with severe symptoms may benefit from a move to a warm climate. Various vasodilator agents are valuable in the nonspecific symptomatic approach to therapy. Phenoxybenzamine hydrochloride (Dibenzyline), an adrenergic blocking agent, may be tried in an initial dose of 10 mg twice daily. The dose is slowly increased to 10 mg four times a day, if tolerated and required. The patient should be cautioned regarding sudden postural changes because orthostatic hypotension is a bothersome side reaction. Reserpine may have a salutary effect in a dose of 0.25 to 0.5 mg daily by mouth. Intra-arterial administration of reserpine has been utilized,[8,9] but its efficacy is uncertain.[10] Since hemodynamic effects of intra-arterial reserpine are short-lived, its usefulness appears limited to treatment of severe acute ischemic attacks associated with skin ulcerations.[2] This drug should generally be avoided in patients with a history of depression; other agents may be effective alternatives. In particular, methyldopa, 250 mg three or four times daily, or guanethidine, 10 to 40 mg daily, are worthy of trial. Nitroglycerine ointment, 2%, is helpful in some patients. The ointment is spread on the hands in a dose beginning with one to two inches of the agent. (This dose can be measured with the applicator provided with the preparation.) It is used three or four times daily in gradually increasing amounts. The patient should be cautioned about nitroglycerine-induced headaches, which may occur early in use; headaches usually disappear as the drug is continued.

Other drugs and therapeutic modalities have been recently recommended for trial. Prazosin HCl in gradually increasing doses is salutary in some patients.[11] Stanozolol, an anabolic steroid, has similarly met with some success.[12] Toxic side reactions include masculinizing effects and hepatic abnormalities; these can be lessened by using the agent on an intermittent basis. Calcium-channel blocking agents such as nifedipine represent a new concept in the therapeutic approach to this disorder.[13] Relief of vasospasm was found excellent in both short and long-term studies. Further evaluation of these agents is indicated with the likelihood they will prove useful in Raynaud's management. Improvement in severity and frequency of Raynaud's phenomenon and associated ulcerations has also been described in some patients with plasmapheresis.[14] In some patients biofeedback may be useful as an adjunctive or primary therapeutic modality.

Sympathectomy should be considered in patients with severe disease who do not respond to a conservative medical regimen. This procedure is usually more effective in patients with Raynaud's disease than in those with Raynaud's phenomenon, in whom an underlying disorder is present. Prior improvement with stellate ganglion block should be demonstrated before sympathectomy is considered.

Specific therapy directed to the associated disorder often has a beneficial effect on the vascular symptoms of patients with Raynaud's phenomenon. Corticosteroids are particularly effective in patients with associated connective tissue disease; their use should be reserved, however, for severe cases not controlled by more conservative measures. Management of Raynaud's phenomenon secondary to non-connective tissue diseases should be directed to the underlying medical problem in addition to symptomatic measures.

OTHER SMALL VESSEL DISEASE

Other vascular abnormalities may be associated with connective tissue disease. *Livedo reticularis* is characterized by a peculiar mottled appearance of the skin (Fig. 13-2). The condition is usually benign and produces few or no symptoms. *Acrocyanosis* is manifested as a persistently cool extremity with bluish discoloration. Mild ulceration is a complicating finding in severe disease. *Erythermalgia* is an interesting and distressing disorder characterized by red, hot extremities that are extremely painful. The condition may be idiopathic or secondary in etiology. Symptoms are often relieved by elevating the extremities or by immersing them in cold water. Aspirin is frequently beneficial.

Figure 13-2. Livedo reticularis. Note mottled appearance of skin. (Courtesy, Dr. B. Michel)

THROMBOPHLEBITIS

Thrombophlebitis occurs more frequently in patients with connective tissue diseases, particularly in systemic lupus erythematosus. Sometimes phlebitis is the initial manifestation of the underlying disease. Both superficial and deep phlebitis occur and attacks may be isolated single occurrences or recurrent. Thrombophlebitis occurs more frequently with long-term corticosteroid therapy, possibly related to changes in mechanisms of coagulation. Patients with Behçet's syndrome not infrequently have recurrent thrombophlebitis as a major manifestation of their disorder. In addition to commonly involved areas, renal vein and inferior vena caval thrombosis have been described. Management of the thrombophlebitis associated with connective tissue disease is similar to that for idiopathic thrombophlebitis and includes rest, heat and the use of anticoagulants. Unfortunately, both the acute attack and prevention of recurrences may be more recalcitrant to therapy than phlebitis related to other causes. Vena caval ligation or insertion of a vena caval umbrella may be indicated in recurrent cases associated with pulmonary emboli not controlled by long-term anticoagulant therapy. Control of the underlying disorder may be beneficial but is not always effective. The use of anticoagulant therapy in patients with connective tissue disease is complicated by the frequent associated use of anti-inflammatory agents that augment the anticoagulant effect or predispose to gastrointestinal bleeding.

SYSTEMIC VASCULITIS

Patients with systemic connective tissue disease may have ischemic changes due to vasculitis of small or large vessels.[15,16] Such lesions are characteristic of periarteritis nodosa and the various forms of allergic angiitis. Similar lesions may be a complication in patients with systemic lupus erythematosus and rheumatoid arthritis, with or without a history of steroid therapy. Symptoms and signs are variable and depend on the size and location of the involved vessel. Involvement of large vessels of the extremities results in severe rest pain and claudication and a cool, cyanotic skin. Small vessel involvement produces focal areas of skin infarction with lesions strikingly similar in appearance to those seen in subacute bacterial endocarditis. Splinter hemorrhages beneath the nails and paronychial infarctions are common (Fig. 10-10). Involvement of vasa nervosum may result in ischemic neuropathy. Mononeuritis multiplex is particularly characteristic. In this syndrome, scattered large nerves such as the peroneal, radial and median nerves are involved. Onset of symptoms is often sudden with the patient complaining of foot-drop (Fig. 13-3) or wrist-drop.

Steroid therapy is presently the most effective agent available for management. Dosage required to control the inflammatory changes is often large; doses of prednisone as high as 80 to 120 mg per day in divided

Figure 13-3. Right foot-drop due to necrotizing vasculitis with ischemic neuropathy. Purpuric lesions of the skin are readily apparent.

doses are not unusual. Immunosuppressive therapy has been recommended for management of severely involved patients.[17,18] Some patients with vasculitis associated with systemic lupus erythematosus or rheumatoid arthritis benefit from the use of antimalarial drugs in addition to steroids. Hydroxychloroquine (Plaquenil) is given in a dose of 200 mg BID for three or four months, following which a daily maintenance dose of 200 mg daily is instituted. Appropriate periodic eye examinations should be carried out to avoid ophthalmic side reactions. D-penicillamine has been described as useful in the treatment of vasculitis associated with rheumatoid arthritis.[19,20]

The clinical features of necrotizing vasculitis may be simulated by patients with atrial myxoma or idiopathic retroperitoneal fibrosis. Atrial myxoma is associated with both cardiac and extracardiac manifestations.[21-24] Cardiac findings may simulate ischemic or valvular heart disease. Murmurs are frequently noted but may be intermittent depending on variations in tumor position and size. Congestive heart failure, myocarditis, and pericarditis are seen. Syncopal episodes occur as the tumor blocks blood flow to the periphery. A second set of clinical manifestations is the result of embolic phenomena, related to the friable nature of the tumor. Recurrent tumor embolization leads to intermittent pain in the extremities, Raynaud's phenomenon and cerebrovascular accidents. Systemic manifestations are common and likely to be confused with connective tissue diseases such as necrotizing vasculitis or systemic lupus erythematosus. Fever, myalgias, arthralgias, anemia, elevated erythrocyte sedimentation rate, and hypergammaglobulinemia are common. Aneurysm formation is frequent, particularly in the cerebral circulation, and may simulate aneurysms seen with necrotizing vasculitis. Tumor emboli may induce vasculitic change, possibly related to an antigenic stimulus initiated and perpetuated by tumor tissue.[21,24]

The diagnosis should be suspected in patients with atypical features of necrotizing vasculitis or other systemic connective tissue disease. The disease may present an especially difficult diagnostic challenge when cardiac manifestations are minimal or absent. Echocardiography represents a noninvasive diagnostic modality which has largely replaced cardiac catheterization and angiography in tumor demonstration.

Idiopathic retroperitoneal fibrosis is a rare disorder which is more commonly recognized as a cause of obstructive uropathy.[25,26] Less well known is its association with various connective tissue diseases and auto-immune disorders. Pathologic evidence of necrotizing vasculitis may be present. Protean clinical manifestations include fever, arthralgias, myalgias, weight loss, anemia, elevated erythrocyte sedimentation rate, Raynaud's phenomenon, and pericarditis. Diagnosis is based on an awareness of this entity as a diagnostic possibility. Intravenous pyelography, abdominal sonograms and computed tomography provide confirmation of the diagnosis.

Thrombotic Thrombocytopenic Purpura

This syndrome is characterized by thrombocytopenia, microangiopathic hemolytic anemia, fluctuating neurologic abnormalities, renal disease, and fever. Hemorrhagic complications and diverse central nervous system manifestations are predominant findings. Studies of the peripheral blood reveal changes consistent with microangiopathic anemia with burr cells and helmet-shaped red cell fragments. Diffuse intravascular coagulation may be a secondary complication of this disorder. Although joint symptoms are not a characteristic component of this syndrome, the multisystem presentation not infrequently leads to confusion with other connective tissue diseases. The prognosis in patients with this disorder has improved considerably with use of various agents which appear to be effective in many patients. Therapy includes use of corticosteroids, anti-platelet aggregation drugs such as dipyridamole and aspirin, exchange transfusions with whole blood, plasmapheresis, and splenectomy when indicated.

TEMPORAL ARTERITIS (CRANIAL ARTERITIS, GIANT CELL ARTERITIS)

Temporal arteritis is characterized by granulomatous inflammation of vessels associated with systemic constitutional symptoms and ischemic vascular changes.[27] The disease occurs most frequently in persons over 50 years of age. Although temporal arteries are involved most frequently, the process may affect other large arteries, such as the carotid, subclavian, femoral, coronary, renal and mesenteric vessels. Onset of symptoms may be acute or insidious. Throbbing headaches are associated with tenderness and swelling of the temporal arteries. The vessels are nodular to palpation (Fig. 13-4) and the overlying skin is erythematous. Pulsations may dis-

Figure 13-4. Temporal (cranial) arteritis. Note thickened enlarged vessels bilaterally, best seen over the lateral aspects of the forehead. (Courtesy, Dr. A. Mackenzie)

appear as the disease progresses. Malaise, anorexia, fever and weight loss are frequent findings. Symptoms of polymyalgia rheumatica (see Chapter 9) occur in a high percentage of patients. Muscle pain involving the shoulders, hips and trunk may be severe. Limitation of function is due to pain rather than weakness. Ischemic changes may lead to claudication in the jaws and extremities. Involvement of vessels to the eye results in symptoms of transient diplopia or loss of vision, which may be irreversible.

Laboratory findings reveal mild anemia and leukocytosis. The erythrocyte sedimentation rate is characteristically elevated, often exceeding 80 to 100 mm/hour. Nonspecific changes in plasma proteins are often present with an increase in alpha-2 globulins and plasma fibrinogen; circulating immune complexes have been described.[28] Mildly abnormal liver function studies have been noted in up to one-third of patients.[29] Protein and liver function abnormalities are of value in supporting a diagnosis in patients with normal or only slightly elevated erythrocyte sedimentation rates. Temporal artery biopsy is the most important diagnostic procedure. Pathologic findings include intimal proliferation with narrowing of the lumen. Thrombosis is often present and the internal elastic lamina is disrupted. Inflammatory infiltrates with lymphocytes and foreign-body giant cells are seen (Fig. 13-5). When feasible, temporal artery biopsy should be performed on the nondominant side in order to avoid interference with this vessel which might be useful for a vascular shunt procedure in the treatment of

Figure 13-5. Cross section of temporal artery from patient with temporal (cranial) arteritis. Intimal proliferation is associated with inflammatory infiltrates of lymphocytes and foreign-body giant cells in the vessel wall. (Hematoxylin, and eosin) (Courtesy, Dr. A. Mackenzie)

arteriosclerotic cerebrovascular disease in later years. Temporal arteriography performed prior to biopsy may provide diagnostic information and help in selecting the optimal site for biopsy.[30] A positive study reveals stenotic and dilated segments of the vessel. Although useful in selected instances, technical difficulties and false-positive and false-negative results significantly limit its diagnostic value.[31]

Although temporal arteritis is a self-limited disease, early diagnosis is important because the risk of blindness is significant. Steroid treatment is effective in preventing blindness and in suppressing local and systemic symptoms (see Chapter 19).

TAKAYASU'S DISEASE (AORTIC ARCH ARTERITIS, PULSELESS DISEASE)

This syndrome is characterized by vasculitis of large elastic arteries. In contrast to temporal arteritis, it is primarily a disease of young females. Pulses are absent in the neck, head and upper extremities. Blood pressure in the arms is usually unobtainable. Claudication of the upper extremities is common. Many patients have systemic symptoms such as malaise, fever, anorexia and weight loss. In some patients these systemic manifestations antedate objective changes in the pulses (prepulseless phase). Ischemic manifestations elsewhere lead to cerebrovascular insufficiency, jaw claudication, angina, and myocardial infarction.

Laboratory studies reveal an elevated erythrocyte sedimentation rate during acute phases of the disease. Mild anemia and leukocytosis are common. Angiograms show irregular segmental stenosis localized to large arteries near their origin. Echocardiography, which may demonstrate aortic luminal changes, represents an attractive non-invasive diagnostic procedure for study of patients with this disease.[32] Corticosteroid therapy is frequently beneficial. Surgery to correct chronic vascular occlusion may be indicated.

KAWASAKI DISEASE (MUCOCUTANEOUS LYMPH NODE SYNDROME, INFANTILE POLYARTERITIS)

This entity, first described in 1974, is characterized by fever, conjunctivitis, fissuring of the lips, reddening of the oropharyngeal mucosa and strawberry tongue, reddening of the palms and soles, edema of the hands and feet with desquamation of skin of the finger tips, a polymorphous rash primarily on the trunk, and acute swelling of cervical lymph nodes.[33] Although described most commonly in children, it has also been reported in adults.[34] In addition to the major characteristics described above, patients may have myopericarditis, aseptic meningitis, diarrhea, arthralgias, or arthritis. Laboratory studies are characterized by a marked leukocytosis. Tests for serum antinuclear antibody and rheumatoid factor are negative. Serum IgE levels may be elevated. Clinical findings are strikingly similar to those seen in patients with toxic shock syndrome and a possible relationship may exist between the two entities.

Although most patients recover completely after a period of weeks to months, sudden death due to coronary arteritis with aneurysms and thrombotic occlusion is a dreaded complication of the disorder.[35] Aspirin appears to be the therapy of choice at present, for its general anti-inflammatory and antipyretic effect, as well as for a suggestive benefit in the prevention of coronary vasculitis due possibly to its anti-platelet aggregation effect. Corticosteroid therapy has not been uniformly helpful and, in one study, appeared to have an adverse effect.[35]

CASE HISTORIES

History 13-1.   Idiopathic Raynaud's Disease

R.S., a 50-year-old white female, was first seen for rheumatologic evaluation in December, 1970. She gave a history of color changes in the hands beginning approximately 15 years prior. Fingers of both hands became white or blue with mild exposure to cold temperatures. Erythema of the fingers developed with rewarming. Color changes were associated with some itching and paresthesia of involved areas. She gave no history of joint symptoms nor any history of frostbite or injury to the hands. There were no ancillary symptoms of hair loss, pleurisy, skin rash, drug allergy, sun sensitivity, dry mouth or dry eyes, alopecia or dysphagia. The patient had been in otherwise generally good health and no chronic intake of medications was noted. On physical examination, blood pressure was 110/70 mm Hg. The skin of the hands and feet was cold and had a mottled red appearance. Exposure of the hands to cold running water induced pallor. No thickening of the skin of the hands or feet was seen. Peripheral pulses and joints were normal. Cervical spine motions were full and nonpainful. Thoracic outlet maneuvers were negative.

Urinalysis, hematocrit, white blood cell count and differential, erythrocyte sedimentation rate and serologic test for syphilis were normal or negative. Serum protein electrophoresis was normal, as were serum protein-bound iodine, calcium and phosphorus studies. Serum uric acid was 4.6 mg/100 ml and serum studies for rheumatoid factor, antinuclear antibody, cryoglobulins and cold agglutinins were negative. No cryofibrinogens were seen. Roentgenograms of the chest and hands were unremarkable. A diagnosis of idiopathic Raynaud's disease was made on the basis of the long history of color changes in the absence of any secondary disorder. The patient was placed on therapy with reserpine, 0.5 mg daily at night, with moderately good relief of symptoms. In addition, she was instructed to keep her hands and body warm. The patient has shown no subsequent evidence of underlying systemic disease on repeated clinical and laboratory study.

Discussion: This patient demonstrated characteristic color changes of Raynaud's disease. Repeated clinical examination and laboratory studies failed to reveal the presence of any systemic disorder. Prolonged observation is often required before a diagnosis of idiopathic Raynaud's disease can be made with assurance, because Raynaud's phenomenon may precede other clinical manifestations of associated diseases by months or years. Prognosis in this patient was good and she could be reassured regarding the relatively benign nature of her disorder.

History 13-2.   Raynaud's Phenomenon Secondary to Systemic Lupus Erythematosus

F.R., a 68-year-old white female, was seen in consultation in January, 1974. The patient was in good health until four weeks previously, when she noted sudden discoloration of the fingertips with associated numbness of the hands. Discoloration was characterized by a persistent cyanosis at the distal aspects of the second and third fingers of the right hand and the second finger of the left hand. Symptoms were aggravated by exposure to cold, at which time the involved digits would become white. There were no other notable symptoms and the patient considered herself in good health otherwise. The patient was taking no medications. System review revealed no evidence of arthritis, myalgia, pleurisy, sun sensitivity, hair loss, dryness of the eyes or mouth, drug allergy or skin rash. Past medical history was noncontributory.

Hematocrit was 36%, white blood cell count was 3600/mm³ with a normal differential, and urinalysis was normal. Routine serologic test for syphilis was weakly positive; FTA-Abs study was negative. Serum rheumatoid factor study was negative, but serum antinuclear antibody was present in a titer of 1:1000. LE cell determinations were consistently positive. Prothrombin time was normal but partial thromboplastin time was prolonged. Reticulocyte count was 1.1% and Coombs test was negative. Creatinine clearance was 83 ml/min. Total serum hemolytic complement was 60% of normal. A diagnosis of systemic lupus erythematosus was made. The patient was placed on prednisone, 10 mg BID, with moderately good relief of vascular symptoms.

Discussion: Raynaud's phenomenon was the initial clinical manifestation of systemic lupus erythematosus in this patient. Multiple laboratory abnormalities related to systemic lupus erythematosus were present. Subsequent studies revealed the presence of circulating anticoagulant as an explanation for her prolonged partial thromboplastin time. Vascular symptoms are a frequent manifestation of systemic lupus erythematosus, as this case well illustrates.

History 13-3.   Raynaud's Phenomenon Secondary to Scleroderma

M.R., a 47-year-old white female, was first seen in consultation in January, 1972. She was in good health until March, 1969, at which time she noted color changes in both hands on exposure to cold. Pallor and whitening of the hands was followed by blue discoloration. Color changes involved several fingers of each hand and were associated with numbness and tingling. The patient did not seek medical help for this complaint until approximately six months later when she noted progressive tightening of the skin of her hands and forearms with limitation in finger range-of-motion. The skin of the hands had become darker and she noted a grating sensation when she flexed her right middle finger. System review was negative for symptoms of dysphagia, hair loss, sun sensitivity, drug allergy, pleurisy or dryness of the mouth or eyes.

Physical examination revealed blood pressure 130/80 mm Hg. The skin over both hands and forearms was erythematous and blanched slightly on pressure. Moderate thickening of the skin of the hands and forearms, and resorption of the tips of several fingers were noted. Telangiectases were absent.

Hematocrit was 39%, the white blood cell count was 6300/mm^3 with a normal differential, the erythrocyte sedimentation rate was 12 mm/hour (Wintrobe) and urinalysis was normal. Serum rheumatoid factor test was negative. Serum antinuclear antibody titer was positive 1:20. Roentgenograms of the chest showed interstitial fibrosis at the bases of both lungs. Pulmonary function studies were normal. Barium swallow and roentgenograms of the upper gastrointestinal tract were unremarkable. Roentgenograms of the hands revealed resorption of several ungual tufts. Electrocardiogram was normal. Histopathologic study of skin obtained by punch biopsy from the dorsal aspect of the left distal forearm revealed thinning of the epidermis, loss of rete pegs and atrophy of dorsal appendages. A diagnosis of scleroderma was made on the basis of the clinical and pathologic findings.

The patient was placed on reserpine, 0.5 mg daily, for treatment of her Raynaud's phenomenon. In addition, she was advised to avoid cold exposure, to use gloves and to dress warmly. Improvement in the Raynaud's phenomenon was noted over a period of several weeks. She was also placed on potassium para-aminobenzoate (Potaba) in progressively increasing doses to 12 g daily. Therapy was associated with softening of involved areas of skin over a period of six months. The dose of potassium para-aminobenzoate was slowly reduced and discontinued over the subsequent two years. No change in the pulmonary interstitial fibrosis was noted. The patient was maintained on no specific therapy except for reserpine, which she used during the winter to control the Raynaud's symptoms. There was no clinical or laboratory evidence of further progression of her disease.

Discussion: Raynaud's phenomenon was the initial clinical manifestation of scleroderma in this patient. Underlying associated disease states must always be excluded when patients appear initially with Raynaud's phenomenon. Clinical and laboratory evidence of the primary disorder is often absent for a long period of time.

REFERENCES

1. DeTakats, G. and Fowler, E. F.: Raynaud's phenomenon. JAMA 179:108, 1962.
2. Blunt, R. J. and Porter, J. M.: Raynaud syndrome. Semin Arth Rheum 10:282, 1981.
3. Goyle, K. B. and Dormandy, J. A.: Abnormal blood viscosity in Raynaud's phenomenon. Lancet, June 19, 1976, p. 1317.
4. Maricq, H. R. and LeRoy, E. C.: Patterns of finger capillary abnormalities in

connective tissue disease by "wide-field" microscopy. Arthritis Rheum 16:619, 1973.

5. Maricq, H. R., Spencer-Greene, G. and LeRoy, E. C.: Skin capillary abnormalities as indicators of organ involvement in scleroderma (systemic sclerosis), Raynaud's syndrome, and dermatomyositis. Am J Med 61:862, 1976.

6. Maricq, H. R. et al.: Diagnostic potential of in vivo capillary microscopy in scleroderma and related disorders. Arthritis Rheum 23:183, 1980.

7. Marshall, A. J., Roberts, C. J. C. and Barritt, D. W.: Raynaud's phenomenon as a side effect of beta blockers in hypertension. Br J Med 2:1498, 1976.

8. McFayden, I. S., Housley, E. and MacPherson, A. I. S.: Intra-arterial reserpine administration in Raynaud syndrome. Arch Int Med 132:526, 1973.

9. Paolino, J. et al.: Arteriographic evaluation of intra-arterial reserpine in Raynaud's phenomenon. Arthritis Rheum 15:448, 1972.

10. Siegel, R. C. and Fries, J. F.: Double-blind cross-over study of intra-arterial reserpine and saline in scleroderma. Arthritis Rheum 15:454, 1972.

11. Waldo, R.: Prazocin relieves Raynaud's vasospasm. JAMA 241:1037, 1979.

12. Jarrett, P. E. M., Moreland, M. and Browse, N. Z.: Treatment of Raynaud's phenomenon by fibrinolytic enhancement. Br Med J 2:523, 1978.

13. Kahan, A. et al.: Nifedipine and Raynaud's phenomenon. Ann Int Med 94:546, 1981.

14. O'Reilly, M. J. G. et al.: Controlled trial of plasma exchange in treatment of Raynaud's syndrome. Br Med J 1:113, 1974.

15. DePalma, R. G., Moskowitz, R. W. and Holden, W. D.: Peripheral ischemia and collagen disease. Arch Surg 105:313, 1972.

16. Bywaters, E. G. L. and Scott, J. T.: The natural history of vascular lesions in rheumatoid arthritis. J Chron Dis 16:905, 1963.

17. Leib, E. S., Restivo, C. and Paulus, H. E.: Immunosuppressive and corticosteroid therapy of polyarteritis nodosa. Am J Med 67:941, 1979.

18. Fauci, A. S., Doppman, J. L. and Wolff, S. M.: Cyclophosphamide-induced remission in advanced polyarteritis nodosa. Am J Med 64:890, 1978.

19. Jaffe, I. A.: Rheumatoid arthritis with penicillamine. Ann Int Med 61:556, 1964.

20. Jaffe, I. A.: The treatment of rheumatoid arthritis and necrotizing vasculitis with penicillamine. Arthritis Rheum 13:436, 1970.

21. Huston, K., Combs, J., Lie, J. and Giuliani, E.: Left atrial myxoma simulating peripheral vasculitis. Mayo Clinic Proc 53:752, 1978.

22. Bulkley, B. H. and Hutchins, G. M.: Atrial myxomas: a fifty year review. Am Heart J 97:639, 1979.

23. Sutton, M. G. S. et al.: Atrial myxomas. A review of clinical experience in 40 patients. Mayo Clinic Proc 55:371, 1980.

24. Byrd, W. E., Matthews, O. P. and Hunt, R. E.: Left atrial myxoma presenting as a systemic vasculitis. Arthritis Rheum 23:240, 1980.

25. Jones, E. A. and Alexander, M. K.: Idiopathic retroperitoneal fibrosis associated with an arteritis. Ann Rheum Dis 25:356, 1966.

26. Zabetakis, P., Novich, R., Matarese, R. et al.: Idiopathic retroperitoneal fibrosis: a systemic connective tissue disease. J Urol 122:100, 1979.

27. Healey, L. A., Parker, F. and Wilske, K. R.: Polymyalgia rheumatica and giant cell arteritis. Arthritis Rheum 14:138, 1971.

28. Papaioannou, C. C. et al.: Circulating immune complexes in giant cell arteritis and polymyalgia rheumatica. Arthritis Rheum 23:1021, 1980.

29. Hunder, G. G. et al.: Daily and alternate-day corticosteroid regimens in treatment of giant cell arteritis: comparison in a prospective study. Ann Int Med 82:613, 1975.

30. Gillianders, L. A., Strachan, R. W. and Blair, D. W.: Temporal arteriography: a new technique for the investigation of giant cell arteritis and polymyalgia rheumatica. Ann Rheum Dis 28:267, 1969.

31. Sewell, J. R. et al.: Combined temporal arteriography and selective biopsy in suspected giant cell arteritis. Ann Rheum Dis 39:124, 1980.

32. Tanaka, H. et al.: Echocardiographic findings in patients with aortitis syndrome. Angiology 30:620, 1979.

33. Kawasaki, T. et al.: A new infantile acute febrile mucocutaneous lymph node syndrome (MLNS) prevailing in Japan. Pediatrics 54:271, 1974.
34. Milgrom, H. et al.: Kawasaki's disease in the healthy young adults. Ann Int Med 92:467, 1980.
35. Kato, H., Koike, S. and Yokoyama, T.: Kawasaki's disease: effect of treatment on coronary artery involvement. Pediatrics 63:175, 1979.

CHAPTER 14

EYE DISEASE AND ARTHRITIS

Ocular abnormalities are common to many of the rheumatic disorders. In some patients, such as those with ankylosing spondylitis, juvenile rheumatoid arthritis, or Reiter's syndrome, eye manifestations may precede musculoskeletal symptoms by periods of months to years. In other disorders, such as adult rheumatoid arthritis, the occurrence of eye disease tends to parallel the underlying disease process, and is seen more often in patients with severe disease of prolonged duration. In some musculoskeletal diseases, such as Sjögren's syndrome and Behçet's syndrome, ocular manifestations are prominent and classic components of the basic disease process. To complicate differential diagnosis, ocular abnormalities in patients with connective tissue disease may be related to therapeutic agents used in management.

Knowledge of eye manifestations of connective tissue disease is important in differential diagnosis. In addition, since such involvement may represent a significant threat to the patient's vision, early detection and treatment is vital to prevention or reversal of visual loss.

The following states in which eye disease may be associated with connective tissue disorders will be discussed:

> Adult rheumatoid arthritis
> Juvenile rheumatoid arthritis
> Sjögren's syndrome
> Seronegative spondarthropathy (ankylosing spondylitis, Reiter's syndrome, enteropathic arthropathy)
> Systemic lupus erythematosus
> Vasculitis
> Relapsing polychondritis, Behçet's syndrome
> Sarcoidosis
> Drug-related abnormalities

ADULT RHEUMATOID ARTHRITIS

Scleritis and episcleritis, important ocular manifestations of patients with rheumatoid arthritis, are generally seen in patients with more severe disease of prolonged duration.[1] Histopathologic findings are similar to rheumatoid nodules seen elsewhere on the body and reveal varying degrees of fibrinoid necrosis, epithelioid cells with palisading, and inflammation. Episcleritis, the milder of these entities, is characterized by congestion of episcleral vessels and infiltration of episcleral tissues by inflammatory cells (Fig. 14-1). Slightly elevated, painful, tender nodular lesions are noted. In most patients, episcleritis is a self-limited disorder but resolution may be hastened by treatment with topical corticosteroids.

Necrotizing and nodular forms of scleritis are associated with redness and severe ocular pain. Although the lesions may be self-limiting, loss of vision may occur especially when the process is complicated by uveitis, keratitis, or cataract formation. Scleromalacia perforans, a form of necrotizing scleritis, is characterized by minimal to absent inflammatory symptoms (Fig. 14-2). The dark uveal tract may be readily seen through the thin sclera; uveal prolapse may occur with minimal trauma to the globe. Although uveitis may occur secondary to scleritis, *anterior uveitis alone is seen no more frequently in rheumatoid arthritis patients than in the general population.*

Keratitis or sclerokeratitis involving the limbus or the cornea are further eye complications seen in patients with rheumatoid arthritis. Corneal ulcers

Figure 14-1.   Episcleritis. Increased vascularity and congestion are seen involving the superficial layers at the nasal portion of the eye (courtesy, The Arthritis Foundation).

Figure 14-2. Scleromalacia perforans. Scleral thinning and conjunctival injection are seen. The dark uveal tissue is readily visible through the thinned sclera (courtesy, The Arthritis Foundation).

seen as a manifestation of this process may be particularly threatening because of the risk of perforation.

Keratoconjunctivitis sicca (dry eye, sicca syndrome) is commonly seen in patients with rheumatoid arthritis, and is a classic component of the triad of dry eyes, dry mouth, and connective tissue disease characteristic of Sjögren's syndrome. A detailed discussion of eye problems associated with sicca syndrome is provided later in this chapter.

Management. As noted, episcleritis is usually self-limited and no specific therapy may be required. Not infrequently, however, topical steroids are of value in symptomatic relief and earlier resolution of symptoms. Scleritis is frequently difficult to control. Topical therapy with corticosteroids is safe and may be of benefit. Subconjunctival corticosteroid injection, on the other hand, is contraindicated in the presence of scleritis; steroid-induced atrophy may add significantly to the risk of scleral perforation. Systemic therapy including nonsteroidal anti-inflammatory agents, or prednisone may be indicated. Immunosuppressive drugs have been utilized with some apparent success in particularly intractable cases. Scleral grafting may be required to bridge defects. Keratitic ulcers may require lamellar grafting in efforts to improve vision and avoid perforation. In most patients with these disorders, ophthalmologic consultation should be sought for diagnosis and guidance in management.

JUVENILE RHEUMATOID ARTHRITIS

Uveitis, band keratopathy, and secondary cataract formation represent the classic triad of eye abnormalities seen in patients with juvenile rheumatoid arthritis.[2] In contrast to patients with adult form rheumatoid arthritis, the incidence of primary anterior uveitis is increased in patients with juvenile forms of the disease. The iritis is subacute or chronic, and frequently bilateral and recurrent. Secondary complications include synechiae (adhesions between the iris, cornea, and lens) and secondary glaucoma. Interestingly, uveitis is seen most commonly in patients with oligo- or pauci-articular forms of the disease, and there is a strong correlation with a positive serum antinuclear factor.[3] In most children eye symptoms tend to be silent or minimal; few patients complain of pain, photophobia, or decreased visual acuity. Accordingly it is extremely important that children with juvenile rheumatoid arthritis be examined on a regular basis for silent uveitis. In patients with pauci-articular disease, examination at a minimum of six-month intervals is recommended. In patients who have a history of uveitis, more frequent repeat examinations at three month intervals should be carried out.

Figure 14-3.   Band keratopathy. A white band-like opacity is readily seen across the interpalpebral fissure as a result of calcium deposition beneath the corneal epithelium (courtesy, the Arthritis Foundation).

As previously noted, additional eye complications seen in patients with juvenile rheumatoid arthritis are band keratopathy and secondary cataract formation. In band keratopathy calcium deposited beneath the corneal epithelium appears as a band-like opacity located in horizontal fashion across the interpalpebral fissure (Fig. 14-3). Slit lamp exam is required to detect the early lesion; eventually, however, the opacity becomes visible to the naked eye. Cataract formation is seen in over 20% of patients as a further complication of chronic uveitis.[2]

Management. Uveitis is treated with topical corticosteroids and mydriatic/cycloplegics. Systemic corticosteroids are at times indicated although glaucoma and cataract formation may be enhanced. Immunosuppressive therapy for intractable disease is under study. Band keratopathy may respond to applications of topically applied sodium versenate solution as a chelating agent. Unfortunately, despite therapy, uveitis, cataract formation, and glaucoma may lead to eventual loss of vision.

SJÖGREN'S SYNDROME

Sjögren's syndrome is characterized by keratoconjunctivitis sicca, dry mouth (xerostomia), and an associated connective tissue disease (see Chapter 7). Commonly noted eye symptoms include burning, photophobia and a foreign body sensation. Tears tend to be more mucoid and often contain epithelial debris. Filamentary keratitis and corneal surface pitting are common; corneal ulceration may progress to perforation. Irregular staining of the cornea and conjunctiva is noted when Rose Bengal solution is introduced into the eye. Dryness of the eyes can be confirmed by use of the Schirmer test which demonstrates decreased tear formation and wetting of filter paper introduced into the lower eyelid (Fig. 7-2). Wetting less than 5 mm over a period of five minutes is considered definitely abnormal.

Management. Patients with mild sicca syndrome benefit from use of artificial tears used as frequently as necessary during the day. Mucolytic agents such as acetylcysteine are helpful in decreasing tear viscosity. Occlusion of the lacrimal punctae is helpful in tear conservation. A soft contact lens helps to maintain eye moisture, but secondary infection is a hazard. Tarsorrhaphy for lid closure may be necessary in severe cases. A conjunctival flap may be necessary to preserve the surface and prevent further ulceration.

SERONEGATIVE SPONDARTHROPATHIES

Acute anterior uveitis is seen with increased frequency in patients with seronegative spondarthropathies such as ankylosing spondylitis, Reiter's syndrome, and arthritis associated with inflammatory bowel disease. Not infrequently, iritis precedes musculoskeletal manifestations by many months or years. Eye involvement is associated with ocular pain, redness, and photophobia. Secondary complications include anterior and posterior synechiae, glaucoma, and cataracts. Uveitis usually responds to treatment with topical steroids, cycloplegics, and mydriatics. Systemic and/or subconjunctival corticosteroids are at times indicated for severe iritis. Relapses are unfortunately common.

SYSTEMIC LUPUS ERYTHEMATOSUS

Retinal lesions, including cotton-wool exudates, hemorrhages, and edema, are the most common eye manifestations of systemic lupus erythematosus.[4] The cotton-wool exudates are similar to those seen in retinopathies observed with other disorders such as hypertension and diabetes mellitus. Pathologic study of the lesions reveals thickening of nerve fiber layers in aggregates known as cytoid bodies. They appear due to focal ischemia and represent microinfarcts of the retina. Hemorrhages are frequently noted independent of hypertension. Retinal disease frequently parallels systemic disease activity.

VASCULITIS

Polyarteritis nodosa is associated with a number of external and internal eye manifestations. Subconjunctival hemorrhage and sclerokeratitis have been observed. Uveitis is uncommon.

Ischemic optic neuritis is a dreaded complication of cranial (temporal) arteritis (see Chapter 13). Sudden loss of vision occurs when branches of the ophthalmic artery which supply the optic nerve are affected. Central retinal artery occlusion occurs but is much less frequent. Transient episodes of partial or total visual loss (amaurosis fugax) may occur episodically prior to more sustained visual loss. Ocular complications can usually be prevented by early and adequate treatment with high dose systemic corticosteroids (see Chapter 19). Aggressive treatment of the underlying disorder is indicated since ocular damage, once it occurs, is rarely reversible.

Wegener's granulomatosis is associated with proptosis and lid edema.[5] Other ocular manifestations include scleritis, episcleritis, vasculitis of vessels to the retina or optic nerve, and keratitis. Treatment with corticosteroids and immunosuppressive drugs is recommended (see Chapter 19).

RELAPSING POLYCHONDRITIS; BEHÇET'S SYNDROME

Ocular involvement is seen in over half the cases of patients with relapsing polychondritis, a disorder characterized by inflammation and destruction of cartilage (see Chapter 8). Most common complications include conjunctivitis, episcleritis, and iritis.

The classic manifestations of Behçet's syndrome are recurrent oral and genital aphthous ulcers, and uveitis. Anterior and posterior uveal involvement is seen. Eye symptoms frequently occur independent of other systemic manifestations of this disorder, and not infrequently may be the presenting finding. Local treatment of the uveitis is effective in mild cases. More severe disease requires consideration of systemic therapy including corticosteroids and immunosuppressive agents.

SARCOIDOSIS

Granulomatous uveitis is the most common eye complication seen in patients with sarcoid. The anterior uveal tract is most often involved, although inflammation of the posterior uveal tract (the choroid) may be seen. Synechial adhesions and cataract formation complicate the inflammatory process. Optic neuritis and retinal perivasculitis are further manifestations of the disease. Involvement of the lacrimal glands may lead to clinical changes of keratoconjunctivitis similar to those seen in Sjögren's syndrome.

DRUG-RELATED ABNORMALITIES

Therapeutic agents used in treatment of connective tissue diseases may cause iatrogenic ocular complications. Ocular toxicity has been described in association with several of the nonsteroidal anti-inflammatory agents, notably indomethacin[6-8] and ibuprofen.[9-11] Findings reported with indomethacin include decreased vision, corneal deposits, constricted visual fields, night-blindness, pigmentary changes of the fundus, and abnormal electrodiagnostic tests. Despite these reports, significant eye toxicity has not proved to be a clinical problem with use of this agent over many years. Nevertheless it would be prudent to discontinue its use and request eye examination in patients complaining of unexplained ocular symptoms during its administration. Toxic amblyopia has been described in patients receiving ibuprofen; its etiology is uncertain.[9] Transient scotomata and enlargement of the blind spot appear reversible when the drug is stopped. Although amblyopia has not been seen in later studies on larger series of patients,[10,11] the drug should be discontinued in any patient noting unusual eye symptomatology. Systemic corticosteroid therapy may lead to premature cataract formation, seen most characteristically in the posterior subcapsular region of the lens.[12,13] This complication appears dose related and occurs more frequently in patients receiving 10 mg of prednisone or more daily for a prolonged period of time. Cataract regression is unlikely even after cessation of corticosteroid therapy; cataract extraction is indicated if vision is significantly impaired.

Corticosteroids may induce glaucoma, more likely to occur with topical use as opposed to systemic administration. This complication in response to steroids appears to be inherited as an autosomal recessive trait.

Systemic administration of gold-containing agents may be associated with corneal deposition of gold (chrysiasis). Conjunctivitis, keratitis, and corneal ulcers have been infrequently described.

Significant eye toxicity may be seen with prolonged use of antimalarial drugs such as chloroquine or hydroxychloroquine. Pigment epithelium and inner retinal layers are involved. The patient may complain of night blindness and various degrees of loss of visual acuity. Constriction of visual fields to a red target is observed early; visual loss at time of such finding appears to be reversible.[14] In contrast, visual field loss to a white target is a late sign and visual loss usually irreversible. Abnormal responses to testing with Ishihara color plates is a helpful study to screen patients for antimalarial eye toxicity. Pigmentary mottling in the area of the macula is seen late in the course of toxicity; a bull's eye lesion is characteristic. Early toxic macular changes may be difficult to differentiate from senile macular degeneration. As noted in Chapter 19, retinal toxicity to antimalarial agents appears dose-related. Cautious use of this agent and periodic eye examinations are essential if this damaging complication is to be avoided.

Corneal deposits which probably represent intracellular deposition of antimalarial drug are commonly seen early in the course of therapy. These deposits disappear within weeks or months after therapy is discontinued and do not result in permanent damage to the eye.

REFERENCES

1. McGavin, D. D. et al.: Episcleritis and scleritis. A study of their clinical manifestations and association with rheumatoid arthritis. Br J Ophthal 60:192, 1976.
2. Chylak, L. T., Jr. et al.: Ocular manifestations of juvenile rheumatoid arthritis. Am J Ophthal 79:1026, 1975.
3. Schaller, J. G. et al.: The association of antinuclear antibodies with the chronic iridocylitis of juvenile rheumatoid arthritis (Still's disease). Arthritis Rheum 20:224, 1977.
4. Gold, D. H., Morris, D. A. and Henkind, P.: Ocular findings in systemic lupus erythematosus. Br J Ophthal 56:800, 1972.
5. Haynes, B. F. et al.: The ocular manifestations of Wegener's granulomatosis. Fifteen years (sic) experience and review of the literature. Am J Med 63:131, 1977.
6. Burns, C. A.: Ocular effects of indomethacin. Slit lamp and electroretinographic (ERG) study. (In: Abstracts of papers presented at the Sectional Meetings of the Association for Research in Ophthalmology; Mid-Western Section, 1-2 April 1966, Chicago, Illinois.) Invest Ophthal 5:325, 1966.
7. Burns, C. A.: Indomethacin, reduced retinal sensitivity, and corneal deposits. Am J Ophthal 66:825, 1968.
8. Henkes, H. E., Lith, G. H. van, and Canta, L. R.: Indomethacin retinopathy. Am J Ophthal 73:846, 1972.
9. Collum, L. M. and Bowan, D. I.: Ocular side effects of Ibuprofen. Br J Ophthal 55:472, 1971.
10. Melluish, J. W. et al.: Ibuprofen and visual function. Arch Ophthal 93:781, 1975.
11. Williamson, J. and Sturrock, R. D.: An ophthalmic study of ibuprofen in rheumatoid conditions. Current Med Res and Opinion 4:128, 1976.

12. Black, R. L. et al.: Posterior subcapsular cataracts induced by corticosteroids in patients with rheumatoid arthritis. JAMA 174:166, 1960.
13. Crews, S. J.: Posterior subcapsular lens opacities in patients on long-term corticosteroid therapy. Br Med J 1(5346):1644, 1963.
14. Young, P. et al.: The apparent elimination of chloroquine retinopathy. Arthritis Rheum 15:464, 1972.

CHAPTER 15

LOCALIZED MUSCULOSKELETAL SYNDROMES

Localized musculoskeletal symptoms may be a manifestation of relatively circumscribed disorders or systemic disease. Accurate delineation of the problem is required for most effective therapy. When due to benign disease, the patient's anxiety regarding the presence of a more generalized disorder can be appropriately allayed. In other cases, the symptoms serve as a clue to the diagnosis of a more serious illness.

BURSITIS

Bursae are closed sacs lined with synovial-like cells. Interposed between bony prominences and tendons or muscles, they facilitate motion. Numerous bursae are present throughout the body and may be the site of localized inflammation, frequently associated with amorphous deposits of calcium. Among the bursae most commonly affected are the subdeltoid and subacromial bursae at the shoulder, the olecranon bursa at the elbow, the greater trochanteric bursa at the lateral aspect of the hip and the anserine bursa at the medial aspect of the upper tibia. Other bursae frequently involved are those related to the Achilles tendon, the ischial tuberosity, the first metatarsophalangeal joint and the prepatellar area.

Patients with shoulder bursitis usually give a history of acute pain and limitation of motion. The shoulder is tender to palpation; pain with passive motion may be excruciating. Although roentgenographic study often reveals evidence of calcification (Fig. 15-1), such deposits are frequently absent. Many cases of shoulder bursitis are associated with a concomitant inflammation of the tendon of the supraspinatus muscle. Bursitis of the shoulder may represent a secondary reaction to tendinitis, when tendinous deposits of calcium rupture into underlying bursae. Symptoms specifically related to shoulder bursitis must be differentiated from inflammation of shoulder area tendons and from tears of the musculotendinous rotator cuff (see following).

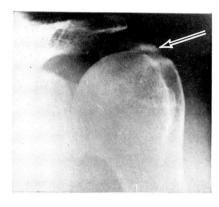

Figure 15-1. Roentgenogram of the shoulder from a patient with recurrent attacks of acute bursitis shows a large calcific deposit (arrow). (Courtesy, Dr. V. Goldberg)

Olecranon bursitis produces swelling, pain, heat and redness at the posterior aspect of the elbow. Although most frequently a manifestation of chronic nonspecific trauma, it is also seen in association with connective tissue diseases or gout. Septic bursitis must always be excluded. Olecranon bursal effusions have also been described in uremic patients secondary to trauma and to uremic toxins as a component of uremic polyserositis.[1] Further, in patients on hemodialysis, increased pressure within bursal vessels as a result of arteriovenous anastomosis, and anticoagulant effects of heparin predispose to hemorrhagic effusions. Patients with greater trochanteric bursitis complain of pain and tenderness at the lateral aspect of the hip; pain is exaggerated by weight-bearing. Hip motion is usually normal, which helps to differentiate this entity from intrinsic disorders of the hip joint. Ischial bursitis involves the bursa between the gluteus maximus muscle and ischial tuberosity. Patients with inflammation of the anserine bursa have pain at the medial aspect of the knee, with localized tenderness readily demonstrable at the upper end of the medial tibial plateau. Prepatellar bursitis causes pain and swelling at the anterior aspect of the knee. Chronic trauma associated with occupations that require frequent kneeling is an important etiologic factor in many cases. Achilles bursitis involves the bursa at the lower end of the attachment of the Achilles tendon to the os calcis. Nonspecific cases are often caused by excessively tight shoes. In other cases, symptoms are related to systemic connective tissue diseases such as rheumatoid arthritis and ankylosing spondylitis. Painful bursitis may be seen overlying the first metatarsophalangeal joint at its medial aspect; tight shoes or hallux valgus are often predisposing factors.

Treatment of bursitis varies with the location of the disorder. Mild cases of shoulder bursitis may be managed with heat and mild anti-inflammatory agents such as aspirin or indomethacin. Local injections of various corticosteroid preparations with 1% lidocaine (see Chapter 21) are extremely efficacious and usually provide rapid relief. Septic infection must always be excluded prior to the use of such corticosteroid agents. Physical therapy should be vigorously instituted when diminished pain allows increased joint use. Exercises of several types are utilized: pendulum exercises, for which the patient leans forward and gently rotates the arm in a circle, are helpful. Range of motion may be further aided by stringing a rope over a door or a shower bar; the patient grasps the ends of the rope and uses the good extremity to assist range of motion of the involved extremity. Another valuable exercise involves grasping the hands together behind the neck and forcefully moving the elbows and shoulders posteriorly. Full doses of aspirin, or other non-steroidal anti-inflammatory agents, often aid patients who do not respond to local steroid therapy. Severe cases with large calcium deposits evident on roentgenogram may be aided by "needling" the deposit with an 18-gauge needle under local anesthesia. Lidocaine or saline is used to lavage the involved area, followed by injection of steroid with lidocaine. Some patients who do not respond to conservative measures benefit from a short course of roentgen therapy to the involved area. An exposure dose of 150 rads (ortho voltage) is given every other day for three doses. Large calcific deposits may be recalcitrant to all the foregoing measures and require surgical excision. Fortunately, the need for surgery is not frequent.

Mild cases of bursitis in other areas similarly respond to heat and mild anti-inflammatory agents. Response to local injections of steroid with lidocaine is usually excellent. Non-steroidal anti-inflammatory agents, as described for shoulder bursitis, are often an effective therapeutic alternative. Recurrent bursitis may require excision of the bursa for permanent relief.

TENDINITIS AND TENOSYNOVITIS (TENOVAGINITIS)

Inflammation with resultant pain and tenderness commonly involves tendons (tendinitis) or tendon sheaths (tenosynovitis, tenovaginitis) in the area of the shoulder, elbow, hands and heel. Supraspinatus tendinitis probably results from an abnormal response of the tendon to chronic trauma. Fibrillary changes of degeneration are seen histologically, and secondary calcification is common. Symptoms, differential diagnosis, and management are similar to those described for shoulder bursitis.

Tenosynovitis at the long head of the biceps muscle as the tendon passes through the bicipital groove of the humeral head is common. Pain and tenderness are severe at the anterior aspect of the shoulder. Maximal pain may be reproduced by forced supination of the hand with the elbow in 45° flexion, because the biceps muscle is the primary supinator of the hand in this position. Shoulder motion is often limited. Roentgenographic studies are usually normal. Symptoms respond to local injections of steroid with lidocaine or to non-steroidal anti-inflammatory agents. Surgical excision of the tendon sheath may be indicated if symptoms are chronic.

The common term for inflammation near tendon origins at the elbow (epicondylitis) is tennis elbow. However, symptoms may be idiopathic in origin or related to chronic trauma induced by other activities or occupations that produce stress at the elbow. Strain and tear result from overuse of forearm muscles and attachments. Symptoms occur at either the lateral or medial epicondyle. The extensor muscles to the hand originate at the lateral epicondyle and this area is involved more frequently. Symptoms at the medial epicondyle are caused by involvement of flexor muscle tendons. Roentgenograms may reveal small calcific deposits in symptomatic areas. Management depends on the severity of the symptoms. Mild cases respond to heat, aspirin and the avoidance of activities that cause stress to the involved tendons. Other cases require local injections of steroid with lidocaine into the tender areas of the epicondyle. Injections should generally not be repeated more than every three to six months to avoid chronic damage and atrophy of tissue. Some patients benefit from splinting, which puts the elbow at rest. Other therapeutic approaches include periodic courses of non-steroidal anti-inflammatory agents or roentgen therapy. Recalcitrant cases may require surgery such as fasciotomy.

Tennis elbow symptoms resulting from epicondylitis must be differentiated from other disorders which cause similar symptoms. Tendinitis which involves the distal insertion of the biceps muscle may limit full elbow extension and produce pain throughout the anterior elbow region. Radial nerve entrapment (radial tunnel syndrome) as the nerve courses around the posterior aspect of the humerus produces symptoms of pain and tenderness at the lateral aspect of the elbow.[2]

Tenosynovitis of the abductor pollicis longus and extensor pollicis brevis tendons at the wrist is common (DeQuervain's tenosynovitis). In most patients this disorder is primary and related to chronic nonspecific trauma. However, it may be associated with systemic connective tissue disease. The patient complains of pain with use of the thumb or wrist. Physical examination reveals severe tenderness and occasionally signs of inflammation over the tendon. Tenderness is usually maximal in the "snuff-box" area between the tendons of the abductor pollicis longus and extensor pollicis brevis muscles. Maximal pain is induced by forced ulnar deviation after the thumb has been placed in the palm of the hand and grasped by the fingers (Finkelstein's sign) (Fig. 15-2). Treatment with local injection of steroid and lidocaine usually results in satisfying relief. Activities that might have precipitated the tenosynovitis should be avoided. Chronic low-grade symptoms may require splinting for various periods of time.

Tendinitis or tenosynovitis of the hands occurs as a primary disorder resulting from chronic nonspecific trauma or from inflammatory changes produced by the connective tissue diseases, particularly rheumatoid arthritis. Flexor tendons are affected most often. Involvement of the thumbs (snapping thumbs) is common. Examination reveals tenderness and a sensation of crepitus as the tendon moves. Swelling, which is often present, may be

Figure 15-2. Finkelstein's sign. Acute pain and tenderness were localized to the "snuff-box" area when forced ulnar deviation was performed. Symptoms of tenosynovitis were relieved by local injection of steroid and lidocaine.

diffuse or localized in the form of a nodule. Locking, in which the patient is able to flex the involved finger but unable to bring it back to its original position, occurs with chronic lesions. This symptom has given rise to the term "trigger finger." Locking results when the flexor muscles pull the tendon through the tendon sheath and the extensor muscles are unable to return the tendons to their original position. Patients often localize the locking to the finger area, but close observation usually reveals that the trouble site is at the distal palmar crease where the palmar fascia is tight and the tendon most subject to impingement.

Locking may occur if inflammation or fibrosis of the sheath causes stricture. In patients with rheumatoid arthritis, locking is related to diffuse rheumatoid inflammation of the sheath, of the tendon or both. In addition, rheumatoid patients may have locking when rheumatoid nodule formation on the sheath or tendon restricts tendon motion.

Most patients with tenosynovitis in the hand respond to local injections of steroid with lidocaine into the involved tendon sheath. Stressful activities should be avoided. In patients with chronic tenosynovitis, surgical release of the tendon sheath and removal of any nodules is indicated.

Inflammation of the Achilles tendon is common. Pathologic changes may result from chronic nonspecific trauma, such as that induced by tight shoes, or may be associated with various connective tissue diseases, especially rheumatoid arthritis, ankylosing spondylitis and Reiter's syndrome. Pain, especially with walking, and localized tenderness are present. Treatment includes removal of local traumatic factors, rest and anti-inflammatory agents. Use of a heel lift lessens muscle pull stresses on the inflamed tendon. Plaster immobilization for a period of weeks may be required if symptoms are persistent. Local injections of steroid with lidocaine directly into the tendon or tendon sheath are to be *avoided* since they predispose to tendon rupture. Injections made into a paratendinous location followed by relative immobilization and avoidance of stressful activity for several days to a week may be cautiously considered in exceptional instances.

ROTATOR CUFF TEAR OF THE SHOULDER

Tears of the musculotendinous rotator cuff of the shoulder most frequently involve the supraspinatus tendon. Partial rupture is more common than complete rupture. A history of injury is usually present; the patient may feel an actual snap, followed by pain and limitation of motion. Tenderness is noted over the greater tuberosity. Symptoms and physical findings may be difficult to differentiate from those of bursitis and tendinitis. Frequently the patient cannot initiate abduction. The tear may be demonstrated by contrast arthrography (Fig. 15-3). Complete rupture requires surgical management. Partial tears usually respond to conservative measures including heat, analgesics, and mild anti-inflammatory agents. A short course of non-steroidal anti-inflammatory therapy is frequently effective. Local steroid therapy is beneficial in selected cases. Physical therapy exercises should be instituted early to maintain range of motion.

ADHESIVE CAPSULITIS OF THE SHOULDER (FROZEN SHOULDER)

Adhesive capsulitis may follow as a sequela of bursitis, tendinitis, or rotator cuff tear when therapy of the acute process has been inadequate or ineffective. Limitation of motion and occasionally pain are severe. An increased frequency of HLA-B27 histocompatibility antigen has been noted.[3] Therapy with analgesic and anti-inflammatory agents is less effective at this stage of shoulder disease. Intensive physical therapy to promote increased range of motion is usually rewarding, although improvement may be slow.

Figure 15-3. Contrast arthrogram of right shoulder in a patient with a rotator cuff tear reveals diffuse spread of dye beyond the normal confines of the shoulder.

Surgical manipulation to release adhesions may be necessary in unresponsive cases.

MULTIPLE CALCIFIC PERIARTHRITIS

Acute episodes of tendinitis or bursitis are frequently associated with deposition of calcium apatite. In most patients, the lesions are localized to one or two joints such as the shoulders or epicondyles of the elbows. Some patients, however, demonstrate multiple areas of calcification of tendons, ligaments or bursae associated with recurrent attacks of acute periarthritis.[4,5] Clinical symptoms resemble acute attacks of gout or pseudogout. Structures in the areas of the shoulders, elbows and hips are commonly involved, but other areas such as the wrists and hands may be affected.

Pain and evidence of inflammation are most notable over the area of calcific deposit. Roentgenograms show mottled calcification in soft tissues at the site of the acute attacks. Aspiration of the affected area reveals a chalky, milky material. On study by phase microscopy, numerous round, globular bodies that have a shiny coin-like appearance are seen. Weakly birefringent particles may be present. Interestingly, the acute attack may be followed by disintegration and gradual disappearance of the calcium deposit.

Whether tendon degeneration precedes calcium deposition is uncertain. It has been suggested that deposition of calcium in these patients may be a primary event related to some systemic disorder. No abnormality in mineral or hormonal metabolism has yet been demonstrated. Treatment is symptomatic. Rapid improvement frequently follows oral administration of non-steroidal anti-inflammatory agents, or administration of corticosteroids orally or by direct local injection. Colchicine administered orally or by intravenous route is efficacious for acute attacks. Splinting of involved areas helps to relieve pain.

A condition somewhat similar to the foregoing has been described in association with periarticular and para-articular deposition of calcium apatite in patients undergoing periodic hemodialysis for chronic renal failure.[6] Colchicine appears to be effective in managing acute attacks. Treatment with aluminum hydroxide gel to reduce serum phosphorus levels is associated with clinical and roentgenologic improvement. Prophylactic use of this agent in patients undergoing periodic hemodialysis is effective in preventing the syndrome.

SHOULDER-HAND SYNDROME (CAUSALGIA, REFLEX DYSTROPHY, SUDECK'S ATROPHY)

This interesting and often distressing syndrome is characterized by pain, swelling and limitation of the hand, wrist and shoulder. Symptoms may be

Figure 15-4. Shoulder-hand syndrome. Note generalized edema of left hand. (Courtesy, the Arthritis Foundation)

unilateral or bilateral. The syndrome is divided into three clinical phases: Phase one is associated with pain, tenderness and diffuse swelling of the hand (Fig. 15-4). Synovitis with localized swelling of proximal interphalangeal and metacarpophalangeal joints and the wrist is common. Shoulder motions are painful and limited. The first phase usually lasts three to six months. In phase two, swelling diminishes but limited movement of the joints of the hand, wrist and shoulder persists. Chronic changes are characteristic of phase three. The skin of the hand becomes cool and atrophic and soft tissue contractures ensue. Wrist motion is limited and adhesive capsulitis leads to a frozen shoulder. Raynaud's phenomenon is common. Radiologic examination reveals bone atrophy with patchy osteoporosis of the hand, wrist and shoulder at any phase of the disorder.

The etiology of this syndrome is unknown. It may result from instability of the autonomic nervous system with an abnormal outflow of neurogenic stimuli from the spinal cord. Many cases are idiopathic. Some cases follow trauma to the involved extremity; the injury may be relatively mild. Other cases are secondary to disorders such as cervical osteoarthritis, cervical disk herniation, esophageal disorders, and diseases of the heart such as chronic angina or myocardial infarction. Less commonly, the syndrome occurs in association with stroke, brain tumor or pulmonary neoplasm.

Management of shoulder-hand syndrome involves prevention as well as treatment. Prolonged immobilization of the upper extremity should be avoided; early mobilization is particularly valuable in patients following myocardial infarction. Mild cases often respond to intensive physical therapy, anti-inflammatory agents such as aspirin and other non-steroidal anti-inflammatory agents, and injection of trigger areas of tenderness with local steroids and lidocaine. More severe cases frequently respond to treatment with oral corticosteroids. Doses of 30 to 60 mg of prednisone or its equivalent are given daily, depending on disease severity. Steroids at these dose levels should be continued until moderate relief is obtained, after which the medication is gradually decreased and finally discontinued as improvement allows. An alternative method of treatment is the use of stellate ganglion blocks with lidocaine, given daily or every other day. Symptomatic response is almost immediate. Therapy should be discontinued if no relief occurs after four such blocks have been given; on the other hand, eight to twelve blocks may be required for complete remission. Pneumothorax is a possible complication of this therapeutic modality. Physical therapy exercises are vital in all cases. In general, the earlier treatment is instituted, the better the results. Resistant cases may respond to surgical sympathectomy. In late, chronic stages of the disease, measures other than physical therapy to maintain range of motion are usually unsuccessful.

Reflex dystrophy is also seen in the lower extremities, although with less frequency. Symptoms and physical findings in the involved foot are similar to those described in cases involving the hand. The foot is diffusely warm, tender and swollen. Therapy with systemic steroids or lumbar sympathetic blocks usually is efficacious.

THORACIC OUTLET SYNDROME

This term is used to describe several neurovascular compression syndromes that produce symptoms in the shoulder and upper extremity. Symptoms include paresthesia, pain, and occasionally swelling of the involved extremity. Muscle weakness may occur and Raynaud's phenomenon is common. Thoracic outlet syndrome may result from several specific mechanisms.

Cervical Rib Syndrome

Approximately 0.5% of individuals have cervical ribs originating from the seventh cervical vertebrae. Musculoskeletal symptoms result from compression of neurovascular structures between the rib and the scalenus anticus muscle. The degree to which symptoms occur depends largely on the size and shape of the rib. Diagnosis is based on clinical symptoms supported by the roentgenographic finding of a prominent cervical rib on the side of the involved extremity. A trial of therapeutic exercises may be helpful in management. Severe cases are managed by surgical resection of the first thoracic and cervical ribs.

Scalenus Anticus Syndrome

Pressure on the neurovascular bundle may be due to compression of the bundle between the scalenus anticus muscle and a normal first rib. Hypertrophy and spastic irritability of the muscle are often present. Pain extends from the neck to the hand, usually in an ulnar distribution. Tiredness or weakness of the extremity may follow. Paresthesia and vasomotor disturbances such as Raynaud's phenomenon are common. Applying pressure over the scalenus anticus muscle reproduces symptoms.

Diagnosis is aided by demonstrating occlusion of radial pulsation by the Adson maneuver (Fig. 15-5). The physician's fingers are held on the radial pulse of the seated patient. The patient takes a deep breath and holds it while fully extending the neck and turning the head toward the involved side. Occlusion of the pulse represents a positive result; in some patients, occlusion occurs only when the head is turned to the opposite side. Since

Figure 15-5. Adson maneuver. Partial or complete occlusion of the radial pulse may occur in patients with cervical rib or scalenus anticus syndromes.

many normal persons demonstrate a transient or persistent diminishing of the pulse by this maneuver, a positive test is merely suggestive and not diagnostic. Auscultation of a systolic bruit just below the proximal and medial portions of the clavicle as the radial pulse decreases and reproduction of symptoms during performance of the maneuver strongly corroborate the diagnosis.

Partial relief of symptoms by injection of a local anesthetic into the scalenus anticus muscle is diagnostically helpful. As in cervical rib syndrome, therapeutic exercises may be useful in relieving symptoms. Resection of the first thoracic rib should be considered in severely symptomatic cases.

Costoclavicular Syndrome

In some patients, neurovascular compression between the clavicle and first rib occurs when the shoulders are braced backward and downward, as in an exaggerated military posture (Fig. 15-6). This position is associated with a diminished radial pulse, but a similar response can be seen in normal people, as with the Adson maneuver. Reproduction of symptoms or demonstration of a loud bruit over the subclavian artery as the pulse diminishes are strong supportive findings. Symptoms are relieved by avoid-

Figure 15-6. Costoclavicular maneuver. Auscultation over the subclavian artery may reveal a systolic bruit.

ing this posture. Resection of the first thoracic rib may be required for relief.

Hyperabduction Syndrome

In this condition, the neurovascular bundle is compressed by the pectoralis minor muscle, the coracoid process, the clavicle and first rib. Symptoms are precipitated by laterally circumducting the arms and clasping the hands over the head (Fig. 15-7). The radial pulse diminishes although positive results are noted frequently in normal individuals. This syndrome is induced by an abnormal persistent hyperabduction position of the extremity. It is particularly apt to occur in some persons during sleep, but is also seen in ballet dancers or mechanics as a result of positioning during occupational activities. Avoidance of hyperabduction is therapeutically indicated.

The diagnosis of thoracic outlet syndrome requires a careful history and physical examination to investigate the presence of various disorders at fault. The specific postural tests for the various syndromes are helpful. At times, a bruit may be heard over partially compressed vessels. Roentgenographic studies of the cervical spine are indicated. Chest roentgenogram is necessary to exclude a tumor of the superior pulmonary sulcus (Pancoast

Figure 15-7.   Hyperabduction maneuver. Partial or complete occlusion of the radial pulse supports a diagnosis of hyperabduction syndrome.

syndrome), which may at times produce similar symptoms. Venograms performed with the upper extremity in the precipitating postural positions may demonstrate compression abnormalities. Nerve conduction velocity studies may demonstrate delayed velocities in the ulnar distribution of the involved extremity.[7,8] Abnormalities noted on electromyographic study are generally less helpful. Cervical myelograms should be considered if symptoms are atypical and cervical disk disease as a cause of symptoms cannot be excluded.

Other diseases that cause pain in the same area, such as cervical degenerative joint disease, cervical disk herniation, and infectious or neoplastic diseases of the lung, should be excluded.

CARPAL TUNNEL SYNDROME

Compression of the median nerve at the wrist occurs when pathologic abnormalities compromise the nerve as it passes under the rigid transverse carpal ligament.[9,10] Paresthesia and pain characteristically involve the first three fingers of the hand; in many patients, however, symptoms are localized to any one or a combination of the first three fingers. Occasionally, symptoms involve the forearm as well, or the ulnar aspect of the hand when branches of the ulnar nerve are affected. Symptoms are often worse at night when the patient sleeps with the hand forcibly flexed; they are also precipitated by long periods of driving, knitting, reading with the hands flexed, or carrying packages. At times, joint swelling occurs. Physical examination early in the disorder is often negative except for a positive Tinel's sign, in which paresthesia of the hand and forearm is precipitated by tapping the median nerve at the wrist. Similar accentuation of symptoms follows holding the wrist in forced flexion or extension. Decreased sensation over the distribution of the median nerve and atrophy of the thenar eminence are associated with late disease.

Carpal tunnel syndrome may have several local or systemic causes. Frequently it is due to chronic trauma sustained by repetitive flexion of the wrists at work. In some patients it results from nerve compression by callus formation or malunion following fracture of the wrist. Benign tumors or tophaceous gouty deposits of monosodium urate are other causes. Not infrequently, carpal tunnel syndrome occurs when wrist structures are compressed by swelling of the tendon sheaths or synovium by rheumatoid arthritis; at times, this syndrome may be the initial manifestation of the rheumatoid state.[9] Other systemic diseases associated with the syndrome include myxedema, polymyalgia rheumatica, amyloidosis, acromegaly, and various hematologic disorders, such as polycythemia vera and the hemolytic anemias. It is seen more frequently in patients with diabetes mellitus, and is a common complaint in pregnant women in association with edema of soft tissues.

Diagnosis is directed not only toward defining the symptoms as carpal tunnel syndrome, but also toward demonstrating the presence of any associated disorder. In most cases, the history and physical findings are typical and strongly support the diagnosis. Roentgenograms of the wrists are indicated to exclude the presence of local pathology. Nerve conduction studies are generally diagnostic; they demonstrate prolonged motor and sensory median nerve conduction velocities across the wrist and a prolonged distal motor latency time. Although positive in most cases, these studies are occasionally normal despite the presence of proved compression.[11] Asymmetric nerve conduction velocities support the diagnosis even when overall velocities are bilaterally within normal limits.

Local injection of steroid with lidocaine into the carpal tunnel area is successful in a high percentage of cases, whether primary or secondary in etiology. A therapeutic trial is valuable when the diagnosis is in doubt. In chronic recurrent cases, a full diagnostic workup to exclude underlying etiologies should be performed. Indicated studies include a complete blood count, erythrocyte sedimentation rate, serum rheumatoid factor and antinuclear factor studies, serum protein electrophoresis (and, later, immunoelectrophoresis), serum uric acid, fasting blood sugar, and thyroxine determinations. When acromegaly is suspected, appropriate diagnostic studies should be performed.

Effective measures are available for management. Although immobilizing the wrist in a splint for several weeks may provide relief, symptoms are more consistently and rapidly relieved by local injections of steroid and lidocaine under the transverse carpal ligament superficial to the median nerve (see Chapter 21). This reduces inflammation and swelling and relieves symptoms for a prolonged time. Occupational stresses that aggravate symptoms should be avoided. Correction of local abnormalities should be considered when feasible. Systemic disorders related to the syndrome should be simultaneously treated. If symptoms are not completely relieved or recur following local steroid injection, a repeat injection may be given. Further recurrence is best treated surgically unless response to management of associated systemic disease is anticipated. Surgical division of the transverse carpal ligament, with or without neurolysis, gives definitive relief in most cases.[11] When surgery has been unduly delayed, muscle weakness and sensory changes may resolve only slowly or persist indefinitely.

It is not unusual to see patients with pain, paresthesia, and weakness of the upper extremity in whom it is difficult to differentiate carpal tunnel syndrome, compression of the ulnar nerve at the elbow, thoracic outlet syndrome and symptoms originating in the cervical spine. Symptoms may actually represent a composite of several entities present at the same time. Special attention to details of history is obviously important. In many cases therapeutic trials directed at various diseases that might be contributing to symptoms is indicated. Local steroid injection into the carpal tunnel area is valuable to exclude carpal tunnel syndrome if diagnostic studies are inconclusive. Similarly, a cervical collar and traction may be tried in excluding symptoms due to disease of the cervical spine. Therapy directed toward thoracic outlet syndrome should be considered in patients unresponsive to these approaches. In some patients, treatment directed at all these entities may be required to bring about significant relief of their symptomatology.

OTHER ENTRAPMENT SYNDROMES

Tarsal tunnel syndrome[12] is an interesting disorder similar to carpal tunnel syndrome. Pain and paresthesia of the foot result from compression of the tibial nerve as it passes behind the medial malleolus. Treatment is similar to that described for carpal tunnel syndrome. Local injections of steroid with lidocaine are usually effective. Surgical decompression may be required in resistant cases.

Suprascapular nerve entrapment leads to shoulder pain and limitation.[13,14] The suprascapular nerve, a mixed sensory and motor nerve, arises from the upper trunk of the brachial plexus and enters the supraspinous fossa through the suprascapular notch, passing below the superior transverse scapular ligament. Branches of the nerve supply the supraspinatus and infraspinatus muscles. Entrapment of the nerve may result from a fracture of the scapula with involvement of the notch and blade of the scapula, or may be caused by traction or compression. Entrapment should be suspected when there is selective wasting of the supraspinatus and infraspinatus muscles associated with weakness of external rotation and of abduction of the shoulder. Pain is noted over the area of nerve distribution. Infiltration of the suprascapular notch with local anesthesia may provide immediate temporary relief of pain, supporting the diagnosis. Nerve conduction studies reveal delayed conduction. Special roentgenograms of the suprascapular notch should be performed to rule out encroachment on the notch caused by an old fracture or fracture callus. Surgical decompression of the nerve, either by excision of the transverse scapular ligament alone, or by excision of the ligament and enlargement of the scapular notch, is usually effective in treatment.

MYOFASCIAL CHEST WALL SYNDROMES

Anterior chest wall pain and tenderness may result from a number of inflammatory conditions affecting chest wall structures.[15-20] *Costochondritis* (costosternal syndrome) results from inflammation of one or more costal cartilages.[15,18] Pain, which may radiate widely, simulates a number of intrathoracic and intra-abdominal disorders. A misdiagnosis of coronary artery disease is not uncommon.[18,20] Chest pain is commonly intermittent and may recur in prolonged episodes for a period of months or years. Palpation of costosternal junctions reproduces the pain. *Tietze's syndrome* is similarly characterized by inflammation of one or more costal cartilages.[16] In addition, there is an enlargement with *swelling* of the involved area. A single costochondral junction, usually the second, is involved in the majority of cases. The etiology of this entity is unknown. Infections or tumors of the underlying rib, or pain from intra-thoracic structures must be excluded in differential diagnosis.

Xiphoidalgia (xiphoid-cartilage syndrome) is associated with tenderness of the xiphoid process of the sternum; pain is aggravated by bending or twisting.[15] Eating may aggravate the syndrome and peptic ulcer disease may be simulated. *Rib-tip syndrome* (slipping rib)[17,19] results from hypermobility of the anterior end of a costal cartilage; the tenth rib is most often involved. Pressure produces pain and a clicking sensation. Pain reproduction brought on by pulling the rib cage anteriorly, with the finger hooked under the ribs at the costal margin helps to confirm the diagnosis.[19]

Although symptoms recur for weeks to years in patients with these myofascial chest wall syndromes, spontaneous remission may occur. Management includes use of local heat, analgesic and anti-inflammatory agents, and reassurance regarding the benign nature of the disease. Injection of involved areas with steroid and lidocaine is often beneficial; multiple, repeat injections may be necessary.

GANGLION

Ganglia are cystic swellings that contain a thick mucinous material. Quite common, they usually occur along tendon sheaths or joint capsules, particularly on the dorsum of the wrist. They may represent synovial membrane herniation through tears in the tendon sheath or retention cysts. The lesions respond well to aspiration and local introduction of steroids. Recurrent cases require surgical excision.

POPLITEAL CYSTS

Cystic tumors of the popliteal space (Baker's cysts) are common. They frequently reflect other primary knee disease, such as rheumatoid arthritis,[21] osteoarthritis, or internal mechanical derangements. Cyst formation is caused by posterior herniation of synovial membrane through the posterior capsule or bursal swelling. Lesions may be large and dissect through fascial planes down the calf. Cysts may be asymptomatic but pain and stiffness are common. Physical examination reveals swelling and tenderness in the popliteal area. Popliteal aneurysms and enlarged popliteal nodes must be excluded in differential diagnosis. Symptoms frequently simulate thrombophlebitis of the calf, although secondary phlebitis may actually be present due to venous compression and hemostasis. Arthrograms of the knee are diagnostic and delineate the presence and extent of cyst formation (Fig. 2-9). Venograms should be performed to exclude the presence of phlebitis if the diagnosis is at all questionable.

The cysts usually respond to local injections of steroid with lidocaine. In patients with rheumatoid arthritis, injection of steroid directly into the knee may alleviate the cyst swelling as well. Surgical ligation of the neck of the cyst followed by excision is required when cysts are large and unresponsive to a conservative therapeutic approach. Treatment directed toward any primary underlying disorder is helpful in eliminating cyst recurrence.

PELLEGRINI-STIEDA SYNDROME

This disorder is characterized by para-articular calcification at the medial aspect of the knee in the area of the medial collateral ligament. Stiffness and pain occur over the area of involvement. Para-articular calcification is seen on roentgenologic study (Fig. 15-8). Various etiologic possibilities include osseous metaplasia, presence of a detached bone fragment, ossification of a hematoma or calcification of soft tissues. Symptoms may simulate those seen in bursitis in this area. Therapy includes use of aspirin or other non-steroidal anti-inflammatory agents. Local injections of corti-

Figure 15-8. Roentgenogram of right knee in patient with Pellegrini-Stieda syndrome. A large para-articular calcification appears at the medial aspect of the femur (arrow). (Courtesy, Dr. V. Goldberg)

costeroids with lidocaine are often helpful. Surgical excision is occasionally indicated.

NIGHT CRAMPS

Many patients complain of cramps of the legs and feet which are unrelated to exertion and which often awaken them from sleep.[22] The etiology of this distressing symptom is unknown and appears unrelated to abnormalities in vascular supply. Extensive walking on cement floors or prolonged sitting may predispose patients to this symptomatology. Symptoms frequently recur in clusters. Avoidance of prolonged sitting, particularly in the evening, or the use of thick crepe-soled shoes in patients whose occupation requires walking on hard floors may be helpful. Quinine or diphenhydramine (Benadryl), administered at night, is often helpful. A warm tub bath at bedtime is beneficial in some patients.

RESTLESS LEG SYNDROME

This syndrome is characterized by painless spontaneous continuous leg movement.[23] In most patients, it is of psychogenic origin. Organic disease states, particularly those associated with neuropathic disease, may be etiologically important in other cases. Therapy is often frustratingly unsuccessful; anti-depressant medications administered at bedtime may be helpful.

SHIN SPLINTS

This terminology is applied to pain and distress in the lower leg associated with activities such as prolonged walking or jogging.[24,25] In mild cases, pain is usually relieved by rest; in more severe cases, pain may be sustained. Pain is usually most prominent over the anterior aspect of the leg; tenderness can be elicited over areas of involvement. Symptoms are thought due to small tears at the origin of involved muscles, or herniation of muscle through fascia. Stress fractures or compartment syndromes associated with ischemia of enclosed muscle compartments must be excluded in differential diagnosis. Shin splints may be avoided or minimized with the use of proper footwear and avoidance of running on hard surfaces.

CASE HISTORIES

History 15-1.   DeQuervain's Stenosing Tenosynovitis

J.R., a 23-year-old black female, was well until February, 1973. At that time she noted pain, slight redness, and swelling at the radial aspect of the left wrist. The patient was a piano major at the Institute of Music and symptoms were aggravated by her routine of three to four hours of piano practice daily. She was seen at the school infirmary where treatment with aspirin, 640 mg QID, splinting of the left wrist, and advice to limit her piano practice was instituted. Symptoms resolved only partially, and acute exacerbations were noted over the ensuing months. Pain and limitation of motion were aggravated by attempts to return to a more full practice schedule in her piano studies. She was referred for evaluation in November, 1973. System review was negative other than her chief complaint, and past medical history was noncontributory.

Physical examination revealed tenderness and slight swelling along the abductor pollicis longus and extensor pollicis brevis tendons. Grip strength was diminished due to pain and the patient had a positive Finkelstein test. The remainder of the joint examination was negative. Laboratory studies revealed normal hematocrit, white blood cell count, serum uric acid and erythrocyte sedimentation rate. Serum rheumatoid factor and antinuclear antibody determinations were negative. No abnormalities were noted on roentgenologic study of both wrists. A diagnosis of DeQuervain's tenosynovitis was made. Local injection of the area with steroid and lidocaine produced excellent relief of symptoms after several days. No recurrence of symptoms was noted despite gradual resumption of piano practice on a limited basis.

Discussion: In this patient DeQuervain's tenosynovitis was probably related to chronic trauma associated with intensive prolonged periods of practice on the piano. Unfortunately, recurrences may be anticipated if chronic trauma is continued. Although a relatively benign disease, this disorder represented a real threat to this patient who had serious goals of achievement as a concert pianist.

History 15-2. Shoulder-hand Syndrome

D.H., a 67-year-old white female, was seen in consultation in December, 1973. She gave a history of radical mastectomy for carcinoma of the left breast in 1969. Metastatic disease to the dorsal spine produced symptoms of spinal cord compression in April, 1973. Decompression laminectomy followed by trans-sphenoidal hypophysectomy provided symptomatic relief. Replacement therapy with cortisone acetate, 25 mg BID by mouth, and l-thyroxine, 0.2 mg daily, was begun. The patient did satisfactorily until December, 1973, when she developed subacute pain and limitation of the right shoulder, and pain and swelling of the right hand. System review was otherwise noncontributory, and past medical history revealed no other significant illnesses.

Physical examination showed extensive limitation of the right shoulder in all directions. The right hand and wrist were diffusely swollen and tender and the proximal interphalangeal and metacarpophalangeal joints of the right hand were slightly swollen. Right hand grasp was weak and fist formation was limited. Cervical spine motions were within normal limits. No other musculoskeletal abnormalities were noted. The remainder of her general physical examination showed no evidence of recurrence of carcinoma.

Hematocrit was 46%, the white blood cell count was 4000/mm³ with a normal differential, the erythrocyte sedimentation rate was 31 mm/hour (Wintrobe) and urinalysis was normal. Serum electrolytes were normal. Fasting blood sugar was 115 mg/100 ml (normal, up to 100 mg/100 ml). Serum calcium was 9.3 mg/100 ml, serum phosphorus, 3.1 mg/100 ml, and serum alkaline phosphatase, 9 King-Armstrong units (normal, 3 to 13 units). Serum glutamic oxaloacetic transaminase and creatine phosphokinase were normal. Serum uric acid, serologic test for syphilis, and studies for serum rheumatoid factor and antinuclear antibody were normal or negative. Serum protein electrophoresis revealed a mild increase in alpha-2 globulin.

Chest roentgenogram showed no abnormalities except for bony changes secondary to previous surgery. Roentgenograms of the shoulders were normal. Hand roentgenograms revealed hypertrophic spur formation at the margins of the distal interphalangeal joints. Cervical spine roentgenograms revealed mild degenerative changes. A diagnosis of right shoulder-hand syndrome was made.

The patient was placed on prednisone, 10 mg QID, and a physical therapy program was instituted. Within 48 hours, symptoms involving the right upper extremity improved greatly. Swelling of the right hand and wrist had diminished, and range of motion of the right shoulder, fingers and wrist was improved. After four days, prednisone dosage was decreased to 30 mg daily. The patient was discharged from the hospital one week later. Physical therapy instructions were given for home use and plans were made for reducing steroid dosage according to clinical response.

Discussion: The history and physical findings in this case were consistent with shoulder-hand syndrome. No specific precipitating cause was noted. The patient had no evidence of recurrence of breast carcinoma. The excellent clinical response to steroid therapy supported the diagnosis. No evidence of other forms of connective tissue disease was detected. Repeated stellate ganglion blocks are an alternative form of therapy when steroid therapy is contraindicated or unsuccessful.

History 15-3. Thoracic Outlet Syndrome

J.S., a 34-year-old white female, was first seen for evaluation in June, 1969. She was well until approximately six months prior, when she noted pain and weakness of the left upper extremity. Pain was aggravated by carrying heavy baskets elevated in front of her, by driving, or by reaching up to shelves. Pain later involved not only the left upper extremity but also the left posterolateral aspect of the cervical spine and the left infrascapular area. Prolonged use of the left arm caused increased pain and tingling of the fourth and fifth fingers of the left hand. Daily activities became severely restricted. Physical examination at the time of consultation revealed normal and equal blood pressures in both arms. There was tenderness over the left brachial plexus and complete occlusion of the left radial artery pulse with Adson's maneuver. Deep tendon reflexes were normal. Several tender trigger areas of spasm of the left shoulder girdle muscles were observed. Sensory examination revealed mild hypalgesia of the medial aspect of the left hand.

Roentgenograms of the chest were normal. Roentgenologic examination of the cervical spine showed mild spondylosis in the area of the C5 and C6 vertebrae. No cervical ribs were seen. Thoracic spine roentgenograms were normal. Laboratory studies including hematocrit, white blood cell count, erythrocyte sedimentation rate, urinalysis, serum electrolytes, serum calcium, phosphorus and alkaline phosphatase, serum uric acid and fasting blood sugar were normal. Routine serologic test for syphilis was negative, as were serum studies for rheumatoid factor and antinuclear antibody. A diagnosis of left thoracic outlet syndrome was made and the patient was placed on therapy with aspirin, 960 mg QID, muscle relaxants, and physical therapy. Intermittent injections with steroid and lidocaine were made into tender trigger areas of muscle spasm.

The patient failed to respond to therapy and had progressive increase in symptoms. She was admitted to hospital for evaluation later in the year. Clinical evaluation revealed normal cervical spine motions. Hyperabduction and Adson maneuvers resulted in a notably diminished left radial pulse. No carotid or subclavian bruits were heard. Nerve conduction studies of the upper extremities and spinal fluid examination were within normal limits. Roentgenograms of the cervical and dorsal spine were unchanged. Cervical myelogram was normal. Venograms of the left upper extremity revealed subclavian vein compression when hyperabduction and Adson maneuvers were performed. The patient was again placed on a full program of conservative therapy which included aspirin, analgesic medications, muscle relaxants, use of a cervical collar, cervical traction and local steroid injections into tender trigger areas. Deep heat was administered to symptomatic regions. Left trans-axillary resection of the first thoracic rib and section of the insertion of the anterior scalene muscle was performed when conservative measures failed to relieve symptoms. The patient had an excellent clinical response.

Discussion: Most patients with various forms of thoracic outlet syndrome will respond to conservative therapeutic measures. Continuous severe or progressive symptoms warrant consideration of surgery, as was eventually performed in this patient. Section of the insertion of the anterior scalene muscle and resection of the first thoracic rib on the side of involvement was associated with excellent relief of symptoms. Diseases of the cervical spine and carpal tunnel syndrome may sometimes simulate symptoms seen with thoracic outlet disorders. These other entities should be excluded by appropriate clinical and laboratory studies before definitive surgical therapy for thoracic outlet syndrome is contemplated.

History 15-4. Carpal Tunnel Syndrome

A.G., an 80-year-old white female, had a history of joint symptoms for many years characterized by mild swelling of the knees, ankles, wrists and proximal interphalangeal joints of the hands. Generalized morning stiffness that lasted two to three hours was a prominent complaint. Treatment with aspirin, 640 mg QID, and indomethacin, 25 mg TID, provided good relief of symptoms. When first seen in consultation in October, 1971, she was particularly troubled by paresthesia and burning sensations in the second and third fingers of the right hand. Physical examination revealed mild swelling of both knees, ankles and the left wrist. The right wrist was moderately swollen and limited in range of motion. Pressure over the right carpal tunnel area produced paresthesia of the second and third fingers. No muscle atrophy was noted and sensory neurologic examination was normal. Elbow and shoulder examinations were unremarkable. Thoracic outlet maneuvers were negative. Cervical spine motions were slightly limited but movement was unassociated with pain. Deep tendon reflexes in the upper extremity were present and equal bilaterally.

Hematocrit was 36%, white blood cell count and differential were normal, and erythrocyte sedimentation rate was 32 mm/hour (Wintrobe). Serum latex fixation test for rheumatoid factor was positive in a titer of 1:160. Serum uric acid was 3.2 mg/100 ml and serum antinuclear antibody was negative. Roentgenograms of the chest were normal. Roentgenograms of the hands and wrists revealed periarticular demineralization of bone and joint space narrowing involving several proximal interphalangeal joints and both wrists. Cervical spine roentgenograms showed mild spur formation. Nerve conduction studies revealed prolonged motor and sensory nerve conduction velocities and a prolonged distal latency time of the median nerve across the right wrist. A diagnosis of rheumatoid arthritis with associated right carpal tunnel syndrome was made.

Local injection of steroid with lidocaine into the right carpal tunnel area produced relief of hand symptoms within 24 hours. Relief lasted approximately three months; at that time symptoms of right carpal tunnel disease recurred. The patient refused definitive surgery for her median nerve compression and was again treated with local injection of steroid. Injections were repeated as required four times over the ensuing two years. Surgery was repeatedly advised and the patient finally acceded. Surgery revealed moderate synovial swelling at the volar aspect of the right wrist with compression of the right median nerve. Histopathologic study of synovium showed nonspecific synovitis consistent with rheumatoid arthritis. The patient had persistent good relief of her carpal tunnel symptoms.

Discussion: Carpal tunnel syndrome was a major manifestation of rheumatoid arthritis in this patient. Conservative therapy with intermittent injections of local steroid is a reasonable interim approach to management while efforts to suppress generalized disease are carried out. Surgical management is indicated when conservative management is ineffective. Prolonged median nerve compression may lead to chronic disability. Delay in surgical decompression is often associated with incomplete postoperative response of symptoms.

History 15-5. Costochondritis

L.P., a 46-year-old white female, was first seen in consultation in November, 1972. She was well until approximately two months prior, when she noted soreness and tenderness of the upper left anterior chest wall. There was no history of trauma and the patient had no other musculoskeletal complaints. Pain was moderately severe and often awakened the patient at night. Therapy with low-dose salicylates gave inconsistent relief. On physical examination no abnormal findings were noted except for marked tenderness in the area of the second and third costochondral junctions of the left anterior chest wall. No swelling was seen. Laboratory studies revealed normal white blood cell count and differential and erythrocyte sedimentation rate. Serum rheumatoid factor and antinuclear antibody studies were negative, and serum uric acid was 3.4 mg/100 ml. Roentgenograms of the chest and rib cage and electrocardiogram were normal. A diagnosis of costochondritis was made.

The patient was treated with local injections of steroid and lidocaine into the tender areas of costochondritis. She had almost complete relief of symptoms within 24 hours with sustained improvement for approximately one month. A mild recurrence of similar symptoms occurred at this time and local steroid injections were repeated. The patient was subsequently completely asymptomatic and no evidence of other disease states was noted on followup evaluation.

Discussion: This patient gave a history consistent with costochondritis, characterized by local tenderness of several costochondral areas. She responded well to local steroid therapy and was reassured regarding the benign nature of her symptomatology. Although recurrences are not uncommon, complete remission may be anticipated in most cases after a variable period of time.

REFERENCES

1. Handa, S. P. and Khaliq, S. U.: Swelling of olecranon bursa in uremic patients receiving hemodialysis. Can Med Assoc J 118:812, 1978.
2. Roles, N. C. and Maudsely, R. H.: Radial tunnel syndrome. J Bone Joint Surg 54:499, 1972.
3. Bulgen, D. Y., Hazelman, B. L. and Voak, D.: HLA-B27 and frozen shoulder. Lancet May 15, 1976, p. 1042.
4. McCarty, D. J. and Gatter, R. A.: Recurrent acute inflammation associated with focal apatite crystal deposition. Arthritis Rheum 9:804, 1966.
5. Pinals, R. S. and Short, C. L.: Calcific periarthritis involving multiple sites. Arthritis Rheum 9:566, 1966.
6. Moskowitz, R. W. et al.: Crystal-induced inflammation associated with chronic renal failure treated with periodic hemodialysis. Am J Med 47:450, 1969.

7. Urschel, H. C. and Razzuk, M. A.: Management of the thoracic outlet syndrome. N Eng J Med 286:1140, 1972.
8. Kelley, T. R.: Thoracic outlet syndrome: current concepts of treatment. Ann Surg 190:657, 1979.
9. Phalen, G. S.: The carpal-tunnel syndrome. J Bone Joint Surg 48A:211, 1966.
10. Chamberlain, M. A. and Corbett, M.: Carpal tunnel syndrome in early rheumatoid arthritis. Ann Rheum Dis 29:149, 1970.
11. Harris, C. M. et al.: The surgical treatment of the carpal-tunnel syndrome correlated with preoperative nerve-conduction studies. J Bone Joint Surg 61A:93, 1979.
12. Lloyd, K. and Agarwal, A.: Tarsal-tunnel syndrome, a presenting feature of rheumatoid arthritis. Br Med J 3:32, 1970.
13. Clein, L. J.: Suprascapular entrapment neuropathy. J Neurosurg 43:337, 1975.
14. Garcia, G. and McQueen, D.: Bilateral suprascapular-nerve entrapment syndrome. J Bone Joint Surg 63A:491, 1981.
15. Wehrmacher, W.: The painful anterior chest wall syndromes. Med Clin N Am 42:111, 1958.
16. Levey, G. S. and Calabro, J. J.: Tietze's syndrome. A report of two cases and review of the literature. Arthritis Rheum 5:261, 1962.
17. McBeath, A. A. and Keene, J. S.: The rib-tip syndrome. J Bone Joint Surg 57A:795, 1975.
18. Wolf, E. and Stern, S.: Costosternal syndrome: its frequency and importance in differential diagnosis of coronary heart disease. Arch Int Med 136:189, 1976.
19. Heinz, G. J. and Zavala, D. C.: Slipping rib syndrome: diagnosis using the "hooking maneuver." JAMA 237:794, 1977.
20. Epstein, S. E., Gerber, L. H. and Borer, J. S.: Chest wall syndrome: a common cause of unexplained cardiac pain. JAMA 241:2793, 1979.
21. Jayson, M. I. V. et al.: Popliteal and calf cysts in rheumatoid arthritis. Ann Rheum Dis 31:9, 1972.
22. Ayres, S. and Mihan, R.: Nocturnal leg cramps (systremma). South Med J 67:1308, 1974.
23. Lee, H. B.: Cramp in the elderly. Br Med J 2:1259, 1976.
24. Slocum, D. B.: The shin splint syndrome. Am J Surg 114:875, 1967.
25. Baugher, W. H. et al.: Injuries of the musculoskeletal system in runners. Contemp Ortho 1:46, 1979.

CHAPTER 16

NECK PAIN

Neck pain is a common complaint. Although most frequently due to local disease, it may reflect a number of systemic disorders.

DIFFERENTIAL DIAGNOSIS

Fibrositis (myofascitis) is a common cause of neck distress (see Chapter 9). Stiffness and pain on motion may be severe. Onset of symptoms is usually subacute and they may become increasingly severe. Continuous low-grade symptoms are associated with more severe exacerbations of acute pain. The patient will often describe localized areas of maximal pain from which more diffuse pain and stiffness seem to radiate. Symptoms are most prominent in the posterior and posterolateral cervical areas and at the upper aspects of the trapezius muscles. Muscle spasm and pain limit cervical spine motion. Symptoms can frequently be reproduced or exaggerated by applying pressure over localized trigger areas of pain. The cervical myofascial syndrome is frequently caused by chronic tension that causes continuous muscle spasm. A vicious cycle occurs, because spasm causes pain and pain causes more spasm. Although essentially a benign disorder, this syndrome can be quite disabling. Systemic disorders that produce similar symptomatology and physical findings must be differentiated.

Degenerative joint disease of the cervical spine is characterized by degeneration of intervertebral disks and osteophytic spur formation from the vertebral bodies (Fig. 16-1). In addition, a true osteoarthritis of the articulating apophyseal joints between vertebrae often exists (Fig. 16-1). Localized and radicular pain and stiffness are the usual symptoms. Localized pain results from spasm and secondary inflammatory reactions. Radicular pain occurs when nerve roots are compressed by degenerative spurs or by a prolapsed degenerated disk as the roots exit through the vertebral foramina. Paresthesia and weakness of areas of the extremities innervated by these roots are common. Deep tendon reflexes in the upper extremity may

Figure 16-1.   Degenerative joint disease of cervical spine. Note narrowing of the intervertebral disk spaces between C5-C6 and C6-C7 vertebrae (arrows). Osteophytic spur formation is seen at the anterior and posterior aspects of these vertebral bodies. Apophyseal joints reveal narrowing and sclerosis.

be diminished. Large posterior spurs cause spinal cord compression. In these cases, hyperactive deep tendon reflexes and pathologic reflexes such as the Babinski are seen in the lower extremities. If the anterior spinal artery is compressed, a central cord syndrome results. Compression of the vertebral arteries by spurs may also compromise the blood supply to the brain, causing transient symptoms of vertigo and visual impairment. Neck motion is usually limited by the osteoarthritic joint changes and by associated pain and spasm.

Herniated intervertebral cervical disks produce pain similar to that caused by degenerative joint disease. Symptoms vary depending upon whether protrusion of disk material occurs posteriorly or laterally. Disk herniation frequently occurs in association with degenerative changes typical of osteoarthritis, but it may occur separately. As in cervical osteoarthritis, spinal cord compression can result from posteriorly protruded disks. Neurologic symptoms due to cervical degenerative joint disease or herniated disk may be simulated by brachial plexus neuritis, in which severe acute pain in the neck and shoulder is followed by weakness and atrophy of involved muscles.[1]

Involvement of the cervical spine is common in patients with *rheumatoid arthritis;* it occurs so frequently in juvenile rheumatoid arthritis (JRA) that its presence is a clue to diagnosis. Roentgenologic changes in JRA are characterized by atlantoaxial subluxation and a tendency toward ankylosis of apophyseal joints (Fig. 16-2). Atlantoaxial subluxation is also

Figure 16-2. Lateral roentgenogram of cervical spine, juvenile rheumatoid arthritis. Irregularities in contour of the C5 and C6 vertebrae are associated with fusion of the upper apophyseal joints. (Courtesy, Dr. V. Goldberg)

Figure 16-3. Lateral tomogram, cervical spine. Atlantoaxial subluxation (arrow) in a patient with rheumatoid arthritis.

common in adults with rheumatoid arthritis of the cervical spine (Fig. 16-3).[2] Inflammatory erosions in bone may result in partial or complete dissolution of the odontoid process. Subluxation may go undetected if only routine lateral roentgenograms are obtained. Lateral roentgenograms taken with the neck in gentle flexion are necessary for complete evaluation. However, these should be performed only with great care if clinical symptoms suggestive of neurologic compression are present. Lateral tomograms (Fig. 16-3), and cineradiograms help to demonstrate detailed abnormalities that might be present. The atlanto-odontoid interval in adults should not exceed 3.0 mm and should be constant in neutral, flexion, and extension positions. Perhaps of more functional importance is the interval measured from the posterior aspect of the odontoid to the interlaminar cortex at the posterior aspect of the spinal canal. Compromise of this interval results in compression of the cord as it courses through the canal. The length of this interval is variable and depends on the overall size of the individual, with normal measurements of up to 26 mm observed. Neurologic manifestations of cord compression rarely occur with a spinal canal dimension greater than 16 mm at the C1 level.[3] In contrast, the posterior spinal canal diameter at the C3 and lower vertebral levels normally measures up to 16 mm, with pathologic compression of the cord more likely at intervals of 13 mm or less.

Rheumatoid changes in the cervical spine produce local pain and spasm. Occipital headaches are common and the patient may hear a clunking noise when flexing the head. Severe cases are associated with neurologic signs and symptoms due to compression of vascular and neurologic structures. Upper extremity weakness and long tract signs may be present. Quadriplegia may occur but is fortunately uncommon.

Ankylosing spondylitis most commonly produces symptoms in the low back and sacroiliac areas (see Chapter 17). However, upward progression

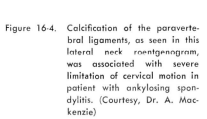

Figure 16-4. Calcification of the paravertebral ligaments, as seen in this lateral neck roentgenogram, was associated with severe limitation of cervical motion in patient with ankylosing spondylitis. (Courtesy, Dr. A. Mackenzie)

Figure 16-5.   Diffuse lytic lesions of the cervical spine caused by bony metastases from a carcinoma of the breast.

of the disease into the dorsal and cervical spine is common. The patient complains of pain and stiffness. Cervical spine motions are limited. Roentgenograms show calcification and ossification of paravertebral ligaments (Fig. 16-4).

Metastatic carcinoma of the cervical spine is usually characterized by severe, continuous pain. In its early stages it may simulate nonspecific myofascial syndrome or degenerative joint disease. Careful evaluation of neck roentgenograms is important in differential diagnosis (Fig. 16-5).

Benign local tumors that arise in bone or neurologic structures must be excluded as a cause of neck pain. Bone tumors such as giant cell tumor and osteochondroma are fortunately uncommon; hemangiomas and osteoid osteomas are more frequent. Roentgenograms may reveal vertical striations and partial vertebral collapse when hemangioma is present. Osteoid osteomas are characterized by an area of sclerotic bone that surrounds a small central radiolucent nidus. Tomograms help in diagnosis. Pain is severe, especially at night. Aspirin provides dramatic relief of symptoms. Removal of the central nidus is associated with lasting relief.

Tumors of nerve tissue origin, such as neurofibromas and meningiomas, may cause severe neck symptoms. Radiating pain related to motion is common. Myelograms are often necessary for diagnosis.

Osteoporosis occurs earliest and most severely in the dorsal and lumbar spine, but cervical spine involvement often occurs as the disease progresses. This disorder most frequently affects older patients. Symptoms may be vague and nonspecific. Diagnosis is based on roentgenographic findings of decreased bone density, "fishmouth" deformities of the vertebral bodies and, when changes are severe, vertebral collapse and fracture.

Whiplash injury occurs most commonly after automobile accidents. The patient usually gives a history of being in a car that was hit suddenly from behind by a second vehicle. This results in a forceful movement of the neck forward with posterior recoil. Neck pain and spasm may occur shortly after injury, but symptoms may be delayed for several days to a week. Symptoms include neck pain, stiffness and limitation of motion; they often spread to the upper trapezius muscle, causing pain and spasm. Neck roentgenograms are often negative; straightening of the cervical spine due to spasm may be noted.

Temporal arteritis (cranial arteritis, giant cell arteritis), a disease of older age, is associated with severe temporal headaches and polymyalgia rheumatica (see Chapter 13). The occipital vessels are also commonly affected, which may cause pain in the occipital and upper cervical regions. The temporal arteries are usually tender, nodular and irregular. Aching and stiffness in the shoulders and hips, fever, weight loss and depression are common associated findings. Laboratory studies show an elevated erythrocyte sedimentation rate, anemia, and a reversal of the albumin/globulin ratio.

DIAGNOSTIC STUDIES

History and physical examination will often define whether the basic problem is local or systemic. All patients should have adequate radiologic examination of the neck, with PA, lateral and oblique views. Oblique views are extremely important to adequately view foraminal openings through which nerve roots exit (Fig. 16-6). Lateral views in flexion and extension are necessary to demonstrate vertebral body subluxation and lesions in the odontoid area. They should be performed with caution. Spot films and tomograms (Fig. 16-3) allow further characterization of sus-

Figure 16-6. Oblique view of cervical spine reveals narrowing of foraminal spaces by osteophytic spurs of degenerative joint disease. Changes are most marked at the C3-C4 foramen (arrow).

pected pathologic changes. Cineradiography is helpful in detailing functional structural abnormalities, but it is not frequently required. Computed tomography (CT) allows visualization of the spine in cross section, the optimal plane of study.[4,5] Although structural size makes this technique somewhat less useful in the cervical than lumbar spine, this radiologic technique holds promise for major advances in noninvasive diagnosis. Abnormalities which may be visualized include bulging of the annulus, ligamentous hypertrophy, degenerative changes of the articular facet joints, and spinal stenosis.

Spinal fluid examination should be performed when myelopathy is present. Manometric studies to evaluate patency of the subarachnoid space should be considered when intracranial lesions can be reasonably excluded. Subsequently, cervical myelography may be indicated.

The foregoing routine studies will usually be adequate in the diagnosis of degenerative joint disease, cervical disk disease, metastatic carcinoma, rheumatoid arthritis, ankylosing spondylitis and osteoporosis. Negative studies are reassuring to those patients whose symptoms are related to myofascial syndrome. Other studies may be indicated to exclude systemic disease; these include erythrocyte sedimentation rate, rheumatoid factor test, serum alkaline phosphatase, and roentgenograms of the lumbar spine and sacroiliac joints. Temporal artery biopsy and arteriograms should be performed when temporal arteritis is suspected.

THERAPY

Symptomatic Measures

Conservative symptomatic measures may be instituted even before a specific diagnosis has been made. Aspirin, 640 to 960 mg four times a day, may relieve pain and inflammation. Other non-steroidal anti-inflammatory agents are similarly helpful. Local heat applied as hot packs, a warm shower, or heating pad similarly relieve pain and spasm. Mild analgesics such as acetaminophen, 300 to 600 mg, or propoxyphene hydrochloride, 65 mg, used on a PRN or regular basis are helpful. A soft cervical collar limits excessive motion and protects against irritation of neurologic structures. Tranquilizers such as diazepam (Valium), 5 mg TID, provide various degrees of relief from spasm and associated pain.

Specific Therapeutic Measures

Patients with *fibrositis* should avoid tension-producing factors if possible. The patient should be reassured that no serious underlying disease exists and that a reasonable amount of relief can be obtained by simple conservative measures. Emotional support is an important element of the therapeutic approach. Aspirin in maximally tolerated dosage should be instituted in addition to mild analgesics. Non-steroidal anti-inflammatory agents may be similarly beneficial in treating acute episodes. Local injections of trigger point areas of pain and spasm with steroids and lidocaine are frequently effective; several areas may have to be injected. Injections should be repeated after several weeks if certain areas have been missed or symptoms are relieved incompletely. Heat and mild range-of-motion exercises are advisable. Tranquilizers help to relieve tension.

A soft cervical collar limits neck motion. This should be worn throughout the night and as frequently as possible during the day when symptoms are severe. Use of the collar can be gradually decreased as symptoms improve. Cervical traction is instituted by the physical therapist and instructions given for home use. Traction should be utilized at least 20 minutes twice a day when symptoms are severe.

Management of *cervical degenerative joint disease* and *herniated cervical disk* is similar to the program outlined for fibrositis syndrome. Therapeutic measures include analgesic and anti-inflammatory agents and muscle relaxants. Heat, use of a cervical collar, and traction are beneficial. Local steroid and lidocaine injections relieve muscle spasm. Surgery should be considered when symptoms are severe and not responding well to a conservative medical program over a reasonable period of time. Anterior fusion has less morbidity and a shorter convalescence than fusion performed by a posterior approach. Posterior fusion and laminectomy may be required, however, in patients with cord compression.

The usual therapeutic programs for *rheumatoid arthritis* and *ankylosing spondylitis* should be instituted in patients with neck pain due to these disorders (see Chapter 19). However, severe involvement of the spine in rheumatoid arthritis requires additional special measures to prevent cord compression. A soft cervical collar should be worn at night and as much as possible throughout the day. It is particularly important to wear the collar when driving because even mild neck injuries may result in severe neurologic damage. A more firm cervical collar made of leather or plastic is required in severe cases. Cervical fusion should be considered if neurologic involvement is severe; unfortunately, failure of fusion is not uncommon. Patients with ankylosing spondylitis find great relief from the newer nonsteroidal anti-inflammatory agents (see Chapter 19). Physical therapy measures are extremely important.

Patients with *metastatic carcinoma* to bone may obtain relief from radiation therapy if the tumors are radiation-sensitive. Appropriate therapy to the primary tumor is indicated when feasible. A cervical collar helps to avoid damage to neurologic structures.

Surgery is usually necessary in the management of benign *local tumors.* Hemangiomas of bone frequently respond to radiation therapy. Failure to rapidly diagnose and treat local neoplasms may result in irreversible neurologic defects.

Although *osteoporosis* is frequently difficult to treat, presently accepted methods of management are worthy of trial. Elemental calcium, up to 1 g daily, and vitamin D, 50,000 IU once or twice weekly have been described as helpful.[6] Studies suggest that estrogens may prevent postmenopausal osteoporosis with at least temporary retardation of bone loss.[7,8] In a placebo-controlled double-blind trial of two years' duration, estrogen combined with a progestational agent led to a gain in bone mineral content, not seen with vitamin D or fluoride administration.[8] The combination of estrogen with sequential gestagen reduced estrogen-related endometrial hyperplasia, reducing the risk of endometrial cancer. Sodium fluoride therapy has been advocated for use, but its administration for this purpose remains investigational.[9] *Whiplash* syndrome is treated by measures similar to those described for fibrositis syndrome. Unfortunately, ongoing litigation often obscures therapeutic results until an adequate settlement has been made.

Prednisone, 15 mg QID, usually relieves symptoms of *temporal arteritis* rapidly, often within two or three days. A good response supports the diagnosis. Steroid therapy is valuable not only in relieving headache and polymalgia but also in preventing blindness that can occur as a complication of vasculitis involving the ophthalmic artery and vessels to the optic nerve.

CASE HISTORIES

History 16-1.   Cervical Spine Degenerative Joint Disease

C. G., a 54-year-old white male, was first seen in consultation in December, 1967, with the chief complaint of acute pain in the right side of the neck of several weeks' duration. Pain radiated down the arm to the wrist and was associated with paresthesia. Pain was also prominent over the dorsal aspect of the right shoulder. Past history revealed a short bout of similar distress in 1962, which had been treated with cervical traction and a soft cervical collar. The symptoms had resolved completely after several weeks, but the patient was troubled with recurrent episodes of neck pain over the ensuing years. On physical examination at time of consultation, cervical spine motions were moderately limited by pain and spasm. Tenderness was present over the right posterior cervical muscles and lateral flexion of the neck to the right produced paresthesia of the right upper extremity. The right grip was diminished in strength and sensation was diminished over the dorsolateral aspect of the forearm. Deep tendon reflexes were normal.

Cervical spine roentgenograms revealed moderately severe degeneration of the C5-C6 and C6-C7 disks. Severe spur formation compromised the intervertebral foramina in the C5-C6 and C6-C7 areas bilaterally. Symptoms and radiologic findings were consistent with a diagnosis of cervical degenerative joint disease. The patient was treated with cervical collar, cervical traction, aspirin, 640 mg QID, and propoxyphene hydrochloride, 65 mg, as needed for pain. Symptoms progressively improved over a period of several weeks and objective neurologic abnormalities disappeared.

Discussion: Cervical degenerative joint disease is a common disorder. In most patients, symptoms are minimal and objective neurologic findings absent. However, acute symptoms may be associated with major disability. Intensive therapy with neck immobilization and traction and the use of mild anti-inflammatory agents and analgesics helps to relieve distress. More serious disorders as a cause of this pain syndrome should be routinely excluded.

History 16-2.   Metastatic Carcinoma of the Cervical Spine

S.R., a 73-year-old white male, was first seen in consultation in December, 1970. The patient had a long history of cervical spine pain of mild to moderate degree. Roentgenograms of the cervical spine performed several years earlier had revealed extensive changes of degenerative joint disease. The patient had been treated intermittently with a cervical collar, cervical traction, aspirin, and mild analgesics with good relief. Several months prior to referral the patient had noted increased pain in the cervical spine. The symptoms were considered an exacerbation of his cervical degenerative joint disease; x-rays of the cervical spine were not obtained. Therapy with aspirin, analgesics, cervical collar and cervical traction were again instituted. Symptoms did not respond to this program of management and the patient was referred for evaluation.

System review was significant in that the patient had suffered a 15-pound weight loss over the previous two months. On physical examination there was slight tenderness over the cervical spine, and cervical spine motions were moderately limited. Cardiorespiratory examination revealed a Grade 2/6 systolic ejection murmur. Prostatic enlargement without nodules or tenderness was noted. Cervical spine roentgenograms taken at this time revealed multiple lytic lesions consistent with metastatic carcinoma. Additional roentgenographic studies revealed destructive bone lesions in the left rib cage and infiltrative changes at the apical segment of the left lower lobe of the lung.

Hematocrit was 40%, white blood cell count was 7900/mm³ with a normal differential, the serum alkaline phosphatase and acid phosphatase values were within normal limits, and tuberculin skin test was positive. Rib biopsy was performed under local anesthesia. Histopathologic study revealed metastatic, poorly differentiated adenocarcinoma. The bone lesions were considered to be metastatic from a primary adenocarcinoma of the lung. The patient was treated with radiation therapy to the cervical spine, with no improvement in pain. A large left pleural effusion, noted on subsequent chest roentgenograms, was treated with instillation of 5-fluorouracil into the pleural cavity. The patient had a progressive downhill course and died after the thirty-sixth hospital day.

Discussion: Pain is a prominent component of the clinical presentation of metastatic carcinoma of the spine. In this patient, recent cervical spine symptoms were attributed to degenerative joint disease that had been demonstrated previously. A notable increase in symptoms associated with a 15-pound weight loss suggested the presence of a more serious disorder. The presence of degenerative joint disease is often a "red herring" in the clinical evaluation of patients with symptoms related to the musculoskeletal system.

History 16-3.   Temporal (Cranial) Arteritis

M.S., a 70-year-old white female, was first seen in December, 1966, for evaluation of pain and swelling of the proximal interphalangeal and metacarpophalangeal joints of the hands, both knees and ankles. Physical examination and laboratory studies were consistent with a diagnosis of rheumatoid arthritis and the patient was placed on a conservative program of aspirin, analgesics and physical therapy. The patient responded well with little progression of joint manifestations. In December, 1967, she noted moderately severe pain in the left side of her neck and scalp. Pain was aggravated by applying pressure to involved areas. The patient increased her dose of aspirin, which provided partial relief of symptoms. She was seen in the office in January, 1968, when pain in the posterior cervical area and over the posterior aspect of the scalp became more severe. She now complained of pain and tenderness in the left temporal area as well. Examination revealed tenderness to palpation over the posterior cervical spine, the posterior aspect of the scalp and the left temporal region. Temporal artery pulsations were normal and no thickening of the vessels was noted. The patient was admitted to hospital for general studies and temporal artery biopsy.

Erythrocyte sedimentation rate was 48 mm/hour (Wintrobe). Hematocrit was 36%, white blood cell count was 12,600/mm³, and urinalysis was normal. Serum protein electrophoresis revealed a slight elevation in gamma globulin. Roentgenograms of the skull and cervical spine showed mild degenerative arthritis. Left temporal artery biopsy was performed. Histopathologic examination showed intimal proliferation and an inflammatory infiltration of the vessel wall with mononuclear and giant cells. A diagnosis of temporal arteritis was made. The patient was begun on prednisone therapy, 15 mg Q6H. Symptoms responded rapidly over 36 hours. The patient was subsequently maintained on progressively lower doses of prednisone for several years. After this time, her symptoms completely resolved and no further therapy was required.

Discussion: Early symptoms of temporal arteritis in this patient consisted of pain in the posterior cervical and occipital areas. Only after a period of one month did symptoms occur in the temporal area as well. The posterior cervical and occipital areas are occasionally the site of prominent symptomatology in patients with temporal arteritis.

REFERENCES

1. Bocevich, B. B.: Paralytic brachial neuritis. J Bone Joint Surg 58A:262, 1976.
2. Mathews, J. A.: Atlanto-axial subluxation in rheumatoid arthritis. A 5-year follow up study. Ann Rheum Dis 33:526, 1974.
3. Bohlman, H.: Atlanto-axial subluxation (abstract). Orthopaedic Transactions 1:3, 1978.
4. Kirkaldy-Willis, W. H., Wedge, J. H., Yong-Hin, G. et al.: Pathology and pathogenesis of lumbar spondylosis and stenosis. Spine 3:319, 1978.
5. Glenn, W. V., Rhodes, M. L., Altschuler, E. M. et al.: Multiplanar display computerized body tomography applications in the lumbar spine. Spine 4:282, 1979.
6. Hahn, T. J. and Hahn, B. H.: Osteopenia in patients with rheumatic diseases: principles of diagnosis and therapy. Sem Arth Rheum 6:165, 1976.
7. Lindsay, R. et al.: Long-term prevention of postmenopausal osteoporosis by estrogen. Lancet, May 15, 1976.
8. Christiansen, C. et al.: Prevention of early postmenopausal bone loss: controlled 2-year study in 315 normal females. Eur J Clin Invest 10:273, 1980.
9. Jowsey, J. et al.: Effect of combined therapy with sodium fluoride, vitamin D and calcium in osteoporosis. Am J Med 53:43, 1972.

CHAPTER 17

LOW BACK PAIN

Diagnosis and treatment of low back pain often tax the ingenuity of the physician. Although in many patients a diagnosis can be made after appropriate history, physical examination and laboratory studies, a specific diagnosis is not always possible and management must be based on an empiric symptomatic approach.

DIFFERENTIAL DIAGNOSIS

One of the most common causes of low back pain is *abnormal posture*. In most cases, the postural defect is functional; in others, structural bony changes result in fixed postural abnormalities. In the latter, secondary degenerative changes are often noted on roentgenographic examination; the postural abnormalities are not readily reversible. Pain associated with functional postural abnormalities is usually relatively mild and results from muscular imbalance and spasm. In patients with fixed changes, severe pain may result from compression of nerve roots; this tends to occur especially when secondary degenerative changes are severe.

Herniation of a nucleus pulposus in the lumbar area is a common cause of low back pain. Unfortunately, this diagnosis is often overused as a "wastebasket" diagnosis when studies are inconclusive. Pain may be acute or chronic. Acute pain results from posterior or lateral herniation of a nucleus pulposus causing compression of contiguous neurologic structures. Chronic symptoms usually result from degeneration of the annulus fibrosus with eventual prolapse or protrusion of degenerated material. In the latter cases, degenerative changes in the vertebral body and apophyseal joints are a common associated finding.

The patient complains of low back pain. Spasm and tenderness of associated muscles are noted in the involved area. Radicular pain in the distribution of the sciatic nerve is often prominent. Straight-leg-raising is limited due to muscle spasm and nerve root irritation. The patient walks with a list, and secondary functional scoliosis is common. Chronic com-

Figure 17-1. Osteoarthritis of lumbar spine. Note florid spur formation, narrowed disk spaces and sclerosis of apophyseal joints. (Courtesy, Dr. F. Bishko)

pression of nerve roots results in neurologic abnormalities such as loss of reflexes, muscle weakness and sensory deficits.

Low back pain may result from *primary degenerative joint disease* of the spine. Degenerative changes are characterized by osteophyte spur formation of the vertebral bodies, degeneration of the annulus fibrosus with eventual prolapse, and joint space narrowing and spur formation involving the apophyseal joints (Fig. 17-1). Pain is usually subacute or chronic; acute symptoms occur if nerve root compression complicates the picture. Clinical findings are generally similar to those described in patients with herniated nucleus pulposus.

Diffuse idiopathic skeletal hyperostosis (DISH, ankylosing hyperostosis, Forestier's disease) is characterized by a flowing ligamentous ossification along the anterolateral aspect of the vertebral bodies[1-3] (Fig. 17-2). The dorsal spine is most commonly involved (Fig. 17-2B), but all spine levels may be affected. Although anatomic abnormalities are often striking, pain is usually surprisingly minimal or absent and limitation of spine motion less than anticipated. Extraspinal manifestations are common[1] and include bony "whiskering," ligamentous calcification, prominent olecranon and calcaneal spurs, and degenerative arthritis in peripheral joints. The presence of an increased frequency of HLA-B27 antigen in these patients has not been confirmed.[3]

Differential diagnosis between DISH syndrome and ordinary degenera-

A   B

Figure 17-2. Diffuse idiopathic skeletal hyperostosis (DISH). A. Lumbar spine. Flowing ligamentous ossification and spur-like formation are seen along the anterior aspect of the vertebral bodies. Disk spaces are preserved. B. Dorsal spine. Similar changes are noted in a roentgenogram of the dorsal spine. (Courtesy, Dr. J. Wisnieski)

tive joint disease of the spine is not always readily made. Osteophyte formation characteristic of degenerative joint disease may co-exist with DISH syndrome, and the possibility that this syndrome represents a variant of osteoarthritis has not been excluded. Resnick and co-workers[1] have suggested specific criteria to allow differentiation of this disorder from other diseases of the spine. Criteria in favor of a diagnosis of diffuse idiopathic skeletal hyperostosis include flowing ossification along at least four contiguous vertebral bodies, preservation of disk space, absence of vacuum phenomena or vertebral body marginal sclerosis, and absence of apophyseal joint ankylosis or sacroiliac joint erosions or fusion. Diffuse radiographic findings involving both the spine and extraspinal structures suggest a generalized disorder of ossification rather than a localized spinal disease.

Spondylolysis, a defect in the pars interarticularis of the neural arch (Fig. 17-3A), may be congenital or acquired and traumatic in origin. Symptoms are not usually common unless *spondylolisthesis,* a forward displacement of one vertebra on the other, ensues (Fig. 17-3B). The latter condition may be asymptomatic, but mild to moderate pain and spasm are not uncommon. Symptoms resemble those seen in herniated disk disease and, in fact, secondary disk disease may also develop. Vertebral displacement is usually anterior. Posterior displacement may compress the cauda equina; fortunately, this is uncommon. Spondylolisthesis sometimes occurs in the

A

Figure 17-3A. Spondylolysis, lumbar spine. A defect (arrow) is seen in the pars interarticularis in this oblique roentgenographic view. (Courtesy, Dr. V. Goldberg)

B

Figure 17-3B. Spondylolisthesis. Early forward displacement of L5 vertebra on S1 is seen. A defect, seen in the pars interarticularis (arrow), was better demonstrated on oblique roentgenographic view. (Courtesy, Dr. V. Goldberg) absence of spondylolysis. Displacement in these cases results from a congenitally large pedicle or from severe degenerative joint disease of the apophyseal joints with dislocation.

Spinal stenosis is characterized by a decrease in the sagittal diameter of the spinal canal.[4,5] Such stenosis is most commonly due to combined factors which operate to diminish canal size. Congenital narrowing alone is generally not symptomatic. It does, however, result in reduction of reserve so that secondary factors cause further compromise of the canal, nerve entrapment, and neurologic manifestations. Commonly associated acquired contributing factors include degenerative spurs, disk herniation, ligamentous hypertrophy, and spondylolisthesis. Other factors which may lead to stenosis include trauma, or fibrosis following laminectomy. Less commonly, spinal stenosis is associated with metabolically induced bone enlargement in patients with Paget's disease or fluorosis.[6] Pain may be constant or intermittent and is usually present in one or both legs in addition to the back. Often it is made worse by exercise and resembles intermittent claudication. Of interest is worsening of symptoms by hyperextension of the back, and relief by flexion. Sensory disturbances may be present and motor power in the legs impaired.

Osteoporosis produces mild to moderate pain that usually parallels the degree of disease (Fig. 17-4). Pain may be continuous, increasing with activity. Compression fracture should be suspected when there is a sudden increase in pain with or without a history of trauma. Trauma may be mild, such as a slight fall, tripping or stressful motion. Neurologic abnormalities occur when structural changes associated with fracture produce compression of adjoining neurologic structures.

Primary bone disease such as *multiple myeloma* is a cause of persistent low back pain (Fig. 17-5). *Metastatic carcinoma* frequently involves the

Figure 17-4. Osteoporosis of spine. All vertebrae appear extensively demineralized. Additional diagnostic features include accentuation of cortical bone outlines and codfish deformities.

Figure 17-5.   Lesions of multiple myeloma seen on lateral spine roentgenogram. Note demineralized appearance of vertebral bodies and compression fracture.

lower spine (Fig. 17-6). Pain, usually persistent, is present at rest and aggravated by motion. Night pain is common.

Paget's disease frequently involves the spine and pelvis. Pain resembles that seen in several other low back disorders. The diagnosis depends on demonstrating typical radiologic changes characterized by sclerosis and a coarsening of the trabecular pattern of bone (Fig. 17-7). The serum alkaline phosphatase level is characteristically elevated. Superimposition of an osteogenic sarcoma should be considered in the presence of severe pain.

Initial symptoms in *ankylosing spondylitis* characteristically involve the area of the sacroiliac joints and lumbosacral spine.[7] This disease, most

6-4-70

Figure 17-6.   Metastatic carcinoma, lumbar spine. Complete collapse of L3 vertebra is associated with metastases to other areas (arrows). (Courtesy, the Arthritis Foundation)

Figure 17-7. Paget's disease, lumbar spine. Sclerosis and a coarsening of the trabecular pattern are seen in the lower lumbar vertebrae. (Courtesy, Dr. V. Goldberg)

commonly seen in young males, may cause very mild symptoms with minimal or absent objective findings early in its course. A diagnosis of malingering or psychiatric illness is often entertained when stiffness and pain are present in the absence of positive physical and laboratory findings. Analysis of the history in patients with this disorder has defined factors which are helpful in differentiating back pain produced by spondylitis from back pain due to other causes.[8] These factors are back discomfort that begins before age 40, is insidious in onset, persists for more than 3 months, is associated with morning stiffness, and improves with exercise. Low back symptoms are often accompanied by pain in a sciatic distribution to the buttocks and knees. Sciatic pain not infrequently alternates from side to side. Peripheral joint involvement occurs in one-third of patients. Heel pain is common. As the disease progresses, pain, stiffness and limitation of motion involve the dorsal and cervical spine. Chest pain occurs when costovertebral joints are affected. Systemic manifestations include pericarditis, cardiac conduction abnormalities, aortic insufficiency and iritis. Physical examination shows tenderness and limitation of affected areas of the spine and spasm of paravertebral muscles. Chest expansion may be severely limited. Progression of the disease leads to severe kyphosis and forward protrusion of the neck (Fig. 17-8).

Laboratory findings other than roentgenologic changes are frequently minimal. The erythrocyte sedimentation rate is elevated during active disease. Serum studies for rheumatoid factor and antinuclear antibody are negative. However, 90% of patients with ankylosing spondylitis have HLA-B27 histocompatibility antigen.[9] Roentgenologic studies may be negative

Figure 17-8. Ankylosing spondylitis, showing kyphosis and forward protrusion of the neck. (Courtesy, the Arthritis Foundation)

for several years after disease onset, but eventually characteristic changes in the sacroiliac joints and spine appear. Early, sacroiliac joints reveal juxta-articular bony osteoporosis and apparent joint space widening (Fig. 17-9); later, joint space narrowing, sclerosis and fusion appear (Fig. 17-10). Spinal roentgenograms show syndesmophytes or calcified spurs. These spurs lie in a vertical direction, differentiating them from osteophytes of degenerative joint disease, which characteristically lie in a horizontal direction and are less likely to be fused. Granulomatous changes at the antero-superior and anteroinferior aspects of the vertebral bodies produce a squared appearance of the vertebrae (Romanus sign) (Fig. 17-11). Calcification and ossification of paravertebral ligaments lead to classic bamboo spine changes (Figs. 17-10, 17-11). Destructive lesions of intervertebral disks and adjoining vertebral bodies may be seen; these lesions may be confused with tuberculous or pyogenic infection.

Spondylitic changes occur in other disease states, such as psoriasis, ulcerative colitis, regional enteritis, and Reiter's syndrome.[10] Syndesmophyte spur formation in patients with ulcerative colitis and regional enteritis is similar to that seen in idiopathic ankylosing spondylitis. The spurs are usu-

Figure 17-9. Ankylosing spondylitis, pelvic roentgenograms. Sacroiliac joints reveal apparent widening of joint spaces and bony sclerosis.

Figure 17-10. Ankylosing spondylitis. Sacroiliac joints are fused. Calcification of paravertebral ligaments has led to development of bamboo spine.

Figure 17-11. Ankylosing spondylitis. Note squared appearance of vertebrae (Romanus sign) in this lateral lumbar roentgenogram. Paravertebral calcification of ligaments is extensive.

ally relatively thin, regular, bilateral and lie close to the intervertebral disk. In patients with psoriasis and Reiter's syndrome, the syndesmophytes tend to be larger, more irregular and are often unilateral.

Osteitis condensans ilii occurs most commonly in young women of childbearing age. Symptoms are characterized by pain and stiffness in the area of the sacroiliac joint. At times, mild radicular pain is present. Polyarthralgia of peripheral joints occurs, and isolated effusions of peripheral joints have been described.[11] Fibrositis symptoms are a common complaint. No increase in the frequency of HLA-B27 has been noted. Radiologic changes are usually easily differentiated from those of ankylosing spondylitis. In osteitis condensans ilii, a condensing sclerosis of iliac bone is seen, and no changes in the sacroiliac joint or sacrum are noted (Fig. 17-12).

Acute spinal infections affect the intervertebral disk spaces or sacroiliac joints.[12,13] Bone involvement is usually secondary. Spinal infection usually emanates from foci elsewhere, such as genitourinary, pulmonary, or cutaneous areas. Radiologic changes may be slow in developing but serial examination eventually reveals gradual destruction of vertebral margins and obliteration of the disk space. Diagnosis is confirmed by culture of aspirates from the disk space. A positive blood culture is helpful in diagnosis, because bacteremia is frequently present.

The most common cause of chronic infection of the spine is *tuberculosis*. Symptoms are often insidious in onset. Systemic evidence of tuberculous

Figure 17-12.   Osteitis condensans ilii. Sclerotic changes involve the iliac sides of both sacroiliac joints.   Oblique views showed that the joints themselves were normal.
(Courtesy, Dr. V. Goldberg)

infection such as fever, chills and night sweats is helpful in diagnosis. A negative tuberculin test militates against the diagnosis; a positive tuberculin test, however, is only supportive and not conclusive. The erythrocyte sedimentation rate is usually elevated. Radiologic examination reveals narrowing of the disk space, the site of initial tuberculous involvement (Fig. 17-13).[14] Soft tissue abscesses are typical. Diagnosis should be pursued by aspiration and culture of the abscessed area. Sacroiliac joint involvement is not uncommon. *Fungal infections* and *brucellosis* cause similar

Figure 17-13.   Tuberculosis of the lumbosacral spine resulted in loss
of the L5-S1 disk space and
destructive changes in contiguous bone.

Figure 17-14. Vertebral epiphysitis (Scheuermann's disease). (Courtesy, Dr. V. Goldberg)

lesions. Diagnosis is based on fungal complement-fixation studies, brucella agglutination titer and culture of involved areas.

Vertebral epiphysitis (Scheuermann's disease) causes back pain in adolescents. It is more common in males and most frequently involves the dorsal spine. Rounding and limitation of the dorsal spine are seen on physical examination. Tight hamstrings are common. Pain may be minimal or absent and the patient's primary complaint is poor posture. The condition is self-limited. Roentgenologic study reveals wedging of the vertebrae, narrow disk spaces and irregular vertebral margins (Fig. 17-14).

Coccygodynia, pain in the area of the coccyx, results from direct trauma with fracture of the coccyx or strain of the sacrococcygeal joint. It may also occur as a result of visceral disease in organs anterior to the area of the coccyx itself. Rectal examination reveals tenderness of the coccyx and associated ligamentous and muscular structures.

Subarachnoid hemorrhage of intracranial origin is an uncommon cause of low back pain but should be considered diagnostically in cases with atypical symptoms. Pain, due to irritation by blood in the spinal fluid, may simulate acute disk herniation or vertebral fracture. Headache and pain and limitation of the cervical spine are frequent associated findings.

Herpes zoster may cause severe low back pain when localized to nerves in this area. The diagnosis is often missed until the characteristic vesicular eruption is seen.

Benign local tumors, such as neurofibroma, meningioma, osteoid osteoma and hemangioma, should be considered in the differential diagnosis of low back pain. Diagnosis requires full use of radiologic techniques including routine roentgenograms, spot films, tomograms, and myelograms. Tomograms are particularly helpful in the diagnosis of osteoid osteoma, which usually involves the posterior aspects of the vertebrae and may not be seen on routine radiologic studies. The typical lesion consists of a zone of dense bone surrounding a small radiolucent nidus. Pain is severe and usually more prominent during the night. Relief of pain by aspirin is often dramatic; this is a helpful diagnostic test.

Although *fractures* of the vertebral bodies are associated most commonly with osteoporosis, they may occur secondary to trauma in otherwise normal spines. Fractures of the posterior elements of the spine are complicated by severe neurologic damage; rapid neurosurgical intervention is indicated. Pathologic fractures occur in patients with metastatic malignancy, primary neoplasms or metabolic bone dyscrasias.

Idiopathic scoliosis is associated with various degrees of back pain. Osteoarthritis, a frequent secondary finding, contributes to the symptomatology. At times, nerve compression with radicular pain is prominent.

Not infrequently, low back pain is a manifestation of *visceral disease,* such as carcinoma of the uterus, kidney, pancreas, or bowel. Large aortic aneurysms that impinge upon the vertebral column cause persistent boring back pain. Adequate investigation of the patient by history and physical examination and appropriate laboratory studies is mandatory, particularly when back symptoms are atypical.

DIAGNOSTIC STUDIES

PA, lateral and oblique roentgenograms of the lumbosacral spine should be performed routinely. Disk disease is not excluded by normal findings, however, since the soft tissue herniation does not show and narrowing of the disk space may appear only late. Oblique views are necessary to demonstrate spondylolysis because the pars interarticularis cannot be outlined adequately in routine PA and lateral views. Spondylolisthesis, a displacement of one vertebra on the other, is best seen on the lateral view. Lesions due to osteoporosis, fracture, metastatic carcinoma, Paget's disease, spondylitis, osteitis condensans ilii, acute or chronic infection, epiphysitis, and scoliosis are usually detected readily. Special oblique views of the sacroiliac joints should be performed in patients suspected of having ankylosing spondylitis when changes on routine PA views are absent or nonspecific. Tomograms may be helpful. Coned-down spot films and tomograms of other areas of the lumbosacral spine are indicated to exclude subtle abnormalities readily missed on routine study.

Computed tomography (CT) promises to play an increasingly important role in the diagnosis of diseases of the spine, especially as resolution of scanners improves.[15,16] Visualization of the spine in horizontal cross section allows optimal evaluation of interspaces, facet articulations, and spinal canal configuration. Demonstrations of degenerative spur formation, and lateral and central spinal stenosis are particularly facilitated; disk herniations can be outlined with increased accuracy.[16] Use of this diagnostic modality may diminish the need for myelograms and allow more detailed non-invasive assessment of spinal disease not readily noted on clinical and routine radiologic examination.

Lumbar myelograms may be necessary in patients with severe persistent disease if the diagnosis cannot be made otherwise. Myelograms are not usually performed in patients with suspected herniated disks unless symptoms are severe and unresponsive to conservative therapy and surgery is being contemplated.

Radioactive scans are helpful in delineating early otherwise nondemonstrable lesions of bone. Diagnoses of bone infections, primary or secondary neoplastic disease, and Paget's disease are particularly facilitated. Attempts to improve diagnostic precision in patients with suspected sacroiliitis have met with variable success.[17-21] Quantitative sacroiliac scintigraphy is performed by measurement of uptake of 99M Technetium labeled phosphates by sacroiliac joints in comparison to uptake over the sacrum. Some studies suggest that this technique accurately separates early cases of sacroiliitis from normal subjects.[17,18] Other studies have been unable to delineate a clear separation of patients with this disease from normals, especially in the presence of early inflammation.[19-21] Normal scintigraphy ratios have been noted in patients with clinically and radiologically demonstrable disease, especially when radiologic changes are advanced. In addition, abnormal scintigraphy ratios have been found in patients without spondylitis. Further studies are needed to assess the value of this technique in the diagnosis of sacroiliitis. It may play a role in monitoring disease activity and response to treatment in known patients with the disorder.

Other studies frequently necessary in diagnosis include chest roentgenogram, complete blood count, erythrocyte sedimentation rate, serum calcium, phosphorus and alkaline phosphatase, serum protein electrophoresis, urine for Bence Jones protein, bone marrow study, and skin testing for tuberculosis and fungal diseases. Histocompatibility antigen studies to demonstrate the presence of HLA-B27 antigen may be diagnostically helpful when ankylosing spondylitis is suspected. Appropriate radiologic studies of viscera are indicated when symptoms are deemed most likely nonosseous in origin. Aortic aneurysms, if calcified, are usually visible on lateral views of the lumbar spine.

THERAPY

Nonspecific therapy with rest and analgesic and anti-inflammatory agents is utilized until a diagnosis is made, when specific measures can then be instituted. The latter vary with the diagnosis, as follows.

Postural low back pain often responds to a program of strengthening exercises for abdominal and spine muscles and directions for better posture. Mild analgesic and anti-inflammatory agents and muscle relaxants are helpful. A lumbosacral corset is valuable for acute or severe symptoms. *Structural abnormalities* such as scoliosis may require corrective immobilization or surgery.

Acute symptoms due to *herniation of a nucleus pulposus* frequently require complete bed rest. Toileting should be limited to use of a bedpan or bedside commode. Rest is aided by pelvic traction, which keeps the patient from moving about excessively and relieves some of the spasm of involved muscles. Pelvic traction is used throughout the day and night. Local heat, such as Hydrocollator packs applied for 30 minutes twice daily, is helpful. Analgesic and anti-inflammatory agents relieve pain and secondary muscle spasm. Occasionally, mild narcotics are required. Muscle spasm is further decreased by the use of tranquilizers such as diazepam, 5 mg three to four times a day. The patient must understand the nature of the disease and the goals of management. Response may be slow; hospitalization to assure complete bed rest may be required. In patients with *degenerative joint disease of the spine,* a similar program of analgesic and anti-inflammatory agents, muscle relaxants, adequate rest, heat, exercise and avoidance of physical stress is indicated. A lumbosacral corset should be prescribed when symptoms require; continued physical therapy must not be neglected.

Management of *spondylolysis and spondylolisthesis* is similar to that described for chronic degenerative joint disease. Surgical fusion with or without prior decompression may be indicated in severe cases.

Treatment of *osteoporosis* is difficult but trial of presently accepted methods of management is worthwhile.[22] Elemental calcium in a dose of 1 g daily, and vitamin D, 50,000 units once or twice a week may be helpful. Periodic evaluation for hypercalcemia and hypercalciuria, possible complications of this regimen, should be performed. Prevention of postmenopausal osteoporosis by estrogens has been described.[23,24] The potential gains of estrogen use must be weighed against the increased risk of cardio-vascular complications and endometrial cancer.[23] Sodium fluoride therapy has been advocated, but its administration for osteoporosis remains *investigational.*[25] Osteomalacia and secondary hyperparathyroidism may develop with this agent unless calcium intake is maintained. Patients should be given a lumbodorsal corset to relieve pain and to prevent vertebral fractures resulting from excessive stress on the spine. Compression fractures are treated with bed rest for four or five days. Analgesic agents including narcotics are usually required temporarily. Progressive ambulation is permitted when pain is diminished or absent and a lumbosacral corset available. The corset should be used during the waking hours and may be needed for a long period of time or indefinitely.

In patients with metastatic *carcinoma* of the spine, roentgenologic therapy may relieve pain. Treatment of the primary neoplasm is indicated when feasible.

Most patients with *Paget's disease* do not require treatment; others respond to full doses of aspirin and mild analgesic drugs. Severe cases may require trials of newer therapeutic agents including diphosphonates,[26] thyrocalcitonin,[27,28] or mithramycin.[29] Sodium etidronate, a diphosphonate, improves clinical, biochemical, and bone-scan abnormalities.[26] A dose of 5 mg/kg body weight/day appears to be safer than higher doses, and is less likely to be associated with complications of diarrhea, bone pain, and non-traumatic fractures. Intermittent courses of therapy based on evidence of biochemical and clinical relapse are recommended. Calcitonin may similarly improve biochemical and clinical abnormalities.[27,28] Formation of neutralizing antibodies may result in drug resistance. Mithramycin, a cyto-toxic antibiotic, produces hypocalcemia and diminishes increased osteoclastic activity.[29] Hepatotoxicity is common, and thrombocytopenia is a major side effect.

Ankylosing spondylitis usually responds well to current programs of management (see Chapter 19). *Osteitis condensans ilii* usually responds to conservative therapy that includes salicylates, heat, and rest. Other non-steroidal anti-inflammatory agents may be similarly beneficial.

Spondylitis of *acute infectious* etiology requires treatment with antibiotic agents directed toward the causative organism. Bed rest and immobilization are often indicated. Surgery is not usually necessary because the involved vertebrae frequently fuse spontaneously. *Tuberculosis* of the spine is treated with appropriate antituberculous regimens, utilizing isoniazid, ethambutol and rifampin. Triple therapy is initially recommended; rifampin can usually be discontinued after a period of three to six months depending on clinical response.[30] Therapy with isoniazid and ethambutol is continued for another six to twelve months or more, with a minimum of 18 to 24 months total therapy recommended. Brace immobilization is indicated to promote fusion. Surgical arthrodesis is sometimes necessary. Drainage of abscesses may be required. Fungous infections are treated with specific antifungal agents if available. Brucellosis usually responds to tetracycline, 500 mg QID, given in combination with streptomycin, 1 g daily for three weeks.

Vertebral epiphysitis (Scheuermann's disease), when symptomatic, is treated conservatively with rest and salicylates. Physical activity should be limited. A lumbodorsal corset or brace may be required for a prolonged period for relief of symptoms and prevention of kyphosis.

Benign *coccygodynia* due to sprain or old fracture will often respond to local injections of steroid with lidocaine. A soft foam rubber pad is advisable for prolonged sitting in patients with chronic symptoms.

Surgery of the offending tumor is usually required for pain relief in patients with *benign local neoplasms*. Orthopedic and neurosurgical consultation should be sought in most cases of *fracture* of the spine. Treatment includes immobilization and appropriate surgical procedures.

Management of *scoliosis* requires extensive evaluation of the nature and etiology of the scoliosis and the structural changes that are present. In younger patients, appropriate extraspinal or intraspinal bracing should be considered. In older patients, management is conservative and similar to that prescribed for degenerative joint disease. Management of low back pain of *visceral origin* is directed to the primary disease process.

CASE HISTORIES

History 17-1. Herniated Nucleus Pulposus

S.C., a 40-year-old white female, was first seen in consultation in September, 1972, with a history of low back pain beginning approximately three years before. Low back symptoms occurred in intermittent episodes that had become progressively more frequent, severe, and prolonged. Pain was worse after sitting for a long period on a soft chair. Past treatment for acute attacks had included pelvic traction, bed rest, heat, and salicylates. Hospital admission was required in September, 1972, for an acute attack of severe low back pain with posterior radiation of pain to the left heel. Symptoms were worse with coughing, sneezing and straining at stool. The patient was unable to perform routine activities. Symptoms were not relieved by therapy with bed rest, pelvic traction, and salicylates instituted at home.

Upon physical examination at the time of consultation, the patient was in acute distress, with pain aggravated by twisting and turning motions of the back. The left sacroiliac area was tender. Flexion of the lumbosacral spine was limited and the patient was able to sit only with pain. Straight-leg-raising was accomplished to 85° on the right side but to only 45° on the left side. Sensory examinations were normal but the left ankle jerk was diminished and slight weakness of left foot dorsiflexion was noted. The remainder of her physical evaluation including pelvic and rectal examination was unremarkable. Routine laboratory studies were normal. Erythrocyte sedimentation rate was 12 mm/hour (Wintrobe). Roentgenograms of the lumbosacral spine revealed narrowing of the L5-S1 interspace. No evidence of spondylitis was seen. A diagnosis of acute herniation of the lumbosacral intervertebral disk was made.

The patient was placed on bed rest. Therapy with continuous pelvic traction, hot packs, aspirin and analgesic medications was instituted. Symptoms gradually improved over the next three to four days and gradual ambulation was begun. The patient improved on this program and was discharged from hospital after ten days. She was instructed in a physical therapy program of exercises to strengthen the abdominal muscles.

Discussion: The history and clinical course in this patient was typical of that seen in patients with herniated nucleus pulposus. Other causes of low back pain were excluded by appropriate clinical and laboratory studies. Most patients with this disorder will respond satisfactorily to an intensive program of conservative therapy. Although treatment at home is often effective, hospitalization is frequently necessary to provide a full program of management.

History 17-2. Spondylolysis and Spondylolisthesis

L.R., a 17-year-old white male, was first seen in consultation in December, 1979. He gave a history of mild back symptoms for several years. He tolerated these without great difficulty until he began work as a clerk in a grocery store six months prior to consultation. Pain, located in the low back, was aggravated by twisting and turning motions. There was no history of morning stiffness, sciatica, heel pain, urethritis, iritis, conjunctivitis, psoriasis or bowel symptoms. There was no family history of arthritis nor back difficulties. Other joints were asymptomatic and his general health was otherwise good. There was no history of back trauma.

On physical examination, abnormal findings were limited to the lumbosacral spine. Flexion was slightly limited and the lower lumbar area was tender. Straight-leg-raising was 85° on the right and 80° on the left. Height was 68″ and chest expansion 3½″. Laboratory studies revealed normal urinalysis and complete blood count. Erythrocyte sedimentation rate was 12 mm/hour (Wintrobe). Serum rheumatoid factor and antinuclear antibody studies were negative. Serum uric acid was 5.5 mg/100 ml. PA, lateral and oblique views of the lumbosacral spine revealed bilateral spondylolysis of L5. Anterior displacement of L5 on S1 was approximately 1 cm. Sclerotic changes were seen bilaterally in the region of the apophyseal joints of the L4-L5 articulation. Sacroiliac joints were roentgenographically normal.

Discussion: This patient complained of back pain aggravated by activity. Initial diagnostic considerations at the time of his examination included ankylosing spondylitis or lumbar disk herniation. Although symptoms were consistent with a diagnosis of spondylolysis and spondylolisthesis, ankylosing spondylitis should still be considered as a diagnostic possibility, because roentgenographic abnormalities may become apparent long after the onset of clinical symptoms in this disease. The patient was placed on a program of aspirin, 640 mg QID as needed for pain, heat, and exercises to strengthen his abdominal muscles. Use of a lumbosacral corset might be considered if he has more acute exacerbations and distress. Clinical observation and followup x-rays will be helpful in determining whether ankylosing spondylitis is present.

History 17-3. Osteoporosis

M.P., an 85-year-old white female, was first seen in consultation in December, 1973, for low back pain that had begun three days earlier. Pain was sudden in onset and radiated from the L4 area of the spine bilaterally in a transverse direction. There was no radiation to the legs. Motion made symptoms worse and walking was painful. History revealed the presence of rheumatoid arthritis of one year's duration, for which she was being treated with aspirin, 960 mg QID and prednisone, 2.5 mg QID.

On physical examination there was evidence of rheumatoid deformities involving the small joints of the hands, both wrists and both knees, with swelling and limitation of motion. The patient lay uncomfortably in bed and was fearful of moving lest she precipitate low back pain. Neurologic examination was within normal limits. There was moderate tenderness to percussion over the L4 area of the spine.

Hematocrit was 34%, white blood cell count was 4700/mm³ and the differential was normal. Serum calcium was 9.9 mg/100 ml and serum phosphorus was 3.7 mg/100 ml. Serum alkaline phosphatase was 9 King-Armstrong units (normal, 3 to 13 units). Serum electrolytes were normal. Erythrocyte sedimentation rate was 22 mm/hour (Wintrobe). Urinalysis was normal except for trace albumin; urine was negative for Bence Jones protein. Serum protein electrophoresis revealed essentially normal findings. Chest roentgenogram was normal. Roentgenograms of the lumbar spine showed moderately severe diffuse osteoporosis and compression of the vertebral body of L4. A diagnosis of vertebral fracture secondary to osteoporosis was made.

The patient was placed on a program of Myochrysine therapy for her rheumatoid arthritis. Gradual decrease in steroid therapy was begun. Indomethacin, 25 mg QID with food, was added as an anti-inflammatory agent. Treatment of the osteoporosis included calcium carbonate 2,500 mg/day (equivalent to 1,000 mg of elemental calcium daily), and vitamin D, 50,000 IU once a week. The patient was maintained on bed rest for several days until a lumbo-dorsal corset was obtained, at which time gradual ambulation was instituted.

Discussion: Osteoporosis is a common complication of steroid treatment in rheumatoid arthritis, likely to be seen earlier and with greater severity in older patients who already have postmenopausal or senile osteoporosis. Vigorous efforts to decrease and discontinue steroid therapy are important in the treatment of the osteoporosis. Other disorders, such as multiple myeloma, hyperparathyroidism and metastatic carcinoma, may produce a similar clinical picture. Accurate diagnosis requires exclusion of these other entities as part of the routine evaluation.

History 17-4. Multiple Myeloma

A.L., a 34-year-old white male, was first seen in January, 1969, for a routine physical examination. He had no specific complaints and system review and past medical history were unremarkable. Clinical and laboratory studies revealed no evidence of significant disease. The patient was seen again for his annual examination in January, 1970. He once again felt in good general health except for a feeling of cracking sensations in the neck and low back. Symptoms were aggravated by long hours of driving in his occupation as a salesman. Physical examination was completely negative. Roentgenograms of the cervical and lumbosacral spine were normal. Symptoms were relieved by use of a firm seat support while driving.

The patient was seen again at annual intervals. He had no notable complaints and routine laboratory studies were normal. In April, 1973, he appeared with a complaint of moderately severe pain and spasm in the muscles of the low back with pain radiating to the left leg. System review revealed dysuria with frequency of urination. He had no eye symptoms nor symptoms in peripheral joints. Physical examination was normal except for the presence of a slightly boggy prostate gland. Lumbosacral spine motions were completely normal. Initial clinical impressions included prostatitis, degenerative disease of the lumbar spine, incomplete Reiter's syndrome, or ankylosing spondylitis.

Urinalysis was normal, hematocrit was 33%, white blood cell count was 3900/mm³ with 45% neutrophils, and erythrocyte sedimentation rate was

44 mm/hour (Wintrobe). Repeat leukocyte counts ranged from 2900 to 4000/mm³. Roentgenograms of the lumbosacral spine were reported to be within normal limits. Hematology consultation was requested to evaluate the leukopenia and anemia. Bone marrow aspiration study revealed numerous plasma cells, many of which were binucleated. Serum protein electrophoresis showed a monoclonal peak in the gamma globulin region. Roentgenographic bone survey revealed numerous punched out lesions in the skull and long bones consistent with multiple myeloma. Retrospective review of his lumbosacral spine films showed early lytic lesions.

Discussion: This patient had a history of intermittent mild low back and neck pain of several years' duration. Clinical examination and laboratory studies, including roentgenograms, were negative for any serious underlying disorder and the patient responded to symptomatic therapy. Diagnostic considerations did not include multiple myeloma. Lumbosacral spine films were initially interpreted as normal. Hematologic abnormalities were the clue to the presence of serious systemic disease.

History 17-5. Acute Leukemia

S.R., a 24-year-old white male, was well until three weeks prior to consultation, at which time he had noted pain in the low back and thighs, and stiffness in the region of the cervical spine. Pain was aggravated by motion and was worse at night. Aspirin, 640 mg TID, provided mild symptomatic help. Approximately two weeks after the onset of symptoms, the patient developed low-grade fever and night sweats. There was no prior history of musculoskeletal symptoms. System review revealed no evidence of Raynaud's phenomenon, conjunctivitis or iritis, urethritis, colitis, or skin rash. He had been treated for gonococcal urethritis six months prior. The patient worked as a car salesman and had not left this area of the country for the previous two years.

On physical examination, blood pressure was 120/90 mm Hg. Temperature was 38° C, pulse was 90/minute, and respirations were 22/minute. The patient appeared pale and acutely ill. He lay quietly in bed and was afraid to move lest he precipitate more severe pain. The remainder of the examination was normal except for decreased mobility of the lumbar spine and tenderness over the sacroiliac joints. No peripheral joint abnormalities were noted. Muscles were strong and nontender. Clinical diagnostic considerations included ankylosing or infectious spondylitis, regional enteritis with spondylitis, vasculitis, or unusual infections such as brucellosis or trichinosis.

Hematocrit was 42%, white blood cell count was 10,200/mm³, and erythrocyte sedimentation rate was 38 mm/hour (Wintrobe). Differential white blood count showed 49% neutrophils, 25% lymphocytes, 5% monocytes, 1% eosinophils, 15% band forms, 1 myelocyte and 4% metamyelocytes. Studies for serum rheumatoid factor and antinuclear antibody and LE cell determinations were negative. Urinalysis, serum electrolytes, fasting blood sugar, serum protein bound iodine and serum calcium and phosphorus studies were normal. Serum alkaline phosphatase was 25 King-Armstrong units (normal, 3 to 13 units). Serum creatine phosphokinase was normal. Heterophile antibody titer was negative. Brucella agglutination, cold agglutinin and febrile agglutinin studies were negative. Australia antigen was absent in the serum. Cultures of blood, throat, and urine were nonrevealing. Roentgenograms of the chest and lumbosacral spine were normal. The patient continued to run a febrile course with temperatures up to 39° C. On the basis of the abnormal differential blood cell count, hematologic consultation was requested. Sternal marrow aspiration study revealed uniform replacement of the marrow with immature blast cells, probably granulocytic in origin. A diagnosis of acute myeloproliferative disease, probably acute granulocytic leukemia, was made.

Discussion: This patient had a history suggestive of primary musculo-skeletal disease. Ankylosing spondylitis was considered on the basis of his severe low back pain and sacroiliac tenderness. Although fever is not common in ankylosing spondylitis, moderate temperature elevation occasionally occurs. Other causes of spondylitis more frequently associated with fever, such as infectious spondylitis or spondylitis associated with regional enteritis or chronic ulcerative colitis, were also considered. Leukemic involvement of the marrow produced symptoms highly suggestive of a primary rheumatic disorder.

The patient was placed on an intensive therapeutic program including pred-nisone, vincristine sulfate, cytosine arabinoside and cyclophosphamide. Re-sponse to therapy was poor, and other antimetabolic agents were added. The patient died from his primary disease about four months later.

History 17-6. Paget's Disease

O.B., a 65-year-old white male, was first seen in consultation in February, 1969. He gave a history of having been well until two years prior, when he noted pain in the low back. Pain was worse in the morning and was associ-ated with moderate stiffness. Pain was not accentuated with cough, sneeze or other strain, and no sciatic radiation of pain was observed. Twisting or turn-ing in bed during the night awakened him at times. There was no history of specific back injury. He was treated with aspirin, 640 mg QID, with little relief. Symptoms continued with slow progression in severity. Further treat-ment with various anti-inflammatory and analgesic agents gave limited help. The patient considered himself to be in otherwise good health. System review was negative and past medical history was noncontributory. The patient had worked as an accountant and was now retired.

On physical examination, abnormal findings were limited to the spine. The lumbar spine was slightly tender to percussion and moderately limited in all directions. Cervical spine motions were also slightly limited. Rectal examina-tion was negative. Hematocrit was 40%, white blood cell count was 9500/mm^3 with a normal differential, erythrocyte sedimentation rate was 18 mm/hour (Wintrobe), and urinalysis was normal. Serum studies for rheumatoid factor and antinuclear antibody were negative. Serum uric acid was 6.1 mg/100 ml. Serum alkaline phosphatase was 36 King-Armstrong units (normal, 3 to 13). Serum calcium, phosphorus and acid phosphatase were normal. Serum pro-tein electrophoresis was within normal limits. Urine was negative for Bence Jones protein. Chest roentgenogram was normal. Roentgenograms of the lumbo-sacral spine and pelvis revealed Paget's changes in the pelvic bones, the proximal end of the left femur, and the third, fourth and fifth lumbar vertebrae. Bone changes were characterized by coarsening of trabecular structure. The patient was placed on therapy with aspirin, 960 mg QID, on a regular basis. Symp-toms were moderately improved but later gradually increased in severity. The patient was begun on therapy with thyrocalcitonin.

Discussion: At first, degenerative joint disease in the lumbar spine was con-sidered the most likely diagnosis for this patient. Radiologic studies revealed severe diffuse bone involvement with Paget's disease. Symptoms were consis-tent with this radiologic finding. Other causes of bone disease such as neo-plasm, multiple myeloma and osteoporosis appeared unlikely on the basis of typical radiologic appearance, general good health and otherwise normal laboratory results. This patient was placed on thyrocalcitonin which had become available at the time he was seen. Presently, sodium etidronate would be con-sidered the drug of first choice by many authorities, based on therapeutic effec-tiveness and ease of administration.

History 17-7.   Ankylosing Spondylitis

M.D., a 32-year-old white male, was first seen for evaluation in January, 1972. He gave a history of low back pain of approximately five years' duration. Low back symptoms were associated with radiation of pain from the low back to both knees. Pain radiation involved the left and right side separately, and at times both sides simultaneously. Morning stiffness lasting 15 to 30 minutes daily had been noted in the low back for the past several years. During the past year the patient had pain and stiffness of the proximal interphalangeal (PIP) joint of the right index finger, and mild stiffness of the PIP joint of the left index finger. No other joint symptoms were noted. The patient was seen by a neurosurgeon who made a clinical diagnosis of herniated disk disease. PA, lateral and oblique roentgenographic views of the lumbosacral spine were read as normal. Lumbar myelogram demonstrated a possible extradural defect at L4-L5 on the right, consistent with a herniated disk. At surgery, minimal abnormalities were noted. The patient was referred for rheumatologic evaluation when low back pain persisted. Review of preoperative roentgenograms of the pelvis and lumbosacral spine revealed that the sacroiliac joints had poorly defined margins and sclerotic borders. The changes were consistent with a diagnosis of ankylosing spondylitis. The patient was placed on buffered aspirin, 640 mg QID, with excellent relief of back pain. He was instructed in a full exercise program for ankylosing spondylitis. In addition, he was advised to have adequate rest and to use a firm mattress and no pillow for sleeping. The patient did well on this program.

Discussion: In this patient, low back pain due to ankylosing spondylitis was initially misdiagnosed as herniated disk disease. Chronic low back pain and morning stiffness associated with incomplete bilateral sciatica are typical findings in patients with ankylosing spondylitis. Roentgenographic changes may be minimal or absent early, in which case the diagnosis remains presumptive. The extradural defect seen on lumbar myelography in this case was equivocal in appearance and did not adequately explain the patient's symptoms.

History 17-8.   Tuberculous Spondylitis

M.L., a 33-year-old Iranian male, was well until November, 1970, when he noted mild but persistent low back pain. Aching was associated with pain radiating into both upper gluteal areas. He attributed his symptoms to physical exertion associated with moving heavy furniture about his office. Low-grade symptoms continued and he was treated with mild analgesic medications. Radiologic examination of the lumbosacral spine was normal. Symptoms were not especially disabling except for occasional mild episodes, at which time he obtained relief by increased rest and regular intake of aspirin. Approximately one year after onset, symptoms became more persistent and severe. In addition to low back pain, morning stiffness lasting 15 to 30 minutes was noted. The patient was referred at that time for rheumatologic evaluation. System review was otherwise negative, except for his low back complaints. There was no associated history of other joint symptoms, Raynaud's phenomenon, psoriasis or other skin rash, iritis, urethritis, pleurisy, alopecia, oral lesions, dry mouth or eyes, or other joint symptoms. He denied symptoms of anorexia, weight loss, fever or night sweats. Past medical history was noncontributory. He had emigrated to the United States from Iran in 1967, following which he had attended college and started his own business.

Physical examination revealed mild limitation of the lumbar spine, with tenderness to percussion over the L5-S1 area. The remainder of his examination was otherwise normal. Initial diagnostic considerations included ankylosing spondylitis or degenerative disease of the intervertebral disk. Hematocrit was 44%, white blood cell count was 8600/mm³ with a normal differential, erythrocyte sedimentation rate was 27 mm/hour (Wintrobe), and urinalysis was normal. Serum electrolytes, calcium, phosphorus, glutamic oxaloacetic transaminase, and serologic test for syphilis were normal or negative. Serum protein electrophoresis showed slight elevation of gamma globulin. Serum alkaline phosphatase was normal. Studies for serum rheumatoid factor, antinuclear antibody, and antibodies to Brucella were negative.

Roentgenograms of the lumbosacral spine revealed a pathologic fracture at the anterior inferior portion of the body of the L5 vertebra. In addition, there was irregular sclerosis of the inferior aspect of the body of L5 and the superior aspect of the body of S1. The L5-S1 interspace was narrowed. A bulging mass was seen in the right parapsoas region. Tuberculin skin test was strongly positive. Skin tests for histoplasmosis and coccidioidomycosis were negative. Urine cultures for tuberculosis were negative. Culture of material obtained by closed needle aspiration of the L5 region was negative for tuberculous infection. Open biopsy of the L5-S1 area was performed by a retroperitoneal approach. Study of biopsy material revealed caseating necrosis and granulomatous inflammation of bone and fibrous connective tissue consistent with tuberculosis. Acid fast stains were negative. Positive cultures for Mycobacterium tuberculosis were subsequently reported.

Discussion: This case demonstrates the insidious manner in which tuberculous spondylitis frequently develops. Symptoms were initially attributed to physical trauma; when evaluated later, they were attributed to ankylosing spondylitis or degenerative disease of the intervertebral disks. Diagnosis was made when the disease was already in advanced state. The patient was treated with isoniazid, ethambutol and rifampin, and a Knight spinal brace was prescribed. Subsequent studies showed progressive healing of the lesion with an excellent clinical response. Rifampin was discontinued after six months and the patient was continued on isoniazid and ethambutol. Therapy for a total of two years led to complete recovery.

History 17-9. Coccygodynia

B.G., a 59-year-old white female, was first seen in consultation in September, 1971. She was in good health until approximately two months previously, when she noted severe pain and tenderness at the base of the spine when sitting. There was no history of trauma to the sacrococcygeal area and no history of joint symptoms elsewhere. Physical examination was negative except for moderate tenderness on pressure over the coccygeal area. Rectal examination revealed a moderately mobile coccyx and tenderness over the coccygeal area and paracoccygeal soft tissue attachments. Pelvic examination was normal. Roentgenograms of the lumbosacral spine were normal. A diagnosis of coccygodynia was made and steroid with lidocaine was injected into the tender area over the coccyx. The patient was advised to use soft chairs or a foam rubber cushion when sitting. The patient had excellent relief of symptoms following local steroid injection. No recurrence of symptoms over a period of several months was noted.

Discussion: This patient had symptoms consistent with coccygodynia characterized by pain in the coccygeal area on sitting and local tenderness to pressure and palpation over the coccygeal area. Frequently, such cases have a prior history of trauma. Although the diagnosis is readily made in most cases, disorders in the pelvic and rectal area and other diseases of bone must be excluded as part of the routine clinical and laboratory evaluation.

REFERENCES

1. Resnick, D., Shaul, S. R. and Robins, J. M.: Diffuse idiopathic skeletal hyperostosis (DISH): Forestier's disease with extraspinal manifestations. Radiology 115:513, 1975.
2. Utsinger, P. D., Resnick, D. and Shapiro, R. F.: Diffuse skeletal abnormalities in Forestier's disease. Arch Int Med 136:763, 1976.
3. Resnick, D., Shapiro, R. F., Weisner, K. B. et al.: Diffuse idiopathic skeletal hyperostosis (DISH) (ankylosing hyperostosis of Forestier and Rotes-Querol). Sem Arth Rheum 7:153, 1978.
4. Kirkaldy-Willis, W. H., Paine, K. W. E., Cauchoix, J. et al.: Lumbar spinal stenosis. Clin Orthop 99:30, 1974.
5. Arnoldi, C. C. et al.: Lumbar spinal stenosis and nerve root entrapment syndromes—definition and classification. Clin Ortho 115:4, 1976.
6. Singh, A. and Joly, S. S.: Endemic fluorosis. Quart J Med 30:357, 1961.
7. Sigler, J. W. et al.: Clinical features of ankylosing spondylitis. Clin Orthop 74: 14, 1971.
8. Calin, A. et al.: Clinical history as a screening test for ankylosing spondylitis. JAMA 237:2613, 1977.
9. Woodrow, J. C.: Histocompatibility antigens and rheumatic diseases. Sem Arth Rheum 6:257, 1977.
10. McEwen, C. et al.: Ankylosing spondylitis and spondylitis accompanying ulcerative colitis, regional enteritis, psoriasis and Reiter's disease: a comparative study. Arthritis Rheum 14:291, 1971.
11. DeBosset, P., Gordon, D. A., Smythe, H. A. et al.: Comparison of osteitis condensans ilii and ankylosing spondylitis in female patients: clinical, radiological and HLA typing characteristics. J Chron Dis 31:171, 1978.
12. Kemp, H. B. S., Jackson, J. W., Jeremiak, J. D. et al.: Pyogenic infections occurring primarily in intervertebral disks. J Bone Joint Surg 55B:698, 1973.
13. Musher, D. M., Thorsteinsson, S. B., Minuth, J. N. et al.: Vertebral osteomyelitis. Arch Int Med 136:105, 1976.
14. Berney, S., Goldstein, M. and Bishko, F.: Clinical and diagnostic features of tuberculous arthritis. Am J Med 53:36, 1972.
15. Glenn, W. V., Rhodes, M. L., Altschuler, E. M. et al.: Multiplanar display computerized body tomography applications in the lumbar spine. Spine 4:282, 1979.
16. Meyer, G. A., Haughton, V. M. and Williams, A. L.: Diagnosis of herniated lumbar disk with computed tomography. N Engl J Med 301:1166, 1979.
17. Russell, A. S., Lentle, B. C. and Percy, J. S.: Investigation of sacro-iliac disease: comparative evaluation of radiological and radionuclide techniques. J Rheumatol 2:45, 1975.
18. Namey, T. C., McIntyre, J., Buse, M. et al.: Nucleographic studies of axial spondyloarthritides. I. Quantitative sacro-iliac scintigraphy in early HLA-B27 associated sacro-iliitis. Arthritis Rheum 20:1058, 1977.
19. Goldberg, R. P., Genant, H. K., Shimshak, R. et al.: Applications and limitations of quantitative sacro-iliac joint scintigraphy. Radiology 128:683, 1978.
20. Ho, G., Sadovnikoff, N., Malhotra, C. M. et al.: Quantitative sacroiliac joint scintigraphy: a critical assessment. Arthritis Rheum 22:837, 1979.
21. Esdaile, J. M., Rosenthall, L., Terkletaub, R. et al.: Prospective evaluation of sacro-iliac scintigraphy in chronic inflammatory back pain. Arthritis Rheum 23:998, 1980.
22. Hahn, E. J. and Hahn, B. H.: Osteopenia in patients with rheumatic diseases: principles of diagnosis and therapy. Sem Arth Rheum 6:165, 1976.
23. Lindsay, R., Aitken, J. M., Anderson, J. B. et al.: Long-term prevention of postmenopausal osteoporosis by estrogen. Lancet, May 15, 1976.
24. Christiansen, C., Christensen, M. S., McNair, P. et al.: Prevention of early postmenopausal bone loss: controlled 2-year study in 315 normal females. Eur J Clin Invest 10:273, 1980.
25. Jowsey, J. et al.: Effect of combined therapy with sodium fluoride, vitamin D and calcium in osteoporosis. Am J Med 53:43, 1972.

11

26. Khairi, M. R. A., Altman, R. D., DeRosa, G. P. et al.: Sodium etidronate in the treatment of Paget's disease of bone. Ann Int Med 87:656, 1977.
27. Haddad, J. F., Birge, S. J. and Avioli, L. V.: Effects of prolonged thyrocalcitonin administration on Paget's disease of bone. N Engl J Med 283:549, 1970.
28. Sturtridge, W. C., Harrison, J. E. and Wilson, D. R.: Long-term treatment of Paget's disease of bone with sodium calcitonin. Can Med Assn J 117:1031, 1977.
29. Lebbin, D., Ryan, W. G. and Schwartz, T. B.: Outpatient treatment of Paget's disease of bone with mithramycin. Ann Int Med 81:635, 1974.
30. Friedman, B. and Kapur, V. N.: Newer knowledge of chemotherapy in treatment of tuberculosis of bone joints. Clin Orthop 97:5, 1973.

CHAPTER 18

THE PAINFUL FOOT

Foot pain of musculoskeletal origin is a common cause of disability. It is frequently the primary complaint of the patient coming into the physician's office. Although often benign and seemingly unimportant, the symptoms are distressing to the patient. Careful study and appropriate therapy to relieve symptoms can be rewarding.

DIFFERENTIAL DIAGNOSIS

The differential diagnosis of foot pain varies with the area of the foot involved. The following diagnostic considerations are divided on the basis of location of symptoms, proceeding from the anterior to the posterior aspect of the foot.

Painful Swollen Great Toe (First Metatarsophalangeal Joint)

Acute gouty arthritis characteristically produces acute pain, tenderness, and swelling of the first metatarsophalangeal (MTP) joint at the base of the great toe. Not all gouty attacks, however, occur in the big toe. In many patients, the first attack occurs in another joint such as the tarsal area, ankle or knee. Similarly, other disorders may cause acute painful swelling of the great toe. A diagnosis of gout, although primarily suspected when acute symptoms develop in this joint, should not be made without considering other possible diagnoses.

The patient with acute gouty arthritis usually gives a rather characteristic history. Acute onset occurring during the night is common. The pain may be so exquisite that even movement of the bed covers or someone walking heavily about the room may increase the already severe throbbing pain. As swelling and inflammation progress, cutaneous changes of inflammation are noted. Skin desquamation occurs as the attack reaches its crest or begins to wane. The inflammation often simulates cellulitis and misdiagnosis is

307

common. On physical examination the inflammation is obvious. Pain and tenderness in gout are likely to be more pronounced medially, in contrast to rheumatoid arthritis, in which tenderness is often maximal at the inferior aspect of the joint.

Pseudogout is characterized by calcifications in hyaline or fibroarticular cartilage and the presence of calcium pyrophosphate crystals in synovial fluid. Acute attacks of crystal-induced arthritis are common. The most common site of attack is the knee. Podagra, or first MTP joint involvement, occurs much less frequently than in true gout.

Rheumatoid arthritis may produce acute inflammation of the metatarsophalangeal joints. Although the first MTP joint is frequently involved, other MTP joints are often affected simultaneously. This is in contrast to gout, in which the acute attack is usually localized to the first MTP joint alone. Acute inflammation of the toes is characteristic of the episodic form of rheumatoid arthritis (see Chapter 8). Acute attacks of pain resolve over several days. A clinical syndrome similar to episodic rheumatoid arthritis is *palindromic rheumatism* (see Chapter 8), which also is characterized by acute attacks of arthritis. Because several connective tissue diseases may simulate palindromic rheumatism during their early phases, diagnosis depends on continued observation.

Acute joint symptoms may result from *trauma*. This often poses a problem in differential diagnosis, because both acute gout and rheumatoid arthritis may be precipitated by trauma. In patients with arthritis due to trauma alone, pain usually develops immediately after the injury and symptoms are proportional to the extent of the injury. In patients in whom gout or rheumatoid inflammation are precipitated by trauma, pain is usually delayed in onset and the severity of symptoms is out of proportion to that anticipated from the injury.

Cellulitis may simulate acute arthritis because it also is characterized by pain, tenderness, increased warmth and swelling. Search for local entry sites of infection should be carried out if this diagnosis is suspected. Blood cultures are frequently positive as a supportive corollary finding. Symptoms respond to appropriate antibiotic therapy based on culture and sensitivity studies.

Pain and swelling in the first MTP joint due to *osteoarthritis* are extremely common; however, symptoms are low-grade and chronic in contrast to the foregoing diseases. Ill-fitting shoes or mild trauma aggravate the symptoms. Roentgenograms reveal joint space narrowing, bony sclerosis, and osteophyte formation. Treatment is usually conservative; well-fitting bunion-last shoes and mild anti-inflammatory drugs are prescribed. Surgery is indicated in patients who do not respond to a conservative program. Excellent relief is anticipated.

Occasionally, acute symptoms may occur with osteoarthritis of the great toe when there is acute inflammation of the overlying bursa. The bursa is usually readily outlined and fluid can be obtained on aspiration. Response to injection of local steroid with lidocaine into the bursa is good.

Symptoms Involving Interphalangeal Joints

Any form of arthritis that affects peripheral joints may involve interphalangeal joints of the toes. Involvement of these joints is particularly characteristic of *psoriatic arthritis,* the arthritis of *ulcerative colitis* and *regional enteritis,* and the arthritis of *Reiter's syndrome.* In patients with these disorders, involvement of the distal and proximal interphalangeal joints, associated with flexor tenosynovitis, produces a characteristic sausage-shaped swelling of the involved digit (Fig. 7-6). The history should specifically include questions concerning skin rash consistent with psoriasis, chronic diarrheal symptoms, or evidence of the typical triad of arthritis, urethritis and conjunctivitis seen in Reiter's syndrome.

Symptoms Involving Other Metatarsophalangeal Joints

These joints may also be involved in any of the systemic arthritides that produce peripheral joint symptoms. *Rheumatoid arthritis* classically involves these joints and may produce severe disability early in the course of the disease. Hammer-toes and subluxation of the joints are common. In addition to the usual systemic management, the use of transverse metatarsal pads inside the shoes or transverse metatarsal bars on the soles aids relief. Pads are usually tried first, because if they give relief, they can be conveniently transferred to various pairs of shoes. If the patient does not respond, transverse metatarsal bars are then prescribed. These often provide more effective relief but have to be placed on each pair of shoes separately. Local injection of steroids is valuable when one or two joints are especially bothersome.

Metatarsal Pain

Morton's metatarsalgia produces severe cramping pains in the anterior part of the foot. Pain is usually precipitated by weight-bearing and walking. The patient gets relief by removing the shoe and rubbing the toes. The syndrome occurs most frequently in the third and fourth interspaces. Etiologic considerations include excessive mobility of the fourth metatarsal,[1] nerve compression between flattened metatarsal heads,[2,3] or impingement of the nerve as it angulates over the transverse tarsal ligament.[2,3] Alternatively, the syndrome may result from ischemia of the plantar nerve induced by traumatic degeneration of the plantar digital artery. Chronic compression and ischemia may eventually lead to fibrosis and neuroma formation.

In uncomplicated Morton's metatarsalgia, pain occurs only on weight-bearing and use. Constant pain suggests the presence of a neuroma, in which case a mass often can be palpated between the metatarsal heads when the heads have been squeezed together.

Therapy of simple metatarsalgia is conservative. Well-fitting shoes and a transverse metatarsal pad or metatarsal bar should be prescribed. Local injection of the tender area with steroids and lidocaine provides relief for acute symptoms. In patients in whom the diagnosis of neuroma is fairly well corroborated and who do not respond to conservative measures, excision of the neuroma should be considered.

Fracture of a metatarsal bone near its neck may occur in the absence of definitive trauma, the so-called *fatigue* or *march fracture*. Fracture most often involves the necks of the second or third metatarsals. The propensity for this site may be related to congenital shortening of the first metatarsal bone, since dorsiflexion then occurs across the necks of the second and third metatarsals. This type of fracture is not uncommon following continual stress on long military marches; thus the name "march fracture." Tenderness is followed by swelling due to callus formation in healing. Roentgenograms of the foot are required for diagnosis, although the frac-

Figure 18-1. Fatigue fracture, second metatarsal bone of left foot. Fracture with callus formation was not visible until several weeks after onset of foot pain.

Figure 18-2. Sudeck's atrophy (post-traumatic osteoporosis). Erythema and edema of the right foot were associated with severe pain. (Courtesy, Dr. F. Bishko)

ture may not be evident until days or weeks following onset of symptoms (Fig. 18-1). Periodic re-examination should be performed if the diagnosis is suspected. The fracture is treated by immobilizing the limb in a plaster cast that extends up to the knee until healing.

Sudeck's atrophy (post-traumatic osteoporosis) is closely related to shoulder-hand syndrome seen in the upper extremity (see Chapter 15). Of unknown etiology, it is characterized by a vasomotor disturbance with hyperemia and atrophy of bone. Precipitating causes include trauma, which is often minimal, local infections, or neoplasm. Pain, edema, and local heat are the earliest manifestations (Fig. 18-2). Later, the skin becomes cold, cyanotic, and atrophic. Severe secondary trophic changes eventually ensue. Roentgenographic studies show a patchy bone atrophy after four to six weeks (Fig. 18-3). Later, the osteoporosis becomes diffuse.

Figure 18-3.   Sudeck's atrophy. Roentgenogram reveals osteoporotic changes throughout tarsal, metatarsal and phalangeal areas.

Mild cases respond to aspirin, analgesic agents, and physical therapy. Contrast baths, warm soaks, or sometimes cold applications are particularly helpful. More severe cases require a trial of systemic corticosteroids such as prednisone in a dose of 30 to 60 mg a day. As symptoms are relieved, the dose is gradually diminished and then discontinued over a period of six to seven weeks. In patients in whom steroids have failed or are contraindicated, a trial of lumbar sympathetic blocks repeated every other day for a series of four to eight injections may be effective. Lumbar sympathectomy should be considered when local blocks are only temporarily successful.

Tarsal Pain

Sudeck's atrophy (see preceding discussion) frequently involves the tarsal as well as metatarsal bones.

Various forms of *flat feet* (pes planus) cause pain in the tarsal area. Weakness, aching and cramps may occur. Flat feet can be classified as flexible (flaccid) type with normal peroneal muscles, rigid type with normal peroneals, and rigid type with spastic peroneals (peroneal spastic flat foot). In all cases, the longitudinal arch is depressed in association with medial prominence of the foot. In the flexible type, the longitudinal arch is depressed with weight-bearing and assumes a normal shape at rest. The joints of the foot may be hypermobile and the Achilles tendon may be short. This type of flat foot is often asymptomatic but may become painful during adolescence. Conservative therapy utilizing arch supports and corrective exercises is usually beneficial. Heat or contrast baths are helpful. In more severe cases, corrective shoes and medial heel wedges are prescribed. Surgery, including tendon transfers and arthrodesis, is occasionally required. Flexible flat foot is common in blacks and the American Indian; in these individuals, this condition can almost be considered physiologic. Symptoms related to anatomy are uncommon and no specific therapy is usually required.

Rigid flat foot with normal peroneal muscles may result secondary to infectious or rheumatoid arthritis or following injury to the tarsal areas. Triple arthrodesis is probably the most satisfactory form of therapy. Rigid flat foot with spastic peroneal muscles is most often due to congenital fusion (coalition) of the tarsal bones. Other cases result secondary to infectious or rheumatoid arthritis or traumatic malalignment of joints. Joint motion is limited and the peroneal muscles are spastic. The spasm probably represents reflex muscle spasm due to pain. Initial therapy should be conservative; arch supports alone are often effective. Immobilization in a plaster cast may be required for management of acute painful episodes. Excision of bony bars early is helpful in certain forms of congenital coalition syndrome. In other cases, treatment by triple arthrodesis must be considered.

Severe pain in the tarsal area may be due to *neuropathic (Charcot) joints*. Although any chronic neuropathy, such as that seen in tabes dorsalis or syringomyelia, may be the cause of this disorder, diabetic neuropathy is the most common etiology. Pain on walking is the earliest symptom; later, pain occurs even at rest. The tarsal area is warm, tender, and swollen. Roentgenograms reveal extensive disorganization of joint structures in the area of involvement. Early changes are characterized by severe bone atrophy; later changes reveal a florid osteoarthritis. Periosteal reaction is common.

Tarsal tunnel syndrome is an entrapment neuropathy of the posterior tibial nerve due to compression as it passes through a tunnel beneath the flexor retinaculum on the medial side of the ankle. Symptoms are characterized by aching, burning, and paresthesia of the plantar surface of the foot. The distal aspect of the foot is more prominently involved, but heel involvement is occasionally noted. Physical examination may reveal sensory loss, but this finding is variable. Tapping of the nerve with the finger or a reflex hammer, or firm rolling pressure at the flexor retinaculum located posterior and inferior to the medial malleolus often produces a positive Tinel sign. Tarsal tunnel compression most commonly results from tenosynovitis of one or more of the tendons passing through the tarsal tunnel, or may be associated with fracture or dislocation of the talus, calcaneus, or medial malleolus. In other patients, no obvious local etiologic factor is present and underlying diseases such as those noted in patients with carpal tunnel syndrome (see Chapter 15) should be investigated. Clinical suspicion of this syndrome may be confirmed by nerve conduction studies. Normal values, however, do not exclude the diagnosis. Symptoms frequently respond well to local injection of a corticosteroid/local anesthetic injection into the region of the tarsal tunnel. A good response is an excellent diagnostic test.

Heel Pain

Plantar fasciitis is a common cause of heel pain. It may be localized or systemic in origin. The etiology of localized fasciitis is primarily mechanical, the result of repeated microtrauma. The origin and insertion of the plantar fascia are such that it acts as a bowstring for the foot. Tension on the fascia exerts a pull at its origin, which eventually leads to an inflammatory periostitis at its attachment to the os calcis. Calcaneal spur formation results from stimulation of bone; accordingly, the calcaneal spur may be secondary to inflammation rather than a primary abnormality.

Pain is the primary symptom of localized fasciitis. Physical examination reveals a tender spot about two inches from the point of the heel. Ossifica-

Figure 18-4. Periosteal reaction with new bone formation involves the attachments of the plantar fascia and Achilles tendon in this patient with ankylosing spondylitis.

tion of the fascia in the form of spur formation may be present on x-ray. Calcaneal spurs are usually asymptomatic and an innocent bystander unless associated with active fasciitis. However, large spurs may contribute secondarily to pain by applying pressure on the plantar tissues.

Fasciitis (calcaneal periostitis) occurs as a manifestation of systemic diseases, particularly in the seronegative spondyloarthropathies such as ankylosing spondylitis (Fig. 18-4) and Reiter's syndrome. Symptoms may be most severe at the heels or they may be diffuse. The periosteal reaction is often less dense than that seen in idiopathic fasciitis; a fluffy periostitis on roentgenogram is characteristic.

Both local and general management are to be considered in the management of plantar fasciitis. Rest with avoidance of excess weight-bearing, and the use of a soft foam-rubber heel pad or cutout is helpful. Local injection with steroid and lidocaine into the point of maximal tenderness is usually effective. Recurrences may be minimized by use of an arch support which relieves pull by the plantar fascia at its origin. Aspirin and some of the newer nonsteroidal anti-inflammatory agents are helpful if symptoms are more chronic; they are particularly useful when fasciitis is associated with a generalized connective tissue disorder.

Calcaneal epiphysitis, a form of osteochondritis, usually occurs in younger patients. The child complains of pain at the back of the heel and usually limps to relieve distress. Roentgenograms reveal areas of osteoporosis interspersed with areas of increased bone density. The disease is usually self-limited and responds to conservative symptomatic measures. In particular, rest, avoidance of excess weight-bearing, the use of foam rubber heel cushions, and mild anti-inflammatory medications are beneficial.

Inflammation of the bursa underlying the Achilles tendon *(Achilles bursitis)* or inflammation of the tendon itself *(Achilles tendinitis)* causes pain at the back of the heel. Inflammation may result from systemic disease or from local trauma, such as that caused by ill-fitting shoes. Diagnostic studies to rule out systemic connective tissue disease should be performed when symptoms are severe and persistent. Similar to plantar fasciitis, symptoms in this area are often an early manifestation of seronegative spondyloarthropathies such as ankylosing spondylitis, Reiter's syndrome, and ulcerative colitis. Patients with achilles bursitis or tendinitis are benefited by the use of a heel lift which diminishes tendon pull in walking. Aspirin and other nonsteroidal anti-inflammatory agents are often helpful. Immobilization for short periods of time is indicated when symptoms are more persistent. Local steroid injections into and around the Achilles tendon are to be avoided because of the risk of promoting acute tendon rupture secondary to steroid-induced tendon atrophy.

Rupture of the Achilles tendon is most commonly exercise-related; it is being seen more frequently in association with intermittent sporadic exercise programs. Symptoms are sudden and characterized by an audible snap, calf pain, and inability to stand up on the toes. Immobilization or complete surgical repair may be necessary, depending on the extent and completeness of the injury.

Post-traumatic osteoporosis (Sudeck's atrophy) may cause heel pain, although, as noted earlier, pain usually occurs throughout the foot. *Paget's disease* is an uncommon cause of heel pain, but it may cause pain at night and after weight-bearing.

Ischemic vascular disease with claudication may cause foot pain. Symptoms are characteristically associated with walking and are relieved readily by standing or sitting. Physical examination demonstrates severely diminished or absent pedal pulses. Trophic changes associated with ischemia are often present. Laboratory evidence of diabetes mellitus or elevated serum lipids is frequently noted.

Neuropathies cause foot pain with burning and dysesthesia. They are usually related to systemic disorders, which should be sought by appropriate clinical and laboratory studies.

Firm nodules may be visualized at the lower end of the Achilles tendon, often associated with the use of high-heeled pumps or loafers.[4] These nodules, commonly called *"pump bumps,"* are usually asymptomatic but may be associated with inflammation if secondary bursitis occurs.

Piezogenic papules are an uncommon cause of pain in the area of the heel.[5] They result from herniations of fat at the medial inferior border of the heel and appear only upon weight-bearing. Weight reduction and use of heel pads or crepe-soled shoes are helpful in management.

CASE HISTORIES

History 18-1.   Gout

S.M.N., a 38-year-old white male, gave a history of joint pains beginning in February, 1970. At that time, on the second day of a skiing excursion, he was awakened during the night by moderately severe pain in the left tarsal area. There was no history of specific trauma. Roentgenographic study of the left foot taken the following morning was normal. He was treated with heat and a walking splint. Symptoms resolved after approximately ten days. He was completely asymptomatic until January, 1972, when he noted tenderness and slight swelling of the left tarsal area several hours following a game of paddleball. He attributed symptoms to a slight twisting injury suffered during the game. Pain and tenderness persisted. Roentgenograms of the foot performed the next morning were normal. Symptoms resolved after several days.

In June, 1973, he noted acute onset of pain in the dorsum of the right tarsal area. There was no history of trauma and the patient had not recently engaged in any athletic activities. Symptoms resolved after several days, but recurred on July 5th, 1973, when he was awakened with soreness and tenderness in the right tarsal area. He attributed his symptoms to a slight twist of the foot suffered while walking to his office that day. The patient was first seen for evaluation at this time. The history was negative for joint symptoms elsewhere. There was no history of renal stones nor family history of gout. The patient considered himself to be in generally good health and system review was otherwise negative. Physical examination was completely normal except for tenderness and a slight increase in temperature over the dorsum of the tarsal area of the right foot. Laboratory studies showed normal hematocrit, white blood cell count and differential, erythrocyte sedimentation rate and urinalysis. Serum rheumatoid factor and antinuclear antibody studies were negative. Serum uric acid was 11.7 mg/100 ml. Repeat serum uric acid study several days later revealed a level of 10.9 mg/100 ml. Twenty-four-hour urinary uric acid excretion was 650 mg on a normal diet. Roentgenograms of both feet were normal. A diagnosis of gouty diathesis with gouty arthritis was made and interval therapy with probenecid and colchicine was instituted. Serum uric acid levels were brought to normal on probenecid 0.5 g/bid, and colchicine discontinued after approximately six months. The patient has been essentially asymptomatic over a number of years of prolonged follow-up.

Discussion: Gouty symptoms in this patient were interpreted for a long while as nonspecific reactions to trauma. Symptoms were disproportionate in severity to the trauma sustained and were usually delayed in onset for several hours after trauma occurred. Gout should be excluded in young males with a history of chronic recurrent tarsalgia or metatarsalgia, particularly when severe pain occurs as a delayed response to mild trauma.

History 18-2.   Fatigue Fracture

H.H., a 46-year-old white male, had had rheumatoid arthritis for approximately 20 years. Past therapy included aspirin, 960 mg QID, indomethacin, 25 mg TID, and, for the previous six years, prednisone in an average dose of 2.5 mg TID. When the patient was first seen in referral in December, 1969, examination revealed rheumatoid swelling and deformities involving the small joints of the hands, left elbow, right knee, and left ankle. Serum rheumatoid factor was positive in a titer of 1:160. Other studies for complicating illness or other forms of connective tissue disease were negative or normal. Hydroxychloroquine, 200 mg BID, was added to his previous therapeutic program. This agent was discontinued after six months when no improvement in symptoms was noted. Gold therapy was instituted but was discontinued when severe bone marrow depression occurred at a total gold dose of 640 mg. Efforts to reduce his prednisone dosage were unsuccessful.

The patient was seen in October, 1972, with the chief complaint of severe tenderness and pain at the lateral aspect of the right foot. This symptom, of relatively recent origin, was aggravated by weight-bearing. There was no history of acute trauma. Examination revealed tenderness and slight swelling at the base of the fifth metatarsal bone. Differential diagnosis included rheumatoid changes at the tarsal-fifth metatarsal area, tendinitis of peroneal tendons, or fatigue fracture. Roentgenograms of both feet revealed moderate periarticular osteoporosis and marginal erosions at the metatarsophalangeal joints, unchanged from previous findings. There was no evidence of fracture. The patient was seen in consultation with an orthopedic consultant who recommended a short-leg plaster cast for relief of symptoms. Following removal of the cast three weeks later, tenderness and pain in the same area were unchanged. Repeat roentgenographic examination now revealed a fracture at the base of the fifth metatarsal bone with fragments in excellent position. The patient was treated with plaster cast immobilization for an additional six weeks. Good callus formation and relief of symptoms were subsequently noted.

Discussion: The clinical features of this patient's foot problem were consistent with fatigue fracture. As in this case, roentgenographic changes consistent with definitive fracture may not develop until several weeks after onset of symptoms. Osteoporotic changes related both to rheumatoid arthritis and to long-term corticosteroid therapy were probably associated with the development of fracture in this patient.

REFERENCES

1. Mann, R. A.: Chapter 15, Diseases of the nerves of the foot. In Mann, R. A. (editor): DuVries' Surgery of the Foot, 4th ed., St. Louis, C. V. Mosby Co., 1978.
2. Kopell, H. P. and Thompson, W. A. L.: Peripheral Entrapment Neuropathies. Huntington, New York, R. E. Krieger, 1976.
3. Curtiss, P. H.: Chapter 17, Neurologic diseases of the foot. In Giannestras, N. J. (editor), Foot Disorders; Medical and Surgical Management, 2nd ed., Philadelphia, Lea & Febiger, 1973.
4. Glick, J. M.: Chapter 7, Traumatic injuries to the soft tissues of the foot and ankle. In Mann, R. A. (editor), DuVries' Surgery of the Foot, 4th ed., St. Louis, C. V. Mosby Co., 1978.
5. Shelley, W. B. and Rawnsley, H. M.: Painful feet due to herniation of fat. JAMA 205:308, 1968.

PART **III**

MANAGEMENT

CHAPTER 19

SPECIFIC TREATMENT OF COMMON RHEUMATOLOGIC DISORDERS

RHEUMATOID ARTHRITIS

Rheumatoid arthritis is a systemic disease that involves not only joints but other areas of the body. A multidisciplinary approach to therapy is required if all facets of disease manifestations and effects are to be adequately managed.

Systemic and Emotional Rest

Bed rest for a prolonged period of the day is required during acute phases of the disease. In patients with subacute or chronic disease, rest periods of 45 to 60 minutes following lunch and 30 to 45 minutes following supper are helpful. Emotional as well as physical rest is important. The home and family situation should be examined to allow maximal emotional support. In severe cases, hospitalization is necessary for adequate physical and emotional rest.

Physical and Occupational Therapy and Supportive Appliances

A regular program of physical and occupational therapy (see Chapter 20) should be specifically prescribed for each patient. Adequate detailed instructions for use of heat and exercises must be given and the importance of the program stressed. Canes, crutches or walkers should be utilized when limited weight-bearing is desirable. Splints are helpful for pain relief and prevention of deformities. Periodic conferences by the physicians and arthritis health professionals involved in the patient's care are valuable. Past treatment programs can be evaluated and future therapeutic goals outlined.

Drug Therapy

Drugs used in the treatment of rheumatoid arthritis can be conveniently divided into short-acting and remittive agents. The short-acting agents are characterized by a rapid onset of action and, similarly, a rapid dissipation of therapeutic effect when discontinued. This group includes salicylates, the newer nonsteroidal anti-inflammatory drugs (NSAID's) and corticosteroids. Remittive agents, on the other hand, are characterized by a latency period of weeks to months before their therapeutic effects become apparent. Various degrees of remission may be induced and are frequently sustained for prolonged periods even after the agents are discontinued. This "remittive" effect may be real, but an apparent prolonged effect resulting from retention of these agents in body tissues for a prolonged period even after drug discontinuation cannot be excluded.

Short-Acting Anti-Rheumatic Drugs

Aspirin and Other Salicylates. Initial drug treatment is begun with a nonsteroidal anti-inflammatory agent administered on a regular basis in properly divided doses. Some of the newer nonsteroidal anti-inflammatory agents have advantage over aspirin in that fewer tablets or capsules need be administered. In addition, some patients tolerate these newer medications with fewer side-reactions. Salicylates, on the other hand, are less costly and their effectiveness has been demonstrated over many decades of use. Accordingly, most rheumatologists still recommend aspirin as the drug of choice in initiating treatment in rheumatoid arthritis. A reasonable starting dose is 640 mg, four to five times daily. The dose is gradually increased until symptoms are relieved or toxicity develops, such as tinnitus or impaired hearing. Determination of blood salicylate levels aids management when response to the usual doses is inadequate; a level of 20 to 30 mg/100 ml should be sought for clinical effectiveness.

Hepatic abnormalities have been noted in association with high blood salicylate levels.[1] Although described more frequently in patients with juvenile rheumatoid arthritis,[2,3] similar salicylate-related hepatic abnormalities have been noted in patients with adult rheumatoid arthritis,[4] systemic lupus erythematosus,[4] and other connective tissue diseases. Elevated serum levels of glutamic oxaloacetic transaminase and, at times, serum alkaline phosphatase are noted. Hepatic abnormalities are more likely to occur with high blood salicylate levels.[3] Abnormalities usually disappear within one to two weeks if the drug is stopped or the dose lowered. In some patients, hepatic function returns to normal even though the drug is continued. Although hepatic abnormalities are not usually clinically significant, close monitoring is advisable.

A reversible effect of salicylates on renal function, characterized by an elevated serum creatinine and blood urea nitrogen, and a diminished creatinine clearance has also recently been described.[5] Seen more commonly in patients with systemic lupus erythematosus,[6] the changes can be explained by inhibition of intrarenal prostaglandin synthesis with resultant fall in renal blood flow. Similar but less marked effects on renal function have been noted in patients with rheumatoid arthritis and even in normal individuals. Abnormalities are more likely to be seen in patients with already compromised renal function, in whom prostaglandin synthesis is increased on a compensatory basis. Recognition of this salicylate effect is of clinical importance since changes in renal function might otherwise be ascribed to the underlying disease process. The salicylate-induced abnormalities clear when the agent is stopped; in many patients, altered function improves even while the drug is continued. Similar effects on renal function have been noted with the newer nonsteroidal anti-inflammatory agents. At present there is no clinical evidence to support a long-term deleterious effect on renal function via this mechanism.

Aspirin is best tolerated when taken with food or antacids. For patients with aspirin intolerance, certain salicylate preparations such as enteric-coated aspirin, aspirin with insoluble alkali, choline salicylate liquid, choline magnesium trisalicylate, time-release salicylate preparations, or salicylsalicylic acid may be better tolerated. Acetylsalicylic acid inhibits platelet aggregation and prolongs bleeding time. This effect appears due to the acetyl group of the aspirin, which irreversibly inactivates prostaglandin synthetase.[7] Salicylate preparations which do not have the acetyl radical, such as sodium salicylate, choline salicylate, choline magnesium trisalicylate, and salicylsalicylic acid have minimal or no effect on platelet aggregation. The non-acetylated salicylates are, accordingly, preparations of choice in patients with bleeding disorders or in whom bleeding may be a problem following procedures such as dental extractions or general surgery.

NSAID's (Nonsteroidal Anti-inflammatory Drugs). If patients do not respond adequately to salicylates in full dosage, or demonstrate intolerance or allergy, one of the newer nonsteroidal anti-inflammatory agents should be considered (Table 19-1).[8,9] These agents share many pharmacologic properties such as the ability to bind to plasma proteins and to inhibit prostaglandin synthesis. In rheumatoid arthritis, these drugs are as efficacious as salicylates in full dosage but may be associated with diminished overall side reactions. A clinical response superior to that of salicylates has been noted, however, in patients with seronegative spondyloarthropathies such as ankylosing spondylitis or psoriatic arthritis. When compared to one another the overall therapeutic effectiveness of these newer agents is similar. Accordingly, selection of which agent to use first in a given patient involves consideration of multiple factors such as number of years experience with the drug, cost, nuances of difference in toxicity, ease of administration in terms of numbers of tablets (capsules) required daily, and history of allergy or other toxicity to chemically related subgroups of agents within this drug classification. Side reactions common to many of these agents include gastrointestinal intolerance, peptic ulceration, rash, dizziness, and eye complaints. Leukopenia and mild decreases in hematocrit have been

TABLE 19-1.   Non-steroidal anti-inflammatory drugs (NSAID's)

	Dose Forms (mg)	Maximum Recommended Adult Daily Dose (mg)	Administration	Approved Indications	Pediatric Use Approved
Indoles, indenes					
Indomethacin (Indocin)	25;50	200	TID,QID	RA,OA,AS,Gout*	No
Sulindac (Clinoril)	150;200	400	BID	RA,OA,AS,Gout	No
Propionic acid derivatives					
Ibuprofen (Motrin)	300;400;600	2400	TID,QID	RA,OA	No
Fenoprofen (Nalfon)	200;300;600	3200	TID,QID	RA,OA	No
Naproxen (Naprosyn)	250;375	1000	BID	RA,OA	No
Pyrrole-acetic acid derivative					
Tolmetin (Tolectin)	200;400	2000**	TID,QID	RA,OA,JRA	Yes
Anthranilic acid derivative					
Meclofenamate (Meclomen)	50;100	400	TID,QID	RA,OA	No

*RA = rheumatoid arthritis; OA = osteoarthritis; AS = ankylosing spondylitis; JRA = juvenile rheumatoid arthritis
**Pediatric dose for children two years or older is 15 mg/kg/day to 30 mg/kg/day

described. Hepatic dysfunction and impairment of renal clearance[10] have been noted, similar to that seen in patients receiving salicylate therapy. Fluid retention may occur and, in a few cases, more severe renal abnormalities including interstitial nephritis, papillary necrosis, acute oliguric renal failure and nephrotic syndrome have been reported.[11-13]

In general, these agents are sufficiently similar in efficacy and toxicity that any may be the first to be prescribed when utilizing this class of drugs. It is useful to consider these agents in terms of chemical similarities, moving from one closely related subgroup to another when lack of response or toxicity is noted. Indomethacin, an indole-acetic acid, and sulindac, an indene-acetic acid, are closely related biochemically. Ibuprofen, fenoprofen, and naproxen are propionic acid derivatives. Tolmetin, a pyrrole-acetic acid derivative, and meclofenamate, an anthranilic acid derivative are generally considered separately. Accordingly, for example, a patient may be begun on indomethacin and response noted. Should the patient not respond or develop toxicity, it would be reasonable to switch to one of the propionic acid derivatives, such as ibuprofen. Subsequent moves to agents in other chemical classes would be initiated depending on clinical response or toxicity. Patients may respond to one agent but not another, even within the same biochemical subgroup. Accordingly, it is not unreasonable to try a number, if not all, of these agents before giving up on the nonsteroidal antiinflammatory drugs as a therapeutic measure.

Generally, these agents should not be used in association with regular doses of salicylates. Their simultaneous use increases gastrointestinal irritation with increased likelihood for gastrointestinal ulceration or bleeding. In addition, diminished blood levels of some of these agents such as indomethacin, ibuprofen, fenoprofen, and meclofenamate have been described when salicylates are added.[14,15] Thus the anti-inflammatory effect achieved with either one used separately may be reduced.

Some specific aspects of each of these agents should be noted. Indomethacin is metabolized chiefly in the liver and should be used with caution, if at all, in patients with liver disease. In some patients, indomethacin causes exacerbation of colitis or regional enteritis. Central nervous system effects are not uncommon and include confusion and loss of concentration, severe pounding headaches, drowsiness, and depression. Initial observations of ocular abnormalities[16] have not been confirmed.[17] Sulindac has the advantage of BID administration since its effective metabolite, the sulfide derivative, has a half-life of 18 hours or more. The propionic acid derivatives, ibuprofen, fenoprofen, and naproxen are similar in efficacy and toxicity. Amblyopia and aseptic meningitis have been noted with ibuprofen administration. The amblyopia, which may occur early in the course of drug administration, is reversible and disappears shortly after discontinuation of the drug. Meningitis has been described as an unusual reaction in patients with systemic lupus erythematosus. The etiology of these unusual

toxic reactions is unknown. Naproxen has the advantage of BID administration, based on its long plasma half-life. Tolmetin, like the other agents,
is an effective anti-rheumatic drug and has been approved for use in patients with juvenile as well as adult rheumatoid arthritis.[18] As with indomethacin and sulindac, central nervous system side effects such as headaches and dizziness have been described. Patients receiving meclofenemate
may experience a troublesome diarrhea, seen in 15% or more of patients
treated. Diarrhea appears early in the course of therapy and disappears
upon drug withdrawal. Indomethacin, sulindac, ibuprofen, naproxen, and
tolmetin have been associated with minimal to absent effects on prothrombin time in patients receiving coumarin. Nevertheless, caution with close
monitoring of prothrombin times should be exercised when these agents
are used in patients on anticoagulant therapy.

A number of other nonsteroidal anti-inflammatory agents are presently
utilized elsewhere throughout the world, or are undergoing basic and clinical trials in the United States. These newer agents include additional drugs
in the propionic acid and fenamate groups, as well as pyrazolones and
phenylacetic acid derivatives. Piroxicam, a benzothiazine derivative, has
an optimum effective dose of 20 mg, which, because of the long half-life
of the drug, is frequently fully effective when given once daily. Divided
doses may be utilized for acute inflammation or to lessen side-effects. Doses
as low as 10 mg/day may be effective in maintenance of disease control;
doses as high as 40 mg/day are beneficial when given for one or two days
in the treatment of acute musculoskeletal problems or gout attacks. Side-
reactions include epigastric distress, abdominal pain and diarrhea, headaches and dizziness, and rash. Overall, these newer agents are similar in
efficacy to those already available. They will be useful for trial in patients
not responsive to or intolerant of presently available nonsteroidal anti-
inflammatory agents.

Phenylbutazone and its closely allied derivative, oxyphenbutazone, are
effective anti-inflammatory agents in patients with rheumatic disorders.
Given the availability of the newer nonsteroidal anti-inflammatory agents
which are generally less toxic, the use of phenylbutazone or oxyphenbutazone for long-term use is less attractive. Side reactions include severe bone
marrow depression with agranulocytosis or aplastic anemia, peptic ulcer
disease, fluid retention, and rash. The prothrombin-lowering effect of coumarin agents is accentuated. Their use should generally be reserved for
treating acute episodes of inflammation for short periods of time. They are
particularly effective in patients with seronegative spondyloarthropathy
such as ankylosing spondylitis and may be considered for use in these patients when symptoms are uncontrolled with other nonsteroidal anti-
inflammatory agents.

Systemic Corticosteroids. Systemic corticosteroid agents are utilized at various stages in the treatment of rheumatoid arthritis, depending on disease severity, socioeconomic needs and response to other agents. In general, systemic corticosteroids should be avoided whenever possible, due to the many severe toxic side effects associated with their use. When utilized, the lowest dose possible should be used for the shortest period of time. Maximal doses for long-term use vary with the age and sex of the patient. If possible, long-term use should be limited to 10 mg prednisone or its equivalent per day in adult males, 7.5 mg per day in premenopausal females and 5 mg per day in menopausal females. Alternate day therapy may be associated with fewer side reactions;[19] unfortunately, it is therapeutically effective in a relatively small number of patients. Prednisolone should be substituted for prednisone in patients with hepatic disease since conversion of prednisone to its active metabolite by the liver may be impaired.

Although systemic corticosteroids should be utilized with caution in patients with rheumatoid arthritis, intra-articular administration of these agents is frequently useful and has limited hazard when used judiciously (see Chapter 21).

Analgesic Agents. Analgesic therapy with propoxyphene hydrochloride (Darvon), 65 mg or acetaminophen, 300 mg given on a regular or PRN basis is a helpful adjunct to anti-inflammatory agents. Acetaminophen in daily doses exceeding 2400-3000 mg/day may be associated with liver toxicity, particularly in patients who already have liver impairment.[20] As a rule, it is wise not to exceed a total acetaminophen intake over 2400 mg/day on a regular basis. Newer analgesic agents, derivatives of the NSAID's, have recently been introduced to the market. These preparations take advantage of the analgesic effects of these agents at lower doses and, when necessary, have been formulated to provide more rapid absorption and onset of action. Agents presently available include zomepirac sodium (Zomax), 100 mg; ibuprofen (Motrin), 400 mg; naproxen sodium (Anaprox), 275 mg; and fenoprofen calcium (Nalfon 200), 200 mg. Adverse reactions to zomepirac sodium include gastrointestinal symptoms such as dyspepsia, abdominal pain and vomiting, and central nervous system reactions such as dizziness and drowsiness. Antacids do not alter absorption of this agent, nor is the prothrombin time affected in patients receiving warfarin. Side-reactions seen with ibuprofen, naproxen sodium and fenoprofen calcium are as described for these agents used for their anti-inflammatory effect. These analgesic preparations should not be used concurrently in patients receiving NSAID's since similar toxic effects are compounded. Pentazocine, 50 mg, may also be considered for analgesic use. It is a narcotic substance and not infrequently associated with dizziness and central nervous system reactions in older patients. This agent, as well as opiates such as codeine, are generally to be avoided in patients with rheumatoid arthritis, although their use is not inappropriate on a temporary basis for acute disease flares.

Remittive Agents and Procedures

In patients who require additional therapy, the use of *antimalarial drugs,* such as hydroxychloroquine (Plaquenil) should be considered.[21,22] Hydroxychloroquine is begun in a dose of 200 mg BID. Response is slow in onset; the drug should be given a three- to six-month trial before being discontinued for lack of effect. When improvement occurs, the dose is decreased to 200 mg once daily. Side effects, such as gastrointestinal upset, rash, headaches, nightmares, and psychic disorientation, may occur but are uncommon. Leukopenia sometimes occurs. Antimalarial medications are contraindicated in patients with psoriasis because psoriatic lesions may be exacerbated.

The toxic reaction of major concern is visual impairment due to the effect of the drug on the retina.[23] Transient changes in visual acuity that occur early in treatment usually resolve and are not important. A baseline ophthalmologic examination should be performed at the outset of treatment and repeated at six-month intervals for the first several years. After two or three years, eye examinations at four-month intervals are advisable. A complete evaluation includes slit lamp and funduscopic examination and studies of visual fields, visual acuity and color vision. A defect in visual fields to a 3-mm red dot is the earliest manifestation of toxicity; visual loss is usually still reversible at this stage. Visual field cuts to a white dot occur late and reversal of visual loss is less likely. Visual abnormalities may worsen even after the drug is discontinued, owing to its prolonged persistence in body tissues. Studies suggest that ocular reactions bear a relationship to daily rate of administration and total cumulative dose.[22] It is recommended that the long-term daily dose for hydroxychloroquine not exceed 7 mg/kg/day. In children, a starting dose of 5 to 7 mg/kg/day is recommended, not to exceed 400 mg/day. Protection of the eyes against bright sunlight and the use of sunglasses may diminish the frequency of toxicity. Older patients are more likely to develop ocular toxicity and the use of lower doses for shorter periods of time is recommended. Chloroquine is considered to have a higher potential for eye toxicity than hydroxychloroquine. Accordingly, the latter is recommended when antimalarial therapy is used.

Quinacrine (atabrine), an acridine dye, has also been described as efficacious in suppressing rheumatoid arthritis inflammation.[24] Ocular changes including scotomas and blind-spot enlargements have been described with use of this drug in doses considerably higher than those recommended for use in connective tissue disease.[25] Prolonged administration in a dose of 100 mg daily for malaria prophylaxis appeared safe although new scotomas of undetermined significance appeared in 3 of 36 individuals studied. Periodic eye examinations as recommended with hydroxychloroquine are prudent although it has been stated that the drug is probably not retinotoxic.[25] An initial dose of 100 mg/day is utilized. Deposits of the drug in the skin produce a reversible yellowish pigmentation, which can be utilized to titer drug dosage. I find it useful to continue the dose at 100 mg/day until the patient has a clinical response or until a deep yellow pigmentation of the skin develops. At this time, the drug is discontinued for two weeks and re-initiated at a dosage schedule of 100 mg/day for six to eight weeks on, and two weeks off. This program diminishes the depth of skin pigmentation which is cosmetically bothersome to some patients. Other side reactions to be monitored include occasional leukopenia and liver function test abnormalities. A lichen planus-like eruption is not uncommon. Deep bluish patchy pigmentation, seen with long-term administration, tends to be more permanent.

Gold therapy is effective in inducing partial or complete remission in many patients with rheumatoid arthritis.[26,27] The most frequently used preparations are gold sodium thiomalate (Myochrysine) and gold sodium thioglucose (Solganal). Gold sodium thiomalate is an aqueous solution; gold sodium thioglucose is prepared as a suspension in oil. Both preparations can be used satisfactorily to initiate and maintain therapy. Some investigators, however, suggest that gold sodium thiomalate be used to initiate therapy since it is more rapidly absorbed, and that the more slowly absorbed gold sodium thioglucose be used for maintenance. A leukocyte count, differential white blood cell count, hematocrit, platelet count and urinalysis should be obtained for baseline study and repeated at weekly intervals for the first 15 to 20 injections. After that time, laboratory studies may be performed following every second or third injection. The gold preparations are administered by intramuscular injection. Aqueous solutions may be given into the deltoid or gluteus muscle regions; oily suspensions are injected into the gluteal region only. Ten mg of gold salt is given the first week, 25 mg the second week, and 50 mg weekly thereafter. In children a maximal weekly dose of 1 mg/kg is recommended, not to exceed 50 mg/week.

Gold therapy is stopped in the presence of clinical side reactions or untoward laboratory abnormalities.[28] Prior to each gold injection, the patient is queried for the presence of stomatitis, metallic taste in the mouth, itching of the skin, rash or diarrhea. Nitritoid vasomotor reactions, characterized by light-headedness, flushing, and syncope, are an unusual type of side reaction that occurs particularly with gold sodium thiomalate. These reactions usually occur almost immediately or within 10 to 15 minutes after drug administration. It is advisable that patients wait in the office for 10 to 15 minutes to avoid injury. Sometimes, mild reactions of this type are eliminated by using a lower dose of the drug. Symptoms may decrease and disappear after five or six injections. In most patients, particularly in those in whom the nitritoid reaction has been severe, use of gold sodium thioglucose is preferred to trials of lower doses or less frequent injections of gold sodium thiomalate.

Adverse reactions to gold are frequent and can occur at any time during treatment.[28] Fortunately most are mild. Rashes are nonspecific in appearance but usually pruritic. Lesions may simulate lichen planus or pityriasis rosea; exfoliative dermatitis occurs but is fortunately rare. Hematologic abnormalities such as leukopenia or eosinophilia are generally mild, but agranulocytosis, thrombocytopenia, and pancytopenia with aplastic anemia are feared, occasional adverse reactions. Eosinophilia is generally transient and without untoward effect; in certain patients, however, it may signal impending severe toxicity in the bone marrow or other organ systems. Renal abnormalities include proteinuria sufficiently severe at times to cause nephrotic syndrome and hematuria. Less common adverse reactions include enterocolitis, cholestatic jaundice, and peripheral neuropathy. Recently, acute pulmonary toxicity with diffuse lung infiltrates has been described.[29] In patients receiving prolonged gold administration, gold deposits (chrysiasis) may be noted in the cornea and, at times, in the lens. These deposits are rarely associated with eye damage.

Symptoms may improve after a total dose of 600 to 800 mg of gold salt has been administered. At least 1 gm of gold salt should be given as a therapeutic trial. If improvement occurs, the maintenance dose can be administered at two-week intervals for several injections, then every three-weeks, and finally once a month to maintain remission. Gold injections are reinstituted at a more frequent interval if exacerbation occurs. Contraindications to gold administration are a history of prior gold reaction, systemic lupus erythematosus, severe hepatic or renal disease, and blood dyscrasias. Mild toxicity is treated by stopping gold therapy. More severe reactions are treated with prednisone in a dose of 20 to 60 mg daily, depending on the type and severity of the reaction. Chelating agents, such as dimercaptopropanol (British anti-Lewisite) or D-penicillamine which increase gold excretion, should be added in cases of severe toxicity.

Auranofin is a new orally active gold-containing compound with remittive anti-inflammatory effects on patients with rheumatoid arthritis. The phase III clinical investigational component of study of this agent is presently being completed and it is likely that it will be approved shortly for use in rheumatoid arthritis. It has the obvious advantage over current gold-containing preparations in that it can be given orally. It is not certain whether its anti-rheumatic activities are specifically related to the gold component of the molecule, or whether its pharmacologic effect resides elsewhere in the agent as constituted. Clinical responses thus far have varied from modest to excellent. Diarrhea and abdominal cramps are common complications and liver function test abnormalities are not infrequent. Additional, less common side reactions include rash, stomatitis, bone marrow suppression and nephropathy. Complications overall, however, appear less frequent and less severe than those seen in patients receiving parenteral gold therapy.

D-penicillamine, a structural analog of the amino acid, cysteine, and a component of the penicillin molecule is similar in effectiveness to gold in the treatment of patients with rheumatoid arthritis.[30–32] A potent chelating agent, it has been used most extensively in the past for treatment of patients with Wilson's disease to chelate copper. The mechanisms whereby it exerts its salutary effect in rheumatoid arthritis are unknown. Possibly operative are effects of the drug on metal-binding, sulfhydryl-disulfide exchange, pyridoxine antagonism, enzyme inhibition and inhibition of collagen cross-linking. Immune complexes are reduced in both serum and synovial fluid. In vitro effects on lymphocyte transformation have been described.

Recommendations regarding the dose and rate of administration of this agent are still in a state of evolution.[31,32] The overall admonition to "go low, go slow" is generally agreed to by most investigators. Therapy is usually initiated at a dose of 250 mg/day. Administration without food, one to one and a half hours after a meal, is recommended to avoid chelation inactivation of the drug by ingested metals. If the patient exhibits no clinical response after 1 to 2 months on this dose, the dose is increased to 500 mg/day and the patient observed once again for a period of another one to two months. Dosage increments of 250 mg at one to two month intervals are made, depending upon response, up to a maximum of 1,000 mg/day total dosage. Alternatively, increments following drug initiation may be made somewhat more frequently in steps of 125 mg added to the previous dose. Although some patients may show a fairly rapid response with clinical improvement after one or two months, the latent period in most patients is usually considerably longer; four to six months may be required before clinical improvement becomes evident. The drug should be discontinued if improvement is not noted at the maximal recommended daily dose. The drug may be administered once a day although it is not uncommon to administer it in BID dosage after a 500 mg/day level has been achieved. Although not yet officially approved for use in children with juvenile rheumatoid arthritis, it has been administered with clinical effectiveness to such patients. Although it is prudent to begin at a lower dose, for example 62.5 mg/day, the overall therapeutic dosage does not appear to be appreciably lower than in adults.

Toxic reactions to penicillamine are common and may be severe.[32] Skin rash, frequently accompanied by pruritus, may occur at any time. Symptoms usually resolve with cessation of the drug or lowering of the dose; concomitant administration of an antihistamine drug is helpful. Bullous lesions indistinguishable from pemphigus have been described. Stomatitis, similar to that seen with gold therapy, is not uncommon. Hypogeusia, diminished taste perception, may occur. Usually the condition is benign and self-limited with clearing over several months despite continuation of the drug. Bone marrow depression with leukopenia, thrombocytopenia, and aplastic anemia is a significant concern. Nephropathy of immune complex origin is characterized by proteinuria, hematuria and eventual nephrotic syndrome. Although some investigators maintain that this agent may be continued despite proteinuria of 1 to 2 g/day, reduction in dose or discontinuation of the drug should be strongly considered when proteinuria is sustained.

A number of unusual auto-immune syndromes have been associated with penicillamine therapy. These include myasthenia gravis,[33] systemic lupus erythematosus,[34] polymyositis,[35] and hemolytic anemia, Goodpasture's syndrome,[36] and thyroiditis. Other complications include cholestatic jaundice,[37] colitis, obliterative bronchiolitis,[38] and breast enlargement. Although drug fever may present a problem in some patients, initiation of therapy in very low doses and the addition of antihistamines or steroids may allow successful use.

Patients receiving this drug should be carefully monitored by clinical and laboratory parameters for symptoms and signs of toxicity. Complete blood counts including white blood cell count, differential, hematocrit and platelet count, and urinalysis should be performed at two-week intervals for the first six months. Laboratory monitoring should be continued at two-week intervals until a steady maximal daily dose is obtained, at which time monthly laboratory studies can be performed. Liver function studies should be performed at two-month intervals during the initiation phase of treatment. Leukopenia below 3,000/cubic mm, or a significant fall in platelet count from the patient's established normal is an indication for immediate discontinuation of the drug. Mild proteinuria may respond to small reductions in daily dosage. The drug should probably be discontinued if proteinuria in excess of 500 mg/24 hours occurs. Mild toxic reactions involving the skin or mucous membranes similarly frequently respond to dosage reduction. Severe reactions may require the addition of corticosteroids for a temporary period of time. The drug should be discontinued in patients who exhibit any of the auto-immune syndromes such as polymyositis or myasthenia gravis.

Systemic *immunosuppressive agents* such as cyclophosphamide,[39-41] chlorambucil, methotrexate[42] and azathioprine[43,44] have been reported beneficial in protracted progressive rheumatoid arthritis. Although only azathioprine is currently FDA approved for use in rheumatoid arthritis, the other agents may be considered on an investigational basis when indicated. The use of these agents should be reserved for patients with chronic progressive, uncontrolled disease who have not responded to more conventional anti-inflammatory and remittive agents, or in whom other agents have been tried and are now contra-indicated because of toxicity. Unwanted drug effects may be serious. Bone marrow suppression and increased bacterial and viral infections may be seen. Drug hypersensitivity with fever and rash, and liver function abnormalities at times producing jaundice occasionally occur with azathioprine, a purine antagonist. The alkylating agents chlorambucil and cyclophosphamide suppress the germplasm, producing amenorrhea and azoospermia. Hair loss is more common in patients receiving cyclophosphamide. Cyclophosphamide also has multiple deleterious effects on the urinary bladder which include acute hemorrhagic cystitis, fibrosis, and late epithelial neoplasm.[45] These side-effects can be diminished by maintenance of a high fluid intake and frequent emptying of the bladder. Chronic long term use of methotrexate, a folic-acid antagonist, may lead to hepatic fibrosis and cirrhosis. It is recommended by a number of investigators that liver biopsy be performed at annual intervals to assess hepatic toxicity which may be otherwise occult and subclinical. Pulmonary infiltrates and fibrosis have also been described. Parenteral administration is associated with less hepatic toxicity since drug concentrations in the liver are diminished.

Increased risk for development of carcinoma and lymphoma have been described with the use of these agents, with the exception of methotrexate. The time lag between onset of drug use and development of neoplasm may be prolonged. This potential for induction of neoplasia represents a significant drawback to use of these drugs. Oral dose recommendations for these agents as described in the literature are variable. Cyclophosphamide appears effective in doses varying from 1.5 to 2.0 mg/kg/day; chlorambucil in a dose of 4 to 6 mg/day; and azathioprine in a dose of 2.0 to 3.0 mg/kg/day. Methotrexate is recommended in a dose of 10 to 15 mg per *week,* given over one day in divided doses. As with other remittive agents, onset of clinical response is slow and trials should extend for three to six months before the agents are considered ineffective. Clinical and laboratory parameters should be closely monitored, with complete blood counts including platelets studied weekly initially and then at two- to four-week intervals. Periodic liver function tests should be obtained. These agents should be used with caution if at all in young patients, especially females in the child-bearing age. Detailed information regarding drug toxicity should be communicated to the patient before drug initiation.

Levamisole is an antihelminthic drug which has recently found clinical use as an immunostimulatory agent. Cell-mediated immunity is altered, with evidence both in vivo and in vitro that lymphocyte function is enhanced. Although clinical improvement in patients with rheumatoid arthritis has been described, serious side reactions including leukopenia with potential for agranulocytosis, thrombocytopenia, and allergic vasculitis have limited its clinical use.[46,47] Rash, gastrointestinal upset, stomatitis, alterations of taste and smell, and a febrile influenza-like illness have also been described. At present, the potential for serious drug toxicity precludes its clinical use on other than an *investigational* basis in management of connective tissue disease.

Major interest has developed in the use of *plasmapheresis, lymphopheresis or combined lymphoplasmapheresis* in the management of rheumatoid arthritis, as well as in other connective tissue diseases and auto-immune disorders.[48–53] These techniques have been used for such diverse conditions as Goodpasture's syndrome, hyperviscosity syndrome, and myasthenia gravis. Beneficial responses have been reported in severely ill patients with acute lupus nephritis who have high levels of circulating immune complexes. In many patients, however, the benefits are not sustained. Studies of the efficacy of these procedures in the treatment of rheumatoid arthritis have shown variable results.[49,50,53] In an uncontrolled study, various degrees of remission were induced in the majority of patients after plasmapheresis or lymphoplasmapheresis; concurrent administration of remittive drugs such as gold or penicillamine appeared to sustain the clinical improvement.[49] Definite, but modest antirheumatic effects of lymphopheresis were also noted in a randomized, double-blind investigation.[53] In another controlled study, however, hospitalization itself was of equal benefit to plasma exchange in the treatment of acute exacerbations of rheumatoid arthritis.[50] Therapeutic effectiveness, if confirmed by further studies, may be related to reduction of circulating antibody and/or immune complexes, removal of a plasma factor or factors which modulate lymphocyte or neutrophil action, or alterations in the cellular immune response related to lymphocyte depletion. Complications of this generally safe procedure include anemia, blood volume shifts, electrolyte imbalance and possible hypocalcemia. Plasmapheresis may result in rapid rebound and overshoot of immune complexes, particularly in LE patients. The addition of cytotoxic drugs as an adjunct to plasmapheresis may have to be considered when this difficulty arises. Costs of plasmapheresis including plasma replacement are extremely high, and less costly plasma substitutes are being considered. Other studies are investigating the potential for return of the patient's own plasma after removal of immune complexes. At present this modality remains investigational in the treatment of patients with rheumatoid arthritis.[52] It may be considered for serious clinical situations such as associated vasculitis or progressive disease unreponsive to other reasonable conventional therapeutic agents.

Surgical Management

Orthopaedic surgery plays a major role in multidisciplinary treatment. Synovectomy may be of value in selected patients to relieve pain and swelling when the inflammatory process is not controlled adequately by medical means. Joints most amenable to this therapeutic modality include the knees and wrists. Surgical procedures for more advanced disease include release of contractures, resection osteotomy, arthrodesis (fusion), and arthroplasty. Arthroplasty with introduction of flexible hinge implants is frequently utilized in patients with disease of the metacarpophalangeal joints. Total joint prostheses are a notable advance in the treatment of severely involved joints. The highest success rate with total joint replacement has been achieved with use of this procedure on the hip. Therapeutic results achieved with total knee replacement are less dramatic, but relief of pain and improvement in range of motion are attainable in a significant number of patients. Total joint procedures for replacement of wrists, ankles, elbows, and shoulders are associated with lower rates of success and await development of more effective prostheses. Complications of total joint replacement include early and late infection, thrombophlebitis and pulmonary embolism, and prosthetic breakage and loosening. Wear has not been a significant problem.

In all patients in whom surgical procedures are to be considered in the management of rheumatoid arthritis, patient selection and preoperative preparation for surgery are extremely important. The patient with rheumatoid arthritis frequently has multiple joints involved so that malfunction of one joint interferes with that of the others. Joint laxity, poor skin integrity particularly in patients receiving steroid therapy, operative bleeding associated with therapeutic agents such as salicylates, and possible impairment of healing in patients receiving steroids, penicillamine, and immunosuppressive agents are important considerations. Postoperative rehabilitation is often strenuous with respect to exercises and ambulation procedures. It is essential that the patient have a detailed clear understanding of the surgical procedure and benefits to be expected. Possible complications must be clearly outlined. Best results can be anticipated in patients who are cooperative and highly motivated, and who understand the disease process and expected results.

ANKYLOSING SPONDYLITIS

Management of ankylosing spondylitis involves a combined program of physical therapy and drugs. Exercises are directed toward maintaining a straight posture and preventing flexion deformity of the spine. Spinal hyperextension and breathing exercises are performed for 10 or 15 repetitions twice daily. Swimming is an excellent exercise to maintain range of motion of the shoulders and hips and movement of respiratory muscles. Heat in the form of a warm tub bath or shower relieves pain and stiffness and allows the patient to exercise more effectively. Patients with severe disease with progressive flexion deformity of the spine are benefited by hyperextension braces.

Drug therapy begins with aspirin, 640 to 960 mg QID. If necessary, the dosage is gradually increased to obtain therapeutic blood salicylate levels of 20 to 30 mg/100 ml. In patients whose response is inadequate, the newer nonsteroidal anti-inflammatory drugs (NSAID's) are particularly efficacious, often exceeding the benefits of full therapeutic doses of salicylates in patients with this disorder. Although at present only indomethacin and sulindac are formally FDA approved for use in this disease, other of the NSAID's are effective and may be utilized. In more severe cases, phenylbutazone or oxyphenbutazone may be considered. These latter agents are generally more effective than other NSAID's in treatment of this disorder, but their increased risk of toxicity including bone marrow suppression, peptic ulceration, fluid retention, and rash generally preclude their use as the agents of first choice. An initial dose of 100 mg QID of either drug is instituted; the dosage is gradually decreased to the minimal daily maintenance dose required to produce reasonable relief of symptoms. A dose of 300 mg daily should rarely be exceeded on a long-term basis. Frequently, 100 to 200 mg daily is adequate for routine administration, with increases to 200 to 400 mg daily for acute episodes. Oral steroids, such as prednisone 2.5 mg TID, are effective in many patients. These agents can be tried if the other drugs give inadequate results or are poorly tolerated. The use of anti-inflammatory agents allows the patients to perform a more adequate exercise program with augmented potential to prevent undesirable deformities. Roentgen therapy to the spine, once used with some frequency, has generally been abandoned due to associated complications of bone marrow aplasia or leukemia.

REITER'S SYNDROME

No specific curative therapy is available for Reiter's syndrome. However, in many patients recurrent episodes of urethritis may be shortened by the use of tetracycline, 250 mg QID, administered over a period of seven to ten days. No controlled evidence exists that antibiotic therapy affects the overall course of the disease. Joint manifestations can usually be satisfactorily managed with aspirin or the newer nonsteroidal anti-inflammatory drugs. Phenylbutazone is similarly effective but is less frequently required with the advent of the newer less toxic agents. Systemic corticosteroids in relatively low doses, such as prednisone 2.5 to 5 mg BID may be efficacious in patients not responding to more conservative agents. Local ophthalmic or systemic corticosteroids are indicated in patients with acute uveitis. Intra-articular injections of steroids may be extremely efficacious in the management of monoarticular or polyarticular joint flares. Immunosuppressive therapy has been described as being helpful but should be reserved for patients with progressive disabling disease.[54]

PSORIATIC ARTHRITIS

Psoriatic arthritis sometimes parallels the course of cutaneous lesions. Vigorous therapy of the psoriasis with crude coal tar and ultraviolet light or with local steroid creams and ointments is indicated. Mild cases of arthritis respond satisfactorily to the use of aspirin in full therapeutic dosage. As in patients with ankylosing spondylitis, the newer nonsteroidal anti-inflammatory agents are particularly effective in patients with psoriatic arthritis. Antimalarial drugs are contraindicated because they may aggravate the psoriatic rash and cause exfoliation. Systemic corticosteroid therapy is beneficial in many patients, but its use should be restricted to patients with severe progressive disease. In contrast, intra-articular injections of steroids judiciously used to control pauci-articular disease can be effective in overall patient management.

Gold therapy has received recent renewed interest in the management of patients with psoriatic arthritis.[55,56] It appears to be an effective agent in a number of patients and is deserving of trial in patients unresponsive to more conservative programs. Although toxic skin rash caused by gold may at times be difficult to differentiate from cutaneous psoriasis, this has not proved a significant problem. D-penicillamine has been tried in this disorder, but controlled studies relative to its efficacy remain to be performed. Response of the arthritis and psoriasis has been noted in patients receiving PUVA therapy (oral 8-methoxypsoralen followed by high-intensity long-wave ultraviolet radiation).[57] This therapeutic program may be considered in patients unresponsive to other agents.

Folic acid antagonists such as methotrexate[58,59] and purine antagonists such as azathioprine[43] and 6-mercaptopurine[60] are beneficial in severe uncontrolled cases of psoriasis and psoriatic arthritis. Serious side reactions preclude their use in all but the more advanced cases. Methotrexate in an oral dose of 10 to 15 mg given in divided doses once a *week* is often effective. Hepatotoxicity and pulmonary fibrosis are major side reactions. Continued use of this drug requires periodic liver biopsy to detect early changes not evident on routine liver function laboratory profiles. Azathioprine, 2.0 to 3.0 mg/kg/day, or 6-mercaptopurine, 1.0 to 1.5 mg/kg/day, are effective alternatives. Physical therapy programs are important in the management of articular changes, as described in patients with rheumatoid arthritis.

GOUT AND PSEUDOGOUT

Gout

Management of gout is divided into treatment of acute gouty attacks and interval treatment designed to prevent recurrent attacks and chronic tophaceous gout.

Treatment of Acute Attacks. Although colchicine is regarded as specific for gout, it may be somewhat effective in other forms of arthritis. With onset of symptoms, one 0.6-mg tablet is given every hour until symptoms are relieved or until gastrointestinal side effects of nausea, vomiting, or diarrhea occur. A maximum of 8 to 10 tablets is administered. Gastrointestinal side effects, if they occur, are usually controlled with paregoric or diphenoxylate hydrochloride. Intravenous colchicine is associated with fewer gastrointestinal side reactions; for this reason, intravenous administration is preferred when gastrointestinal symptoms are particularly to be avoided, as after surgery. A dose of 2 mg is given initially, followed by 1 mg at eight-hour intervals if needed; a daily dose of 4 mg should not be exceeded. Colchicine solutions are highly irritating to veins and soft tissues. The dose should be diluted with 10 ml of sterile saline solution and administered slowly. Infiltration of soft tissues around the vein should be avoided.

The newer nonsteroidal anti-inflammatory drugs (NSAID's) used at maximal dosage levels are effective in treatment of acute gouty attacks. Although only indomethacin and sulindac have been formally approved by the FDA for this use, the other agents in this category appear to be similarly effective. Phenylbutazone and oxyphenbutazone are highly effective in the treatment of acute gouty attacks; the need for use of these agents has, however, been reduced by the availability of the newer nonsteroidal drugs. If phenylbutazone or oxyphenbutazone are utilized, a dose of 400 to 600 mg/day in divided doses is administered for several days, followed by gradually decreasing doses over 6 to 8 days. In general, with any of these agents, a more rapid and complete response is to be anticipated if the drug is begun as soon as possible after onset of the attack.

ACTH gel may be used in the management of acute attacks. The drug is given in a daily intramuscular dose of 40 to 80 mg for two or three days. Oral corticosteroids such as prednisone, 20 to 30 mg daily in divided doses, are often efficacious. The daily dose is then gradually decreased over a period of four to seven days. Acute gouty episodes following cessation of steroid therapy are not uncommon. It is wise to place the patient on maintenance colchicine, 0.6 mg BID, when the prednisone is discontinued. Aspiration of the involved joint followed by intra-articular injection of steroid with lidocaine is an effective therapeutic alternative when larger joints are involved.

Prevention of Recurrent Acute Attacks and Chronic Tophaceous Gout (Interval Therapy). Chronic manifestations of gout can be prevented by treatment programs that reduce the body pool of urates and serum uric acid. Indications for use of a preventive interval program include the presence of tophi, recurrent acute gouty arthritis or significant asymptomatic hyperuricemia. The level at which asymptomatic hyperuricemia should be treated is not universally agreed upon. Consistent hyperuricemia above 10 mg/100 ml probably deserves treatment because acute attacks of gouty arthritis and renal calculi are common. Patients who overexcrete uric acid similarly deserve consideration of an interval program, irrespective of the height of the serum uric acid, since many of these patients will develop renal stones.

In routine cases of gout uncomplicated by urate overexcretion or renal stones, probenecid is the treatment of choice. This drug has a proven record of safety and efficacy and can be taken lifelong with minimal hazard.

Treatment is initiated in a dose of 0.5 g daily. Dosage is gradually increased until the serum uric acid level, checked at periodic intervals, is brought into a normal range. Not all patients should be treated with a standard daily dosage, since the dosage required for adequate control varies. At times, a dose of 2 or 3 g per day is required for adequate results. Sulfinpyrazone (Anturane) is an alternative uricosuric agent for use in patients who are intolerant or allergic to probenecid. One hundred milligrams are approximately equivalent to 0.5 g of probenecid. Patients being treated with probenecid or sulfinpyrazone should avoid salicylate-containing compounds, which nullify the action of the uricosuric agents.

Allopurinol (Zyloprim), a xanthine-oxidase inhibitor, reduces serum uric acid by reducing uric acid formation. The fall in serum uric acid is accompanied by a drop in urinary uric acid excretion. Although it is a relatively safe drug, side effects are more serious than those occurring with uricosuric agents. Side reactions include fever, skin rash, elevations of serum glutamic oxaloacetic transaminase (SGOT), bone marrow depression, vasculitis, granulomatous hepatitis, interstitial nephritis, and diarrhea. Vasculitis and exfoliative dermatitis occur more frequently in patients with impaired renal function. Xanthine stones, secondary to increased xanthine levels, may occasionally occur. Muscle deposits of hypoxanthine, xanthine, and oxypurinol have been described but no serious toxic effects on muscle have been reported. Long-term side effects resulting from inhibition of purine metabolism by this agent are theoretically hazardous; fortunately, none have yet been noted. Despite these considerations, allopurinol is a valuable and useful drug when used in appropriate situations. Indications for the use of allopurinol in the interval treatment of gout include allergy to the usual uricosuric agents, a history of uric acid stones, presence of renal impairment, or urinary uric acid overexcretion. In these situations, allopurinol is the drug of choice. It is given in a starting dose of 200 mg daily. The dose is gradually increased at increments of 100 mg every two to four weeks until the serum uric acid is brought to a normal level. Most patients are controlled on a total daily dose of 300 to 600 mg. The drug has a long duration of action and may be given in one daily morning dose.

Colchicine, 0.6 mg once or twice daily, should be given to patients who are beginning therapy with uricosuric agents or allopurinol, because onset of therapy with these agents may be associated with an increased frequency of acute gouty attacks. Colchicine therapy is continued for approximately six months, at which time it can be discontinued if the gouty attacks have been controlled. Scattered reports suggest that daily colchicine therapy may be associated with decreased male fertility[61] or with induction of congenital birth defects.[62] The drug should probably be discontinued two to three months before attempts at conception to avoid any possible hazard. In patients over 70 years of age who experience acute gouty attacks for the first time, interval therapy with a uricosuric agent or allopurinol is less mandatory. Tophaceous complications, which usually take years to develop, are unlikely to be troublesome. Prophylaxis of acute attacks in these patients can usually be attained by daily use of colchicine alone in a dose of 0.6 mg once or twice daily.

Pseudogout

Therapy of pseudogout syndrome is divided into the management of acute attacks and chronic arthralgia, and the prevention of recurrent acute attacks. Joint aspiration followed by local intra-articular injection of steroids is efficacious for treatment of acute inflammation. In addition to the therapeutic effect of the steroids, prior aspiration is beneficial because offending crystals that perpetuate the inflammation are removed. Short courses of the newer nonsteroidal anti-inflammatory agents or phenylbutazone or systemic corticosteroids are effective therapeutic alternatives. Colchicine, 0.6 mg given orally every hour until nausea, vomiting or diarrhea occur or symptoms are relieved, is effective at times, but less consistently than in the treatment of true gout. Intravenous colchicine, administered in doses as described for acute gouty arthritis and begun early in the course of a pseudogout attack is more consistently effective.[63]

Aspirin or the newer nonsteroidal anti-inflammatory agents are helpful in the management of low-grade chronic arthralgias. Similarly, the NSAID's used in relatively low daily maintenance doses are worthy of trial in the prevention of recurrent attacks. Recently, colchicine, 0.6 mg BID to TID has also been described as effective in diminishing recurrent attacks.[64] Therapy based on removal of calcium deposits has not yet been described.

DEGENERATIVE JOINT DISEASE (OSTEOARTHRITIS)

Osteoarthritis, the most common form of arthritis, is often undertreated owing to the misconception that it is always a benign disease. On the other hand, overtreatment is not unusual when it is misdiagnosed as some other more serious disorder.

Rest of involved joints is important for relief of pain and to delay disease progression. Bed rest is usually unnecessary. Physical therapy with heat and therapeutic exercise is a vital part of the therapy program, as in other types of arthritis.

No specific drug is presently available that consistently prevents or retards the basic degenerative disease process. Drug therapy is directed toward symptomatic relief. Aspirin is the preferred drug for basic management. Doses of 640 to 960 mg, three or four times a day, usually provide analgesic and anti-inflammatry effects. The newer nonsteroidal anti-inflammatory drugs (see rheumatoid arthritis, p. 323) are effective in many patients. Phenylbutazone may be considered for use on a short-term basis to treat acute episodes of symptoms. Long-term daily administration of phenylbutazone may be considered, but careful monitoring for possible side effects is necessary. Analgesic agents which may be considered include propoxyphene hydrochloride, acetaminophen, and the newer analgesic formulations such as zomepirac sodium, ibuprofen, naproxen sodium, and fenoprofen calcium (see p. 327). The latter group of agents are derivatives of the nonsteroidal anti-inflammatory drugs and should not be used with them in combination.

Systemic corticosteroids are contraindicated in the management of osteoarthritis. They are minimally effective and toxic reactions may be severe. Intra-articular corticosteroid injections, on the other hand, are valuable when judiciously used in the treatment of acute episodes (see Chapter 21).

Appropriate supportive appliances are helpful in overall management. Cervical spine symptoms often benefit from use of a soft cervical collar and cervical traction. Traction is usually begun by the physical therapist and the procedure is taught for home use. Involvement of the lumbosacral spine is helped by abdominal muscle strengthening exercises and a lumbosacral corset. Canes, crutches or walkers are required for joint protection when weight-bearing joints are severely affected. Surgical procedures such as debridement, osteotomy, arthrodesis, and partial or total prosthetic replacement should be considered when indicated.

SYSTEMIC LUPUS ERYTHEMATOSUS

The treatment of systemic lupus erythematosus depends on which organ systems are involved. Adequate rest and good general health measures are valuable to increase resistance to stress. Mild cases require little specific therapy. When arthritis is the major manifestation of the disease, management is similar to that described for rheumatoid arthritis, although gold therapy is contraindicated. Severe manifestations of systemic lupus erythematosus, such as severe serositis, vasculitis or renal involvement, require the addition of corticosteroids to the therapeutic program. The dosage depends on the acuteness of the process and the critical nature of the organ involved.

Active progressive renal disease is treated with prednisose, 40 to 60 mg, or its equivalent, daily for weeks or months. The dosage is gradually decreased on the basis of clinical and laboratory response. Urinalysis, quantitative urinary protein, and creatinine clearance studies are important parameters in followup of therapeutic response. A fall in the serum anti-DNA titer and a rise in serum complement indicate improvement. Therapy with immunosuppressive agents, such as azathioprine, 2 mg/kg/day,[65,66] cyclophosphamide, 2 mg/kg/day,[65,67] or chlorambucil, 4 to 8 mg/day,[68] has been described in investigational studies as being beneficial.[69,70] Nitrogen mustard in a dosage of 0.4 mg/kg per course administered intravenously appears to be similarly effective. It may be given as a single dose or in divided doses of 0.1 to 0.2 mg/kg/day. Controversy exists as to whether the immunosuppressive agents provide additional benefit to steroids alone, both with respect to response of renal impairment and overall mortality. Although subsets of patients with systemic lupus erythematosus may be benefited by these agents, parameters of patient selection are as yet unavailable. Possible benefits must be balanced against the potentially severe toxicities of these agents. Although the benefits of these agents in the treatment of lupus nephritis are uncertain, most rheumatologists at present would concur in their use in patients with active progressive renal disease not responding to steroids or in whom toxicity prevents steroid use in effective doses.

Vasculitis is also an indication for high-dose steroid therapy. The dosage should be increased to whatever level necessary to bring this complication under control. Prednisone in doses of 60 to 80 mg per day is usually effective. However, doses of 150 to 200 mg per day or higher may be indicated. Management of central nervous system lupus disease is difficult. Some studies suggest that high dose steroids are not only ineffective in control of this serious complication, but may increase mortality due to side reactions such as intercurrent bacterial or viral infection, or gastrointestinal hemorrhage. Other studies, mainly uncontrolled, suggest that steroids in high doses are helpful. On a practical basis, it is usually clinically difficult for the physician to withhold using high dose steroids and immunosuppressives in patients with deteriorating life-threatening disease unresponsive to less heroic measures.

High dose pulse therapy utilizing methylprednisolone, 1 g intravenously daily for 3 doses, has been associated with clinical and serologic improvement in patients with lupus renal disease.[71] Patients with recent antecedent functional deterioration were particularly benefited. Speculations regarding therapeutic mechanisms include beneficial effects of corticosteroids on cellular immunity, suppression of antibody synthesis with reduced immune complex formation, reduction of inflammation and associated mediators, or alterations in release of vasoactive substances.[72] Corticosteroids might also alter glomerular basement membrane permeability to proteins or change the glomerular plasma flow rate. Recently, improvement in components of lupus other than renal disease have been described with this therapy.[73] Further well-controlled double-blind studies will be necessary to establish the role of this therapeutic modality in the overall management of systemic lupus erythematosus. Complications include steroid pseudorheumatism symptoms following cessation of therapy, and occasional serious infections. Fatalities have been described when rapid administration is combined with furosemide therapy leading to rapid potassium shifts and presumed decrease in peripheral resistance or arrhythmias. It is recommended that the medication be administered by piggyback intravenous route over a period of at least 30 minutes, and that concurrent administration of potent diuretics such as furosemide be avoided.

As noted in the section on management of rheumatoid arthritis (page 333), pheresis therapy has been investigated in the management of patients with various connective tissue diseases.[51–53] Studies to date suggest that various forms of pheresis may be a valuable additional form of therapy in patients with systemic lupus erythematosus with severe deteriorating disease not responsive to conventional treatment, and in whom elevated levels of circulating immune complexes have been demonstrated.[52] Plasmapheresis may be followed by a rapid rebound and overshoot of immune complexes and antibody to greater than pretreatment levels, particularly in patients with SLE. Accordingly it is recommended that cytotoxic drugs be used as an adjunct to plasmapheresis to prevent this rebound phenomenon. Although plasmapheresis improves symptoms such as skin rash, arthralgias and arthritis, its use should be limited to trials in life-threatening lupus. Further, trials should be limited to units equipped for clinical investigation.

Antimalarial drugs, such as hydroxychloroquine (Plaquenil) or quinacrine (Atabrine), are effective in the treatment of the arthritis and skin rash. Hydroxychloroquine is given in a dose of 200 mg BID until clinical response occurs; the dose is then reduced to 200 mg once a day for maintenance therapy. Periodic eye examination is mandatory to avoid irreversible eye toxicity. Atabrine is used in a dose of 100 mg BID for two weeks, followed by 100 mg daily. Yellowing of the skin can be controlled by periodic discontinuation of the drug. Skin rash is further helped by topical steroids. Excessive sun exposure should be avoided if there is a history of sun sensitivity; sun screen lotions are valuable as preventive agents in this regard.

SJÖGREN'S SYNDROME

Treatment of Sjögren's syndrome can be divided into symptomatic treatment and treatment directed towards the basic disease process. Artificial tears are useful in relieving eye dryness. In addition, eye symptoms may be aided by removal of excess abnormal mucus through the use of mucolytic agents such as acetylcysteine. Obliteration of the nasolacrimal punctae allows conservation of tears which are allowed to evaporate rather than drain into the nose. Soft contact lenses protect the dry eye but infection can be a major problem. Dryness of the mouth may lead to early and extensive caries; close dental supervision is recommended. Increased oral fluid intake is helpful. Artificial saliva preparations are newly available but do not always meet with patient acceptance. Treatment of associated connective tissue diseases such as rheumatoid arthritis or systemic lupus erythematosus is carried out in similar fashion to when these diseases occur alone. Joint symptoms frequently respond to nonsteroidal anti-inflammatory agents; plaquenil may be helpful. Gold therapy may be instituted when indicated for chronic joint disease; recent studies suggest that gold reactions are not more common. Corticosteroid therapy should be considered when disease manifestations are severe. Corticosteroids and cytotoxic agents such as cyclophosphamide may produce a dramatic response in patients with pseudolymphoma, particularly when the disease involves the kidneys or lungs. Malignant lymphoma, when present, is treated in usual fashion. Renal tubular acidosis and interstitial nephritis may require therapy with steroids or cytotoxic agents, particularly if impairment of renal function is progressive.

SCLERODERMA (PROGRESSIVE SYSTEMIC SCLEROSIS)

Treatment of scleroderma is difficult since no agent has proven effective for specific therapy. Potassium para-aminobenzoate (Potaba), 12 g daily in divided doses, is helpful in some patients for cutaneous changes and is still recommended by some investigators. The dosage is gradually decreased as response ensues. Favorable effects have been noted occasionally with antimalarial agents, such as hydroxychloroquine. More recently, beneficial effects of D-penicillamine in this disease have been described.[74] The extent and degree of skin thickening was decreased and punch skin biopsies before and after therapy revealed significant decrease in the mean weight of biopsy specimens. Visceral manifestations in penicillamine treated patients were approximately half that in non-penicillamine treated patients, and five-year cumulative survival was somewhat improved. These findings suggest cautious optimism that D-penicillamine therapy might be beneficial in patients with progressive systemic sclerosis. The reported beneficial effects of colchicine therapy, 0.6 mg BID or TID, have not been confirmed. Cytotoxic agents have been described as being efficacious in this disorder but use of these agents remains investigational pending further more definitive well-controlled trials.

Symptomatic measures are beneficial in the treatment of various manifestations of the disease. Rest, maintenance of good nutrition, and an exercise program to avoid soft tissue contractures and joint limitation are important measures. Raynaud's phenomenon may be severe and trials with various agents known to be beneficial are indicated (see Chapter 13). Skin ulcers are difficult to manage, although local steroid applications may hasten healing. The ulcer should be kept clean and trauma avoided. Infection, if present, is treated with appropriate antibiotics.

Dimethylsulfoxide (DMSO), which appears helpful when used locally in the treatment of skin ulcerations, requires further study before its use can be considered other than investigational. Dysphagia caused by involvement of the esophagus may respond to bethanechol chloride (Urecholine). Tablets of 5 to 10 mg are chewed and swallowed 30 minutes before meals. Antacids prevent reflux esophagitis. Elevation of the head of the bed on

6 to 8 inch blocks is also valuable. Severe constipation is aided by the use of high fluid intake and bulk promoting agents. Diuretics lessen skin edema and are worthy of trial when this is a prominent symptom. Joint symptoms respond to mild anti-inflammatory agents, such as aspirin, 640 to 960 mg QID, or one of the newer nonsteroidal anti-inflammatory agents. Use of the latter agents should be approached with caution since functional renal impairment may be associated with their administration. Metoclopramide, which stimulates smooth muscle of the gastrointestinal wall and sphincters by its cholinergic activity,[75] has been studied for its use in improving gastrointestinal motility in patients with scleroderma. Improvement has been limited to absent.

Pulmonary symptoms are the second most common cause of death in scleroderma, after renal failure. In patients in whom symptoms or pulmonary roentgenograms suggest early involvement of the lungs by scleroderma, trials of prednisone in doses of 40 to 60 mg/day in divided doses for 8 to 12 weeks may improve function. Pretreatment and follow-up studies should include routine pulmonary function studies, diffusion capacity analyses and gallium scan. Steroid therapy is ineffective when fibrosis has already developed.

Corticosteroid therapy is beneficial in the treatment of myositis occurring in patients with scleroderma. Renal involvement, looked upon in the past as a harbinger of irreversible renal failure and rapidly impending death may respond to blockade of the renin-angiotensin mechanism.[76,77] Remaining renal function is protected and impairment already present reversed to variable degree. Captopril, an oral angiotensin-converting enzyme inhibitor, rapidly controls blood pressure elevations in patients with scleroderma renal disease and may stabilize renal function when initiated before complete renal failure has occurred. The effectiveness of treatment has been confirmed in a small number of patients for a period of many months. Of interest is the concomitant improvement in Raynaud's phenomenon and cutaneous ulcerations, likely related to cutaneous vasodilatation. Similar improvement in renal function has been demonstrated using other antihypertensive agents, particularly propanolol and minoxidil which are renin inhibitors.[78] These observations support aggressive intervention in the treatment of hypertension in patients with scleroderma renal disease; improvement can be anticipated in a significant number of such patients. In patients in whom renal failure has ensued and in whom hypertension control is unsuccessful despite all other measures, nephrectomy may be considered in management.[79] Renal transplantation has had limited success but can be considered as an alternative to chronic hemodialysis.

POLYMYOSITIS (DERMATOMYOSITIS)

Although previously considered a generally fatal disease, polymyositis can now be effectively treated with corticosteroids in most patients. The average patient usually responds to prednisone, 15 mg QID. Doses as high as 100 mg a day or more may be required, however, in patients with resistant disease. High doses are maintained until the patient has shown significant clinical improvement and serum muscle enzymes are approaching normal values. A decrease in creatinuria is also anticipated, but the response is generally slower than that seen with the enzyme levels. Prednisone dosage is then slowly decreased as clinical response and laboratory parameters allow. A dose of 7.5 to 15 mg/day is usually required for a prolonged period to maintain disease control. Close monitoring of the patient by clinical and laboratory study at regular intervals is important during periods of remission, because elevations in serum enzymes or the urinary creatine-creatinine ratio usually precede and signal a clinical episode. Increased doses of prednisone are then indicated.

Routine use of a low-salt diet, potassium supplements, and antacids are valuable in avoiding steroid side reactions. Periodic examination of stools for occult blood and checks for edema and weight gain are advisable. Precipitation of active clinical diabetes is not uncommon. In those few patients who do not respond to prednisone, immunosuppressive agents such as azathioprine[80–82] and methotrexate[83] may be helpful. Immunosuppressive therapy can be considered when the clinical response to high dose prednisone is inadequate, or when intolerance or side reactions to steroids preclude their use in effective therapeutic doses. The therapeutic efficacy of both azathioprine and methotrexate appear similar. As noted previously (see p. 332), these agents are not without significant hazard and should only be initiated with appropriate indication. Their use, however, may allow successful therapeutic response in otherwise resistant cases. A steroid-sparing effect may diminish the need for use of high dose steroid therapy over a prolonged period of time.

NECROTIZING VASCULITIS

High-dose prednisone therapy is the treatment of choice in the management of various forms of necrotizing vasculitis. The average starting dose is 60 mg per day. Higher doses are required in severe disease and the dosage should be increased to whatever level is required to be effective. Recent studies suggest that immunosuppressive agents such as cyclophosphamide or azathioprine are important adjuncts in the management of patients with these disorders.[84–86] At present, it is reasonable to initiate and continue steroid therapy alone in patients with relatively mild disease who show a good clinical response. Immunosuppressives may be added if the therapeutic response to steroids is limited, or requires unacceptably high steroid doses for a prolonged period. In patients who present with life-threatening disease involving vital visceral organs such as the heart, kidney, or brain, the addition of immunosuppressive agents at the *onset* of therapy is appropriate. In patients with Wegener's granulomatosis, immunosuppressive therapy may be life-saving and should be instituted when the diagnosis is made.[87-89] Cyclophosphamide is the drug of choice based on current experience, but other immunosuppressive agents such as azathioprine and methotrexate have been described as being useful. In patients in whom cyclophosphamide is not tolerated on a long-term basis, other immunosuppressive agents may be tried. Cyclophosphamide therapy should be given intravenously in critically ill patients but can be initiated orally in patients whose disease is less threatening. Prednisone 40 to 60 mg/day, or its equivalent, should be initiated simultaneously with immunosuppressive therapy until disease manifestations are well controlled. The steroid dose may then be reduced, according to clinical response. Cyclophosphamide is recommended orally in a daily dose of 1 to 2 mg/kg of body weight. In critically ill patients, 4 to 8 mg/kg IV is administered daily for 3 days, followed in seven to ten days by oral therapy or repeat intravenous administration. Oral therapy should not be initiated for seven to ten days after intravenous administration since there is a lag period after initiation of treatment before the maximal leukopenic effect of cyclophosphamide is seen.

TEMPORAL (CRANIAL) ARTERITIS AND POLYMYALGIA RHEUMATICA

Although temporal arteritis is a self-limited disease that usually remits spontaneously over a period of two to five years, symptoms may be disabling and blindness may occur in untreated cases. Corticosteroid therapy is effective in relieving symptoms and preventing blindness. Patients in whom a diagnosis of temporal arteritis is made should be considered a medical emergency since visual complications may occur suddenly and without warning. If the diagnosis is strongly suspected, blood should be drawn for baseline laboratory studies to include at a minimum a complete blood count and erythrocyte sedimentation rate. Additional blood for plasma fibrinogen level, serum protein electrophoresis, and liver function studies should be obtained as well if feasible. Although steroid therapy may alter the histopathologic findings on temporal artery biopsy, persistent abnormalities will be diagnostic even though biopsy is obtained several days to a week later. In the absence of a history of visual symptoms, a starting dose of prednisone at a level of 60 mg/day in divided doses, or its equivalent is usually satisfactory. In patients with a history of visual symptoms, however, a dose of 100 to 120 mg/day in divided doses is indicated. The dosage is then gradually decreased at a minimum of two- to four-week intervals, utilizing suppression of symptoms and control of the erythrocyte sedimentation rate as guides to management. After appropriate slow reduction in dose over a period of months, a maintenance dose of prednisone, 5 to 10 mg/day, is frequently required for a period of years until resolution of the basic disease process. Recrudescence of symptoms or increase in erythrocyte sedimentation rate should be managed with temporary increases in the daily steroid dosage. Steroid administration on alternate days, or on a once daily basis is less effective in controlling disease manifestations and is not recommended.[90] Since temporal arteritis is a disease of older persons, special attention must be paid to possible complications of steroid therapy such as diabetes and osteoporosis. In general, the lowest dose possible to maintain control of symptoms and sedimentation rate should be used.

In some patients, steroid administration at effective dosage levels is limited by intolerance, or severe complications such as osteoporosis with multiple compression fractures. In these patients, therapeutic alternatives present a real challenge since no other agent has been shown to be of definite help in suppressing the disease and avoiding eye complications. In such cases it has been recommended that cytotoxic agents be added to the maximal tolerated dose of steroids. This program is investigational but might have to be considered when steroid therapy at an effective level cannot be maintained.

Polymyalgia rheumatica syndrome may be idiopathic or may be associated with temporal arteritis and rarely with carcinoma, lymphoma or rheumatoid arthritis. When present in association with clinical or pathologic evidence of temporal arteritis, treatment is carried out as outlined above. Patients with idiopathic polymyalgia rheumatica in the absence of temporal arteritis can usually be managed with a more conservative program. Therapeutic considerations are complicated, however, by the fact that from 10 to 30% or more of patients with polymyalgia rheumatica will have occult pathologic inflammation of the temporal vessels in the absence of any localizing clinical signs or symptoms.[91–93] Accordingly, I routinely recommend biopsy of a temporal artery to exclude occult vasculitis. Although even this study is not always conclusive in that a small percentage of patients with temporal arteritis will have negative findings on biopsy due to resection of an uninvolved part of the vessel in a disease process characterized by skip lesions, a negative temporal artery biopsy considerably diminishes the likelihood that temporal arteritis is present. It is recommended that a long 3 to 4 cm segment of the artery be resected, and that serial sections of the vessel be studied. In the absence of localizing signs, the temporal artery on the patient's nondominant side should be biopsied to save the dominant side vessel for bypass surgery to the cerebral circulation if indicated in future years for arteriosclerotic disease. Superficial temporal arteriograms may help demonstrate arteritis when the biopsy is negative but the additive yield of this procedure in diagnosis has not been striking.[94]

If histopathologic evidence of vasculitis is absent, the patient can be treated as idiopathic polymyalgia rheumatica. Although some experts recommend that such patients can first be treated with nonsteroidal anti-inflammatory agents, I prefer to use prednisone, 20 to 30 mg/day in divided doses, until symptoms of polymyalgia rheumatica and the erythrocyte sedimentation rate are controlled. The dosage is then gradually reduced to the minimal dose required to suppress symptoms and to maintain an essentially normal erythrocyte sedimentation rate. Some authors recommend an alternative overall course of action in patients with polymyalgia rheumatica in whom clinical signs or symptoms of temporal arteritis are absent. They recommend that prednisone be started in a dose of 15 to 20 mg/day and the patient observed closely. If symptoms and the erythrocyte sedimentation rate are rapidly brought under control over a period of one to two weeks, treatment is continued as idiopathic polymyalgia rheumatica. If symptoms and laboratory abnormalities are not rapidly brought under control, temporal artery biopsy is recommended and the steroid dosage increased to control clinical manifestations. I prefer the first alternative in which temporal artery biopsy is performed on all patients with polymyalgia rheumatica; temporal artery biopsy is a benign procedure and therapy can be more appropriately carried out if evidence of arteritis is detected. In patients with polymyalgia rheumatica associated with other disorders, treatment of the underlying disease may provide symptomatic relief. Additional therapy with salicylates, nonsteroidal anti-inflammatory agents, or steroids is usually necessary.

GONOCOCCAL AND SEPTIC (INFECTIOUS) ARTHRITIS

Gonococcal arthritis responds to appropriate doses of penicillin. In acute cases, daily doses of 6 to 10 million units of aqueous penicillin G are given intravenously. Results are most effective if the daily dosage is divided into equal amounts and given as intermittent rather than continuous infusions. High-dose intravenous therapy is continued until clinical response occurs (usually within three to four days). Amoxicillin in a dose of 500 mg q 8h orally can be substituted when acute symptoms have been brought under control. A total of 10 to 14 days of therapy is usually recommended. Use of amoxicillin throughout the entire course of therapy may be considered in selected instances when parenteral therapy is not feasible and clinical manifestations of the disease are mild. A loading dose of 3.0 g with probenecid 1.0 g is administered, followed by a daily dose of 500 mg q 8h. Close daily supervision is essential to assure appropriate clinical response. Bed rest, use of analgesic agents and splinting of acutely inflamed joints are helpful for symptomatic relief. Heat applications should be used with caution (if at all) because they may potentiate the inflammatory process. For patients who are allergic to penicillin, tetracycline is the drug of choice. A dose of 500 mg QID intravenously for two to three days is followed by 500 mg QID orally for the two-week course of therapy.

Management of septic arthritis requires specific identification of the offending infectious agent followed by institution of appropriate antibiotic therapy. The most commonly involved organisms are the gram-positive

TABLE 19-1. Suggested Treatment Schedules for Management of Septic (Infectious) Arthritis

Drug	Dosage*	Alternative agents†
(1) Therapy before infecting organism has been identified or presumptive diagnosis, no organism eventually isolated		
Adults and older children: Penicillinase-resistant semisynthetic penicillins‡		
Nafcillin	100 mg/kg/day in equal doses q 4-6 h IV	Cefazolin, § 50 mg/kg/day in equal doses q 6-8h IV, or Vancomycin, 2.0 gm/day in equal doses q 6-12h IV, or Clindamycin, 20 to 30 mg/kg/day in equal doses q 4-6h IV, or Erythromycin, 30 to 50 mg/kg/day in equal doses q 4-6h IV
Oxacillin	100 mg/kg/day in equal doses q 4-6 h IV	
Children under age three: Penicillinase-resistant semisynthetic penicillins plus	See above	
Ampicillin‖	150 to 200 mg/kg/day in equal doses q 4-6 h IV	Cefamandole, § 100 to 150 mg/kg/day in equal doses q 4-6h IV, or Chloramphenicol, 25 to 60 mg/kg/day in equal doses q 4-6h IV ¶
(2) Therapy based on gram-stain identification		
Gram-positive cocci		
Penicillinase-resistant semisynthetic penicillins	See above	Cefazolin, § 50 mg/kg/day in equal doses q 6-8h IV, or Vancomycin, 2.0 gm/day in equal doses q 6-12h IV, or Clindamycin, 20 to 30 mg/kg/day in equal doses q 4-6h IV, or Erythromycin, 30 to 50 mg/kg/day in equal doses q 4-6h IV
Gram-negative cocci or coccobacilli		
Adults: Aqueous penicillin G	1.5 to 2.5 million units q 6 h IV	Tetracycline, 250 mg q 6h IV, or Cefoxatin, § 100 to 150 mg/kg/day in equal doses q 4-6h IV

Gram-negative bacilli	Children: Ampicillin‖	150 to 200 mg/kg/day in equal doses q 4-6 h IV	Chloramphenicol, 25 to 60 mg/kg/day in equal doses q 4-6 h IV¶
	Tobramycin	3.0 to 5.0 mg/kg/day in equal doses q 8 h IV	Chloramphenicol 0.5 to 1.0 g q 6 h IV
(3) Therapy based on specific organism identification			
Penicillin-G resistant Staphylococcus aureus	Penicillinase-resistant semisynthetic penicillins	See above	Cefazolin, § 50 mg/kg/day in equal doses q 6-8h IV, or Vancomycin, 2.0 gm/day in equal doses q 6-12h IV, or
Penicillin-G sensitive Staphylococcus aureus	Aqueous penicillin G	1.0 million units q 6 h IV	Clindamycin, 20 to 30 mg/kg/day in equal doses q 4-6h IV, or Erythromycin, 30 to 50 mg/kg/day in equal doses q 4-6h IV
Streptococcus pneumoniae (pneumococcus)	Aqueous penicillin G	600,000 units q 6 h IV	
Streptococcus pyogenes	Aqueous penicillin G	600,000 units q 6 h IV	
Gonococcus	Aqueous penicillin G	1.5 to 2.5 million units q 6 h IV	Tetracycline, 250 mg q 6h IV, or Cefoxatin, § 100 to 150 mg/kg/day in equal doses q 4-6h IV
Hemophilus influenzae	Ampicillin‖	150 to 200 mg/kg/day in equal doses q 4-6 h IV	Cefamandole, § 100 to 150 mg/kg/day in equal doses q 4-6h IV, or Chloramphenicol, 25 to 60 mg/kg/day in equal doses q 4-6h IV ¶
Escherichia coli	Ampicillin	8 to 12 gm daily in equally divided doses q 4 h IV	
Pseudomonas	Tobramycin plus Ticarcillin	3.0 to 5.0 mg/kg/day in equal doses q 8 h IV; 200 to 300 mg/kg/day in equal doses q 4 h IV	New β-lactam antibiotics may prove useful in Pseudomonas and other gram-negative bacillus infections.

*Variation in dosage may be required in the presence of renal or hepatic impairment. DOSES GIVEN FOR ADULTS UNLESS OTHERWISE NOTED.

†If drug allergy or intolerance occurs, or if therapeutic response is inadequate.

‡Add tobramycin, 3.0 to 5.0 mg/kg/day in equal doses q 8 h IV, if trauma, predisposing underlying disease, or malignancy is present.

§Cephalosporins are useful as alternative agents in the absence of major idiosyncratic reactions to penicillin, such as angioneurotic edema, exfoliative dermatitis and anaphylaxis.

¶In neonates, chloramphenicol dose should not exceed 25 mg/kg/day.

‖Regional variations in susceptibility of Hemophilus influenzae to ampicillin have been described.

cocci, Staphylococcus aureus, Streptococcus pneumoniae (pneumococcus) and Streptococcus pyogenes. Less common causes are the gram-negative bacilli, Escherichia coli, Salmonella species and Pseudomonas. The gram-negative coccobacillus Hemophilus influenzae is a common cause of infectious arthritis in infants and children up to age three.

Antibiotic treatment can be divided into four phases: (1) therapy before the infecting organism has been identified, (2) therapy based on gram-stain identification of the etiologic agent, (3) therapy following specific culture identification of the organism and knowledge of the results of sensitivity studies, and (4) therapy based on a presumptive diagnosis of septic arthritis when no offending organism can be identified following all appropriate microbiologic studies. Specific recommendations for therapy in all age groups are given in Table 19-1. The high frequency of infection with Hemophilus influenzae in children under age three is reflected in the programs outlined for this patient population.

Initial therapy is given by parenteral routes in order to rapidly establish high serum and synovial fluid drug concentrations. The daily dose of IV drugs is divided into equal doses, which are administered intermittently. This technique provides high peak activity of the drug. Intra-articular administration is not required because effective concentrations in the synovial fluid are achieved following parenteral administration of most antibiotics.[95] In addition, direct instillations of the drug into the joint may result in a complicating chemical synovitis. A fall in body temperature, drop in the peripheral leukocyte count, and decrease in joint swelling indicate clinical response. Therapeutic response is further monitored by periodic synovial fluid analysis and culture and roentgenologic examination. Paired samples of serum and synovial fluid should be tested for bactericidal activity against the responsible pathogen to monitor dosage requirements. Oral administration of drugs is substituted for parenteral therapy when clinical evidence of synovitis diminishes and inflammatory changes in joint fluid revert toward normal. Antibiotic treatment is continued for a minimum of one to two weeks after clinical and laboratory cure appears to have taken place. Usually, at least four to six weeks of therapy are required. Close observation of the patient is indicated for another several weeks after cessation of antibiotic therapy to detect signs of relapse.

Joint drainage by needle aspiration is performed daily or every other day if synovial fluid rapidly reaccumulates. This procedure keeps the joint cavity relatively free of destructive enzymes elaborated by bacteria and leukocytes. If needle aspiration does not control reaccumulation of fluid, or if clinical response is slow, open surgical drainage is indicated. Open drainage should be instituted even earlier in the course of management if gross pus is observed on initial synovial fluid studies, since repeated aspirations may be inadequate to remove the highly destructive bacteria and proteolytic enzymes. Although a number of orthopaedists continue to recommend immediate open drainage in all cases of septic arthritis, conservative therapy with antibiotics and repeated aspiration is effective in most patients. Morbidity associated with anesthesia and surgery is avoided and rehabilitation hastened. Open drainage should, however, be utilized early in septic arthritis involving the hip, since aspiration is difficult and incomplete. Early consideration of open drainage is advised for septic arthritis in children, no matter which joint is involved.

The involved joint should be placed at complete rest until significant signs of improvement are noted. Use of infected joints may result in more rapid breakdown of cartilage by the addition of mechanical stress. Pain relief is aided by immobilization in a splint. Physical therapy with gentle range-of-motion exercises is instituted when clinical remission allows.

ACUTE OSTEOMYELITIS

Osteomyelitis is most often due to infection with Staphylococcus aureus. Intravenous use of a semisynthetic penicillinase-resistant penicillin is the treatment of choice for initiation of therapy until positive organism identification and sensitivity studies have been completed. Aqueous penicillin G, given intravenously, can then be substituted if the organism is susceptible to this agent. In the presence of infection by other bacterial agents, other antibiotics specifically directed to the offending organism are utilized. Oral therapy can be substituted when the infectious process begins to respond. Periodic roentgenograms, leukocyte counts, erythrocyte sedimentation rates, and blood cultures should be performed in disease followup. As with septic arthritis, antibiotic treatment should be continued for several weeks following clinical and laboratory evidence of cure. Although many patients will respond to a four- to six-week course of therapy, the need for more prolonged antibiotic administration is not uncommon. Close observation for signs and symptoms of relapse is indicated. The erythrocyte sedimentation rate is a particularly useful parameter in evaluating the therapeutic response both during active therapy and in followup observation. Surgical drainage should be initiated in patients who do not respond to a conservative program of management.

The foregoing programs of therapy are suggested methods of management. Alternative programs are effective if based on sound principles of antibiotic usage. Specific recommendations will change as new, more effective antibiotics become available. Drug dosage may have to be lowered to avoid toxicity if renal or hepatic disease cause higher effective drug levels.

REFERENCES

1. Wolfe, J. D., Metzger, A. L. and Goldstein, R. C.: Aspirin hepatitis. Ann Int Med 80:74, 1974.

2. Rich, R. R. and Johnson, J. S.: Salicylate hepatotoxicity in patients with juvenile rheumatoid arthritis. Arthritis Rheum 16:1, 1973.
3. Miller, J. J., III and Weissman, D. B.: Correlations between transaminase concentrations and serum salicylate concentration in juvenile rheumatoid arthritis. Arthritis Rheum 19:115, 1976.
4. Seaman, W. E. and Plotz, P. H.: Effect of aspirin on liver tests in patients with RA or SLE and in normal volunteers. Arthritis Rheum 19:155, 1976.
5. Kimberly, R. P. and Plotz, P. H.: Aspirin-induced depression of renal function. N Eng J Med 296:418, 1977.
6. Kimberly, R. P. et al.: Elevated urinary prostaglandins and the effects of aspirin on renal function in lupus erythematosus. Ann Int Med 89:336, 1978.
7. Roth, G. J., Stanford, N. and Majerus, P. W.: Acetylation of prostaglandin synthetase by aspirin. Proc Natl Acad Sci USA 72:3073, 1975.
8. Huskisson, E. C.: Antiinflammatory drugs. Semin Arth Rheum 7:1, 1977.
9. Simon, L. S. and Mills, J. A.: Non-steroidal antiinflammatory drugs (second of two parts): new non-steroidal antiinflammatory drugs (in: Koch-Weser J: Drug therapy). N Eng J Med 302:1237, 1980.
10. Kimberly, R. P. et al.: Reduction of renal function by newer nonsteroidal antiinflammatory drugs. Am J Med 64:804, 1978.
11. Brezin, J. H. et al.: Reversible renal failure and nephrotic syndrome associated with nonsteroidal anti-inflammatory drugs. N Eng J Med 301:1271, 1979.
12. Walshe, J. J. and Venutuo, R. C.: Acute oliguric renal failure induced by indomethacin: possible mechanism. Ann Int Med 91:47, 1979.
13. Wendland, M. L., Wagoner, R. D. and Holley, K. E.: Renal failure associated with fenoprofen. Mayo Clin Proc 55:103, 1980.
14. Champion, D. et al.: Effect of concurrent aspirin (ASA) administration on serum concentrations of indomethacin (I). Arthritis Rheum 14:375, 1971.
15. Brooks, P. M., Walker, J. J., Bell, M. A., Buchanan, W. W. and Rhymer, A. R.: Indomethacin-aspirin interactions: a clinical appraisal. Br Med J 3:69, 1975.
16. Burns, C. A.: Indomethacin, reduced retinal sensitivity and corneal deposits. Am J Ophthalmol 61:825, 1968.
17. Carr, R. E. and Siegel, I. M.: Retinal function in patients treated with indomethacin. Am J Ophthalmol 75:302, 1973.
18. Levinson, J. E. et al.: Comparison of tolmetin sodium and aspirin in the treatment of juvenile rheumatoid arthritis. J Pediat 91:799, 1977.
19. Carter, M. E. and James, V. H.: Effect of alternate day, single dose, corticosteroid therapy on pituitary-adrenal function. Ann Rheum Dis 31:379, 1972.
20. Licht, H., Seeff, L. B. and Zimmerman, H. J.: Apparent potentiation of acetaminophen hepatotoxicity by alcohol. Ann Int Med 92:511, 1980.
21. Marks, J. S. and Power, B. J.: Is chloroquine obsolete in treatment of rheumatic disease? Lancet 1:371, 1979.
22. Conference proceedings. The place of antimalarials in rheumatology. Ann Rheum Dis 40:323, 1981.
23. Percival, S. P. B. and Meanock, I.: Chloroquine: ophthalmological safety and clinical assessment in rheumatoid arthritis. Br Med J 3:579, 1968.
24. Freedman, A. and Back, F.: Mepacrine and rheumatoid arthritis: preliminary communication. Lancet 2:321, 1952.
25. Dame, L. R.: Effect of atabrine on the human visual system. Am J Ophthalmol 29:1432, 1946.
26. Research Subcommittee of the Empire Rheumatism Council: Gold therapy in rheumatoid arthritis. Report of a multicenter controlled trial. Ann Rheum Dis 19:95, 1960.
27. Sigler, J. W. et al.: Gold salts in the treatment of rheumatoid arthritis. A double-blind study. Ann Int Med 80:21, 1974.
28. Gibbons, R. B.: Complications of chrysotherapy: a review of recent studies. Arch Int Med 139:343, 1979.
29. Podell, T. E. et al.: Pulmonary toxicity with gold therapy. Arthritis Rheum 23:347, 1980.

30. Jaffe, I. A.: The technique of penicillamine administration in rheumatoid arthritis. Arthritis Rheum 18:513, 1975.
31. Tsang, I. K. et al.: D-penicillamine in the treatment of rheumatoid arthritis. Arthritis Rheum 20:666, 1977.
32. Hill, H. F.: Treatment of rheumatoid arthritis with penicillamine. Semin Arth Rheum 6:361, 1977.
33. Bucknall, R. C. et al.: Myasthenia gravis associated with penicillamine treatment for rheumatoid arthritis. Br Med J 1:600, 1975.
34. Crouzet, J. et al.: Lupus induced by D-penicillamine during the treatment of rheumatoid arthritis: two observations and systemic immunologic studies during this treatment. Ann Med Interne 125:71, 1974.
35. Cucher, B. G. and Goldman, A. L.: D-penicillamine-induced polymyositis in rheumatoid arthritis [letter]. Ann Int Med 85:615, 1976.
36. Sternlieb, I., Bennett, B. and Scheinberg, I. H.: D-penicillamine-induced Goodpasture's syndrome in Wilson's disease. Ann Int Med 82:673, 1975.
37. Seibold, J. R., Lynch, C. J. and Medsger, T. A., Jr.: Cholestasis associated with D-penicillamine therapy: case report and review of the literature. Arthritis Rheum 24:554, 1981.
38. Murphy, K. C. et al.: Obliterative bronchiolitis in two rheumatoid arthritis patients treated with penicillamine. Arthritis Rheum 24:557, 1981.
39. Cooperative Clinics Committee of the American Rheumatism Association: A controlled trial of cyclophosphamide in rheumatoid arthritis. N Eng J Med 283:883, 1970.
40. Williams, H. J. et al.: Comparison of high and low dose cyclophosphamide therapy in rheumatoid arthritis. Arthritis Rheum 23:521, 1980.
41. Abel, T. et al.: Rheumatoid vasculitis: effect of cyclophosphamide on the clinical course and levels of circulating immune complexes. Ann Int Med 93:407, 1980.
42. Willkens, R. F., Watson, M. A. and Paxson, C. S.: Low dose pulse methotrexate therapy in rheumatoid arthritis. J Rheumatol 7:501, 1980.
43. Levy, J. et al.: A double-blind controlled evaluation of azathioprine treatment in rheumatoid arthritis and psoriatic arthritis. Arthritis Rheum 15:116, 1972.
44. Dwosh, I. L. et al.: Azathioprine in early rheumatoid arthritis. Comparison with gold and chloroquine. Arthritis Rheum 20:685, 1977.
45. Plotz, P. H. et al.: Bladder complications in patients receiving cyclophosphamide for systemic lupus erythematosus or rheumatoid arthritis. Ann Int Med 91:221, 1979.
46. Runge, L. A. et al.: Treatment of rheumatoid arthritis with levamisole. A controlled trial. Arthritis Rheum 20:1445, 1977.
47. Miller, B. et al.: Double-blind placebo controlled crossover evaluation of levamisole in rheumatoid arthritis. Arthritis Rheum 23:172, 1980.
48. Cardella, C. J.: Plasma exchange—a new approach to immune modulation in rheumatic diseases. J Rheumatol 6:606, 1979.
49. Wallace, D. J. et al.: Plasmapheresis and lymphoplasmapheresis in the management of rheumatoid arthritis. Arthritis Rheum 22:703, 1979.
50. Rothwell, R. S. et al.: A controlled study of plasma exchange in the treatment of severe rheumatoid arthritis. Arthritis Rheum 23:785, 1980.
51. Wallace, D. J. et al.: Advances in the use of therapeutic pheresis for the management of rheumatic diseases. Semin Arth Rheum 10:81, 1980.
52. Jones, J. V. et al.: The role of therapeutic plasmapheresis in the rheumatic diseases. J Lab Clin Med 97:589, 1981.
53. Karsh, J. et al.: Lymphopheresis in rheumatoid arthritis. A randomized trial. Arthritis Rheum 24:867, 1981.
54. Farber, G. A., Forshner, J. G. and O'Quinn, S. E.: Reiter's syndrome. Treatment with methotrexate. JAMA 200:171, 1967.
55. Dorwart, B. et al.: Chrysotherapy in psoriatic arthropathy. Arthritis Rheum 21:513, 1978.
56. Richter, M. B., Kinsella, P. and Corbett, M.: Gold in psoriatic arthropathy. Ann Rheum Dis 39:279, 1980.

57. Perlman, S. G. et al.: Photochemotherapy and psoriatic arthritis: a prospective study. Ann Int Med 91:717, 1979.

58. Black, R. L. et al.: Methotrexate therapy in psoriatic arthritis. JAMA 189:743, 1964.

59. Weinstein, G. D. and Frost, P.: Methotrexate for psoriasis. A new therapeutic schedule. Arch Dermatol 103:33, 1971.

60. Baum, J. et al.: Treatment of psoriatic arthritis with 6-mercaptopurine. Arthritis Rheum 16:139, 1973.

61. Merlin, H. E.: Azoospermia caused by colchicine. Fertil Steril 23:180, 1972.

62. Ferreira, N. R. and Buoniconti, A.: Trisomy after colchicine therapy. Lancet 2:1304, 1968.

63. Tabatabai, M. R. and Cummings, N. A.: Intravenous colchicine in the treatment of acute pseudogout. Arthritis Rheum 23:370, 1980.

64. Spiliotis, T. E.: Colchicine and chronic pseudogout [letter]. Arthritis Rheum 24:862, 1981.

65. Steinberg, A. D., Decker, J. L. and Aptekar, R. G.: Completed ten week trial of cyclophosphamide or azathioprine or placebo in lupus nephritis. Arthritis Rheum 16:572, 1973.

66. Hayslett, J. P. et al.: The effect of azathioprine on lupus glomerulonephritis. Medicine 51:393, 1972.

67. Steinberg, A. D. et al.: Cyclophosphamide in lupus nephritis: a controlled trial. Ann Int Med 75:165, 1971.

68. Epstein, W. V. and Grausz, H.: Favorable outcome in diffuse proliferative glomerulonephritis of systemic lupus erythematosus. Arthritis Rheum 17:129, 1974.

69. Decker, J. L.: Cytotoxic agents in the management of systemic lupus erythematosus. Clin Rheum Dis 1:665, 1975.

70. Ivanova, M. M. et al.: Cyclosphosphamide, azathioprine or chlorambucil for systemic lupus erythematosus nephritis. Arthritis Rheum 22:624, 1979.

71. Kimberly, R. P. et al.: High-dose intravenous methylprednisolone pulse therapy in systemic lupus erythematosus. Am J Med 70:817, 1981.

72. Fan, P. T. et al.: Effect of corticosteroids on human immune response: comparison of one and three daily 1 gm intravenous pulses of methylprednisolone. J Lab Clin Med 91:625, 1978.

73. Eyanson, S. et al.: Methylprednisolone pulse therapy for nonrenal lupus erythematosus. Ann Rheum Dis 39:377, 1980.

74. Steen, V., Medsger, T. A. and Rodnan, G. P.: Beneficial effect of D-penicillamine (DPA) on the course of progressive systemic sclerosis (PSS): a retrospective analysis. Arthritis Rheum 24(Suppl):S82, 1981.

75. Schulze-Delrieu, K.: Metoclopramide (in: Koch-Weser J: Drug therapy). N Eng J Med 305:28, 1981.

76. Clements, P. et al.: Clinical course of four patients with scleroderma renal crisis treated with captopril. Arthritis Rheum 23:662, 1980.

77. D'Angelo, W. A. et al.: Early versus late treatment of scleroderma renal crisis and malignant hypertension with captopril. Arthritis Rheum 23:664, 1980.

78. Lam, M. et al.: Reversal of severe renal failure in systemic sclerosis. Ann Intern Med 89:642, 1978.

79. LeRoy, E. C. and Fleishmann, R. M.: The management of renal scleroderma: experience with dialysis, nephrectomy and transplantation. Am J Med 64:974, 1978.

80. Benson, M. D. and Aldo, M. A.: Azathioprine therapy in polymyositis. Arch Int Med 132:547, 1973.

81. Bunch, T. W. et al.: Azathioprine with prednisone for polymyositis: a controlled, clinical trial. Ann Int Med 92:365, 1980.

82. Bunch, T. W.: Prednisone and azathioprine for polymyositis: a long-term follow-up. Arthritis Rheum 24:45, 1981.

83. Sokoloff, M. C., Goldberg, L. S. and Pearson, C. M.: Treatment of corticosteroid-resistant polymyositis with methotrexate. Lancet 1:14, 1971.

84. Fauci, A. S., Doppman, J. L. and Wolff, S. M.: Cyclophosphamide-induced remissions in advanced polyarteritis nodosa. Am J Med 64:890, 1978.
85. Fauci, A. S. et al.: Cyclophosphamide therapy of severe systemic necrotizing vasculitis. N Eng J Med 301:235, 1979.
86. Leib, E. S., Restivo, C. and Paulus, H. E.: Immunosuppressive and corticosteroid therapy of polyarteritis nodosa. Am J Med 67:941, 1979.
87. Novack, S. N. and Pearson, C. M.: Cyclophosphamide therapy in Wegener's granulomatosis. N Eng J Med 284:938, 1971.
88. Capizzi, R. L. and Bertino, J. R.: Methotrexate therapy of Wegener's granulomatosis. Ann Int Med 74:74, 1971.
89. Wolff, S. M., et al.: Wegener's granulomatosis. Ann Int Med 81:513, 1974.
90. Hunder, G. G. et al.: Daily and alternate-day corticosteroid regimens in treatment of giant cell arteritis: comparison in a prospective study. Ann Int Med 82:613, 1975.
91. Dixon, A. S.-J., Beardwell, C., Kay, A. et al.: Polymyalgia rheumatica and temporal arteritis. Ann Rheum Dis 25:203, 1966.
92. Fauchald, P., Rygvold, O. and Oystese, B.: Temporal arteritis and polymyalgia rheumatica. Clinical and biopsy findings. Ann Int Med 77:845, 1972.
93. Hunder, G. G. and Allen, G. L.: The relationship between polymyalgia rheumatica and temporal arteritis. Geriatrics 28:134, 1973.
94. Sewell, J. R. et al.: Combined temporal arteriography and selective biopsy in suspected giant cell arteritis. Ann Rheum Dis 39:124, 1980.
95. Parker, R. H. and Schmid, F. R.: Antibacterial activity of synovial fluid during therapy of septic arthritis. Arthritis Rheum 14:96, 1971.

CHAPTER **20**

PHYSICAL THERAPY, OCCUPATIONAL THERAPY, AND SUPPORTIVE APPLIANCES

PHYSICAL THERAPY

Patients with connective tissue disorders require careful evaluation by the physical therapist. Joint motion, muscle strength and functional level should be assessed in detail, so that overall goals of treatment can be determined. The specific procedures selected by the therapist to achieve these goals will vary according to the specific problems under consideration.

Joint limitation is treated by a combined program of rest, heat and programmed exercises. Moist heat is generally more beneficial than dry heat due to its greater conductive properties. Deep heat is especially effective in treating periarthritis of the shoulder. Simple measures such as warm soaks, tub baths, and Hydrocollator packs are effective and can be readily used at home on a day-to-day basis. Paraffin applications (Fig. 20-1) are beneficial in the treatment of arthritis of the hand and wrist. Hydrotherapy allows greater ease of movement during exercise because it eliminates the effects of gravity. Hubbard tank therapy is useful when multiple joints are involved.

Although heat therapy is used more commonly, cryotherapy should be considered in certain situations. The temporary anesthetic effect of cold applications is especially valuable in managing patients following reconstructive surgery, since it allows a more pain-free range of motion for exercise.

Heat, followed by exercise, is directed toward maintaining and improving joint mobility. When knees are involved, isometric exercises are generally associated with less pain than isotonic exercises. Isometric exercises are performed by contracting the muscle without moving the joint through its range of motion. During isotonic exercises, the joint moves actively through its range of motion.

Assessment of muscle strength is often difficult in patients who have limited joint range of motion or inflammatory muscle disease. In patients

Figure 20-1. Application of paraffin to hand of patient with rheumatoid arthritis.

with polymyositis, frequent re-evaluations of muscle strength and function and careful grading of exercise programs are required.

Maintenance of functional independence in patients with chronic disease requires careful planning with the patient in order to set realistic goals. Shoulder and knee mobility and good quadriceps strength are especially important. Adaptive equipment and appliances should be selected with care. Canes, crutches or walkers may be used to reduce stress on weight-bearing joints. Improper use of such devices can be not only ineffective but unsafe; instructions regarding their use varies with the disability. In general, a cane should be used in the hand opposite the joint to be protected. Although walkers are ordinarily one of the most stable appliances, they are unsafe on sidewalks and stairs. Modification of hand grips on appliances is often necessary for patients whose hands and wrists are affected by disease.

Cervical or pelvic traction is utilized when a distraction force is indicated. Application can be either intermittent or static; the specific method varies with the individual patient's problem.

OCCUPATIONAL THERAPY

The major goal of occupational therapy in the management of patients with arthritis and related disorders is the attainment of maximal independence in daily activity. Physical capabilities, self-care needs, and psychosocial background are evaluated. Identification of problem areas allows individualization of treatment programs and the setting of realistic goals.

Purposeful activities and exercise are utilized to overcome limitations in joint range of motion and muscle weakness. Craft activities, such as painting, loom weaving and woodworking, provide exercise for specifically involved joints. Strengthening is achieved through antigravity positioning of involved extremities or use of weighted cuffs. Small finger weights, light rubber bands and pliable plastic media are used for similar purposes.

For patients with increasing physical disability, an important aspect of the occupational therapy program is instruction in self-care.[1] The levels of function in bathing, feeding, dressing and hygienic activities are evaluated. Necessary training and assistive devices are then provided to help the patient maintain or regain maximal independence.[1]

For the arthritic patient, bathing is made easier and safer through instructions in transfer and the use of low tub stools, shower seats, nonskid

Figure 20-2. Supportive aids used in occupational therapy. (A) Button hook. (B) Long-handled shoe horn. (C) Long-handled wooden scissors (reachers).

rubber mats and grab rails. Special hydraulic lifts are effective in transferring patients into and out of tubs and showers, but their usefulness is limited by cost factors. Long-handled sponges and brushes are helpful for bathing the lower extremities, particularly when hip and knee flexion is limited.

Various commercial devices are available to facilitate ease in dressing. Velcro fasteners and button aids (Fig. 20-2A) are useful for patients with limited finger movement. When arthritis or proximal girdle weakness prevents normal function of the lower extremities, long-handled shoe horns (Fig. 20-2B), stocking aids, and shoelaces that do not require tying are particularly useful. Long reachers (Fig. 20-2C) to pick items off the floor are valuable. Elevated toilet seats help patients with weakness or limitation of motion in the lower extremities.

Patients can be taught to maintain their general activity level through the use of joint protection and work simplification techniques. These techniques are prophylactic in the early stages of the disease process when deformity is minimal. Kitchen activities, for example, can be made easier with the use of wide-handled utensils (Fig. 20-3A), specially designed knives, forks and spoons (Fig. 20-3B), and lightweight pots and pans. Where possible, sitting instead of standing is encouraged, and work surfaces with adjustable heights should be used. Patients should be shown how to organize their work, daily living, and leisure time to maintain an adequate balance of rest and activity.

A   **B**

Figure 20-3. Special eating utensils. (A) Wide-handled spoon and fork to facilitate grasp. (B) Hinged spoon and fork; curved knife allows cutting with rocker motion.

Figure 20-4.   Elastic wrist splint with Velcro fasteners. Stabilization of the wrist is aided by a volar metal insert.

Figure 20-5.   Specially designed splints. (A) Volar splint for relief of joint pain and maintenance of normal wrist and hand position. (B) Thumb opponens splint.

Throughout the treatment course provided by the occupational therapist, emotional and motivational factors are primary considerations. The patient may require a period of adjusting to his disability before he is ready to participate in purposeful activities or self-care training.

SUPPORTIVE APPLIANCES

Splints

For arthritic patients, resting and dynamic splints can be effective in providing pain relief, support, and the proper positioning of affected muscles and joints. They are most often applied to wrists, hands and knees and are usually worn at night. Splints of various types and sizes are available from commercial sources (Fig. 20-4) or can be individually fabricated by the occupational therapist using thermal plastic materials or plaster bandage (Fig. 20-5).

Foot Appliances

Foot pain can often be partially alleviated by various simple appliances. Transverse metatarsal pads, which take the weight off the metatarsophalangeal joints, are indicated when these joints are symptomatic. They can be built into the longitudinal arch of the shoe or may be inserted as a separate appliance. When metatarsal pads do not provide adequate relief, metatarsophalangeal joint pain may be effectively relieved by placing transverse metatarsal bars on the outer sole of the shoe. Longitudinal arch supports help to prevent pronation deformities of the foot. Lifts are used to correct disparities in leg length. Inversion and eversion deformities of the foot may benefit from the use of appropriate wedging. Molded Space Shoes are helpful in the presence of severe multiple deformities.

Cervical Collars

Collars for partially immobilizing the cervical spine are indicated in the management of various neck disorders. Soft collars are available in many sizes. Rigid plastic collars should be utilized when more complete immobilization is required (Fig. 20-6). Duration of use depends upon the specific problem being treated. In patients who have significant involvement of the cervical spine with rheumatoid arthritis, the collar should be worn as often as possible. Use of the collar is especially important when riding in an automobile, since severe neck injury may occur with relatively slight trauma in case of accident.

Figure 20-6. Plastic cervical collar used for treatment of neck pain in patient with juvenile rheumatoid arthritis.

Back Supports

Disease of the lumbosacral or dorsal spine may require the use of supportive corsets or braces; well-fitting lumbosacral or lumbodorsal corsets respectively are usually sufficient for the treatment of most such disorders. These garments require individualized tailoring by experts familiar with their use. Semirigid stays are added as required. More intensive immobilization may require use of spinal ortheses (braces).

Transcutaneous Nerve Stimulation (TNS)

Transcutaneous nerve stimulation is a modality in which an electrical current is applied through the skin to a peripheral nerve or nerves.[2-7] Pain relief is felt partially due to modulation of nerve synapses or "gates" in feedback neurogenic pain control. Clinical benefits described in various studies are at times difficult to evaluate, and well-demonstrated placebo effects make interpretations of data difficult. Evaluation is further complicated by attempts to compare the many different types of such TNS units available, applied to a heterogeneous group of pain disorders. Instructions as to the proper variation of electric current and frequencies, and which anatomic areas are to be selected for application of leads must be carefully individualized. The eventual role of this modality in pain relief has yet to be determined.

REFERENCES

1. Klinger, J. L. (ed.): Self-help Manual for Patients with Arthritis. 2nd Edition. Prepared by the Allied Health Professions Section of the Arthritis Foundation. (Available from the Arthritis Foundation, 3400 Peachtree Road, NE, Atlanta, Georgia 30326.)
2. Loeser, J. D., Black, R. G. and Christman, A.: Relief of pain by transcutaneous stimulation. J Neurosurg 42:308, 1975.
3. Sternbach, R. A., Ignelzi, R. J., Deems, L. M. et al.: Transcutaneous electrical analgesia: a follow-up analysis. Pain 2:35, 1976.
4. McKelvy, P. L.: Clinical report on the use of specific TNS units. Phys Ther 58: 1474, 1978.
5. Mannheimer, C., Lund, S. and Carlsson, C.: The effect of transcutaneous electrical nerve stimulation (TNS) on joint pain in patients with rheumatoid arthritis. Scand J Rheum 7:13, 1978.
6. Schuster, G. D. and Infante, M. C.: The efficacy of TNS: noninvasive postoperative analgesia. Ortho Rev 8:143, 1979.
7. Mannheimer, C. and Carlsson, C.: The analgesic effect of transcutaneous electrical nerve stimulation (TNS) in patients with rheumatoid arthritis. A comparative study of different pulse patterns. Pain 6:329, 1979.

CHAPTER 21

LOCAL INJECTION THERAPY

INTRA-ARTICULAR THERAPY

Intra-articular therapy is a valuable adjunct to general therapeutic programs in the treatment of arthritis. It is particularly useful in the management of patients with monoarticular or oligoarticular arthritis, or in the management of patients with generalized disease in whom one or two joints are "out of pace" with the clinical progress. In these situations, local therapy allows effective control of a limited number of joints and diminishes the hazard of side reactions associated with more aggressive use of potent systemic medications. Corticosteroid preparations are the most commonly used agents for intra-articular therapy. Immunosuppressive drugs and radioactive substances have also been used in an attempt to provide longer periods of effectiveness.

Corticosteroids

Intra-articular administration of corticosteroids is beneficial and safe when judiciously used.[1,2] Suppression of synovitis in the various noninfectious inflammatory arthritides is often striking. Post-injection studies reveal increased synovial fluid viscosity and hyaluronic acid concentration.[3] It has been suggested that corticosteroids act via stabilization of lysosomal membranes with prevention of release of acid hydrolases.[4] Experiments utilizing leukocyte in contrast to hepatic cell lysosomes have, however, failed to document such stabilization.[5] Relief of symptoms in osteoarthritic joints has also been described,[6–8] although many of these studies have been uncontrolled. It is important to note in this regard that placebo injections with suspending vehicle, sodium chloride, or local anesthetics have been shown to provide relief similar to that seen with corticosteroids.[9,10] The effectiveness of this therapeutic modality in the treatment of patients with osteoarthritis may be related to suppression of the secondary inflammatory response commonly seen in the synovium of patients with this disorder.

Overall, intra-articular steroid therapy is well-accepted as a local adjunct of temporary benefit in the treatment of a variety of rheumatic diseases.[11]

In addition to the general indications outlined above, this therapeutic procedure is valuable in several other clinical situations. It is useful as adjunct therapy while awaiting a response to recently-initiated slow-acting anti-rheumatic remittive drugs such as antimalarials, gold, or D-penicillamine. Physical therapy and rehabilitation may be made more effective by its use in reducing acute or subacute inflammation. Similarly, this procedure is effective in diminishing joint pain and increasing patient cooperation when orthopedic procedures such as serial casting are utilized.

Local steroid injection therapy is not without hazard.[11,12] Corticosteroids have a direct deleterious effect on cartilage.[13-15] Cystic degeneration of hyaline articular cartilage[13] and suppression of proteoglycan[14,15] and collagen[15] synthesis have been described in experimental animals following its use. In addition, the chance for joint destruction is enhanced when pain relief promotes joint overuse; too frequent use may actually promote joint deterioration. Repeated intra-articular corticosteroid injections have resulted in clinical and radiologic findings similar to those seen in neuropathic (Charcot) joints.[16,17] Joint infection is a serious complication that fortunately is uncommon when appropriate aseptic technique is utilized. Other complications are usually minimal. Occasionally local joint inflammation results when the crystalline steroid in suspension causes a crystal-induced synovitis. Some patients experience several days of weakness and malaise. An occasional patient may complain of increased warmth and flushing of the skin. Urticarial reactions are probably caused by allergy to components of the suspending vehicle. Local subcutaneous and peri-articular soft tissue atrophy and depigmentation may occur.[18] Menstrual irregularity and breast tenderness can be noted in women. Joint capsule calcification has been described with use of larger than usual injections of steroid into finger joints.[19] Many of these calcifications resolved after two years' follow-up. Pituitary-adrenal suppression with decreased resistance to stress such as occurs with operative procedures may be seen, particularly if this modality is utilized for simultaneous injection of multiple joints, or if its use is repeated over short-term intervals.[20]

Other complications may be related to local anesthetics used in the injection mixture. Accidental intravenous injection of these agents may produce severe central nervous system or cardiovascular reactions. Central nervous system side-effects include dizziness, visual complaints, slurred speech and convulsions. Cardiovascular responses such as bradycardia, hypotension and cardiorespiratory collapse have been described. Immediate vaso-vagal reactions in patients with vasomotor instability are not uncommon.

As noted, a strict aseptic technique is required to avoid infection. Excess hair should be removed. Cleansing of the injection site with a germicidal

Figure 21-1. Materials for use in intra-articular joint injections.

soap such as hexachlorophene is followed by copious cleansing with alcohol and the application of tincture of iodine. The latter is allowed to dry for several minutes. Alternatively, one may use Betadine or Amphyl. Gloves and sterile drapes are usually not necessary if the procedure is performed by a physician experienced in injection technique. The area to be injected should not be touched after cleansing, except with alcohol sponges. All necessary materials should be available prior to beginning the injection (Fig. 21-1). Disposable syringes and needles are valuable to avoid transmission of infectious agents. A 20-gauge needle is usually satisfactory for larger joints; a 25- or 26-gauge needle is used for small joints. An 18-gauge needle may be required if the synovial fluid is especially viscous. One percent lidocaine is used for local anesthesia and for mixing with the local steroid for injection. Use of anesthetic preparations containing epinephrine should be avoided. In patients with a history of allergy to local anesthetic agents, ethyl chloride spray may be used for surface anesthesia and the steroid may be diluted in sterile normal saline.

Contraindications to corticosteroid therapy should be kept in mind before using it. Local infection in or around the joint is an absolute contraindication. It is inadvisable to use local steroid therapy to treat acute disease that involves a large number of joints; it usually does not provide adequate relief and often only complicates the therapeutic program. Local steroid therapy should be avoided in severely damaged joints that are the site of little or no active inflammatory disease. It should be used with caution, if at all, in areas of fracture because it may impede healing.

Almost all diarthrodial joints may be approached for injection. Injection into some of these joints is difficult and intra-articular therapy should be left to the more experienced rheumatologist or orthopedist. On the other hand, injection into certain commonly involved joints can be accomplished without much difficulty or hazard. Knowledge and experience in this form of therapy adds a most useful procedure to the armamentarium of the physician treating arthritis.

The specific technique for intra-articular injection varies somewhat with the joint involved. If feasible, synovial fluid should first be aspirated to provide fluid for analysis and to lessen joint swelling and distension. However, a small amount of fluid should be allowed to remain to lessen the risk of dislodging the needle from the joint space before the injection itself is completed. In addition, a small amount of fluid allows better diffusion of the therapeutic agent throughout the joint. The amount of steroid injected varies with the agent used and the size of the joint to be treated (see Table 21-1). Preparations containing acetate, acetonide or hexacetonide are long-acting; the therapeutic effect begins after 24 to 48 hours and lasts for weeks to months. Phosphate derivatives have a rapid onset of action and a therapeutic effect lasting 24 to 48 hours. Some preparations contain a combination of short- and long-acting components so that the effect begins rapidly followed by prolonged improvement. Only preparations that are hydrocortisone derivatives are effective for intra-articular use. Unless contraindicated, 1% lidocaine, in a volume equal to the steroid used, is mixed and injected at the same time. This allows better dispersion of the steroid and also allows immediate evaluation of the success of the injection. Specific techniques for injection into commonly treated joints follow.

Interphalangeal and Metacarpophalangeal (MCP) Joints. A small needle is used to avoid unnecessary injury. Usually a 25- or 26-gauge needle is satisfactory. The needle is inserted from a medial or lateral approach on the dorsal aspect of the hand (Fig. 21-2). Although the joint can often be entered readily, it may be possible to inject only a small amount of the steroid into the joint. Periarticular infiltration is added for maximal benefit.

First Carpometacarpal (CMP) Joint. The needle for injection is placed at the dorsal-radial aspect of the hand in the area of the first CMP joint. Once again, it may be difficult to inject the total amount of medication within the joint. Suitable relief can usually be obtained by periarticular injection of some of the agent as well.

Wrist. Injection into the wrist is best performed from a dorsal approach. The needle is directed perpendicularly into the depression normally present at the radiocarpal indentation. The radial styloid is a helpful marker to

TABLE 21-1. Average Doses of Steroid Preparations Used in Local Therapy of Musculoskeletal Disorders

Corticosteroid Preparations (Strength of Preparation in mg/ml)	Average Recommended Doses in ml								
	Shoulders, Knees, Ankles	Wrists, Elbows	PIP, MCP, First CMP, MTP*	Tendinitis, Bursitis	Epicondylitis	Costo-chondritis	Trigger areas	Ganglion	Carpal tunnel
Long-acting									
Dexamethasone acetate 8 mg/ml	1.0–1.5	1.0–1.2	0.3–0.4	1.0–1.2	0.6–1.0	0.3–0.5	0.3–0.5	0.3–0.5	1.0–1.2
Hydrocortisone acetate 25 mg/ml	0.6–1.5	0.6–1.0	0.2–0.4	0.6–1.0	0.6–0.8	0.3–0.4	0.3–0.4	0.4	0.6–1.0
Methylprednisolone acetate 40 mg/ml	0.5–0.75	0.4–0.6	0.1–0.25	0.4–0.5	0.3–0.5	0.2–0.3	0.2–0.3	0.2–0.3	0.4
Prednisolone tertiary butylacetate† 20 mg/ml	1.0–1.2	1.0	0.4–0.5	0.5–1.2	0.5	0.3–0.4	0.3–0.4	0.5	0.6–0.8

Triamcinolone diacetate 40 mg/ml	0.4–0.6	0.4–0.5	0.15	0.4–0.5	0.3	0.2–0.25	0.2–0.25	0.2–0.25	0.4
Triamcinolone acetonide 10 mg/ml	1.0–2.0	1.0	0.3–0.5	1.0–2.0	0.6–1.0	0.3–0.5	0.5–0.6	0.5–0.6	1.0–1.2
Triamcinolone hexacetonide† 20 mg/ml	0.5–1.0	0.5–0.75	0.2–0.3	0.5–1.0	0.3–0.4	0.2–0.3	0.2–0.3	0.2–0.3	0.5–0.75
Short- and long-acting									
Betamethasone sodium phosphate 3 mg/ml plus Betamethasone acetate 3 mg/ml	1.0	0.5–1.0	0.25–0.5	0.5–0.75	0.5	0.2–0.3	0.2–0.3	0.3	0.5–0.75
Short-acting									
Dexamethasone sodium phosphate 4 mg/ml	0.5–0.75	0.5–0.6	0.2–0.25	0.25–0.6	0.3–0.4	0.2–0.3	0.3	0.25–0.3	0.5–0.6

*PIP = proximal interphalangeal joint; MCP = metacarpophalangeal joint; CMP = carpometacarpophalangeal joint; MTP = metatarsophalangeal joint

†Prednisolone tertiary butylacetate, and triamcinolone hexacetonide are somewhat longer lasting in effect than their respective acetate and acetonide derivatives.

Figure 21-2. Injection into proximal interphalangeal joint. (Courtesy, Dr. A. Mackenzie)

Figure 21-3. Injection into lateral aspect of elbow joint. (Courtesy, Dr. A. Mackenzie)

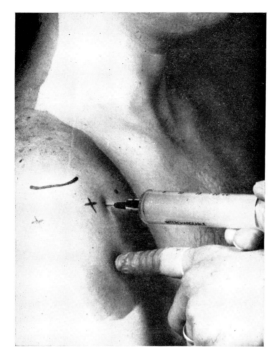

Figure 21-4.   Injection into shoulder joint, anterior approach. (Courtesy, Dr. A. Mackenzie)

Figure 21-5.   Injection into shoulder joint, lateral approach, between acromion process of the scapula and head of humerus.

determine the level for needle insertion. The needle is inserted for a distance of 1 to 2 cm for injection.

Elbow. Injection into the elbow may be difficult unless moderate swelling is present. A lateral approach is generally recommended to avoid injury to the ulnar nerve. With the elbow held at a 90° angle, the needle is inserted just below the lateral epicondyle and outside the olecranon process (Fig. 21-3).

Shoulder. Intra-articular injection of the shoulder joint may be performed from either an anterior or lateral approach. In the anterior approach, the needle is inserted just medial to the head of the humerus below the tip of the coracoid process (Fig. 21-4). In the lateral approach, the needle is inserted between the acromion process of the scapula and the humeral head (Fig. 21-5). Swelling of the shoulder joint usually protrudes anteriorly and the anterior approach is the simpler technique.

Knee. Aspiration and injection into the knee is usually easy when the knee is inflamed and contains increased joint fluid. Injection into osteoarthritic knees is somewhat more difficult because they usually contain little or no excess fluid, and osteophytic spurs that distort the joint margins make it difficult to insert the needle. Injection is usually performed with the patient lying on his back with the knees fully extended. If possible, injection should be made into the suprapatellar pouch to avoid inserting the needle between closely apposing cartilaginous surfaces. The superior tip of the patella is identified and used as a landmark for injection. The injection is made into either the medial or the lateral aspect of the knee. The lateral aspect is usually preferred because it can be approached more conveniently.

Figure 21-6.   Lateral approach for injection, left knee. Note relationship of needle to outline of patella above. (Courtesy, Dr. A. Mackenzie)

The needle is inserted ¾ to 1 inch below the superior aspect of the patella and is directed slightly cephalad to enter the suprapatellar pouch (Fig. 21-6). If no fluid is obtained, the needle is redirected between the posterior surface of the patella and the patellar groove of the femur. An alternative approach may be considered in patients in whom deformity prevents complete knee extension. In these cases, aspiration and injection are accomplished by inserting the needle in an anteroposterior direction lateral or medial to the inferior patellar tendon (Fig. 21-7). The needle passes through the fat pad into the knee joint space between the condyles of the femur and the tibial plateaus.

For popliteal cysts of the knee, aspiration and injection may be performed directly through a posterior approach. Great care must be taken to avoid the popliteal artery. Small popliteal cysts usually respond to intra-articular injection directly into the knee; direct injection into the cyst usually is not required.

Ankle. Intra-articular therapy of the ankle may be difficult if swelling is not great. However, the technique can usually be mastered with experience. The anteromedial approach is the most common. The needle is directed horizontally toward the tibiotalar articulation just above and lateral to the medial malleolus and medial to the extensor hallucis longus tendon (Fig.

Figure 21-7. Anterior approach for knee injection. (Courtesy, Dr. A. Mackenzie)

Figure 21-8. Injection into ankle. (Courtesy, Dr. A. Mackenzie)

21-8). It is well to mark the location of the dorsalis pedis artery so that it can be avoided during injection. Although this artery is usually located lateral to the extensor pollicis longus tendon, its course may be aberrant in some patients. Abrupt entrance of the needle through the capsule and into the joint is usually less obvious as compared to the knee. When joint swelling is greatest laterally, an anterolateral approach should be utilized: the needle is directed toward the tibiotalar articulation from a point 1 to 2 cm medial to the lateral malleolus.

Metatarsophalangeal (MTP) Joints. The MTP joints are readily accessible to local injection therapy. Injection is made from a dorsal or ventral approach, depending on the site of maximal pain and swelling. A 25- or 26-gauge needle is advisable. When direct injection into the joint is difficult or incomplete, injection into surrounding periarticular tissues usually provides effective symptomatic relief.

Immunosuppressive Agents

Intra-articular therapy with alkylating agents, such as nitrogen mustard or triethylenethiophosphoramide (Thio-tepa)[21] has been used to produce a prolonged anti-inflammatory effect on the synovitis of rheumatoid arthritis. Unfortunately, results have been variable and inconsistent. Nitrogen mustard is very irritating to periarticular soft tissues if not injected directly into the joint. Thio-tepa has minimal hazard in this regard. Either agent has potential hazard for bone marrow suppression if used in sufficiently large dosage, a complication more likely to be associated with simultaneous multiple joint injections. These agents, of questionable efficacy and potential risk, are now rarely utilized any longer for suppression of inflammation via the intra-articular route.

Radioactive Agents

Long-term suppression of synovial inflammation has been described with the intra-articular use of radioactive substances such as colloidal [198]Au,[22] colloidal ^{32}P and [90]Yttrium.[23-25] This therapeutic approach, so-called chemical synovectomy, has been suggested as an alternative to surgical synovectomy. Advantages include decreased costs of hospitalization and the ability to follow-up with surgical synovectomy in the event of failure. Therapeutic benefits must be weighed against known and theoretic hazards associated with the use of radioactive agents.[26,27] Radiation emitted by injected particles may irradiate not only the targeted synovium, but also other tissues such as cartilage, regional and distant lymph nodes, other organs of the reticuloendothelial system including the bone marrow, and organs of reproduction. Biological hazards of potential concern include chromosomal abnormalities,[26] leukemia and induction of solid neoplasms.[27] [90]Yttrium is somewhat preferable to the other agents because it drains less to regional lymph nodes and systemic areas.[24,25]

Extra-articular spread of radiation can be lessened by careful attention to injection technique. Except in the case of the knee, where needle position can usually be readily ascertained clinically, roentgen ray contrast medium should be used to check the position of the needle in the joint. Back-flow of radioisotope through the skin and underlying tissues can be avoided by using a three-way system with flushing of the needle with saline prior to removal. The joint to be treated should be injected with intra-articular corticosteroids at an interval of at least two days prior to intra-articular isotope.[28] Use of prior local steroid lessens reactive inflammation to the colloidal agent; more importantly, the short range beta-emission of the colloidal agent is more effective when the effusion has been lessened and the synovium is less thickly inflamed, and leakage of isotope is significantly reduced. Immobilization of the treated joint for 24 hours or more following isotope injection further reduces the amount of radioactivity which may escape.[29]

The use of these agents should be avoided in women of childbearing age and also in men who anticipate having more children. Their use may be considered in patients with monoarticular arthritis or in patients who have one joint out of pace with the clinical progress.

EXTRA-ARTICULAR THERAPY

Local therapy is frequently used in the treatment of disorders involving periarticular soft tissues. Although use of local anesthetics without corticosteroids for this purpose has been advocated by some,[30,31] injection mixtures of a corticosteroid combined with local anesthetic are more commonly employed. The added corticosteroid suspension provides longer lasting benefits, and avoids the need for larger volumes and more frequent injections required when local anesthetics alone are used. Risks associated with use of local anesthetics are accordingly appreciably lessened.

The results obtained with extra-articular injections of corticosteroid/anesthetic mixtures are often dramatic and associated with minimal hazard. The steroid to be injected is usually mixed with 1% lidocaine in a volume one to two times that of the steroid suspension. This technique allows treatment of a wider area of involvement and also lessens the deleterious effect of high concentration of steroid on the tissue. The amount of steroid used varies with the specific agent utilized and the site to be injected (see Table 21-1).

Complications associated with these procedures are similar to those described earlier in this chapter for intra-articular injections. Additional hazards relate to the specific site at which the injection is given. For example, pneumothorax may be a complication of soft tissue injections made into the anterior or posterior chest wall area. Intravascular injection should be carefully avoided when injections are made into sites near large arteries such as at the posterior aspect of the knee, volar aspect of the elbow or in the region of the inguinal ligament. Local atrophy of the skin or depigmentation is more commonly seen than with deep intra-articular injections. Injection of steroid into an inflamed tendon sheath may result in subsequent tendon rupture, especially if the preparation is injected directly into the body of the tendon itself.[32,33] Specific techniques of injection for various disorders follow.

Shoulder area. Local steroids are therapeutically beneficial for shoulder area bursitis, supraspinatus tendinitis, periarthritis, tenosynovitis of the long head of the biceps, and rotator cuff tears. The injection should be made into the points of maximal tenderness. Inflamed subacromial and subdeltoid bursae are injected directly, aiming the needle into the areas of maximal tenderness. For treatment of supraspinatus tendinitis, the needle is inserted just at the anterior aspect of the greater tuberosity of the shoulder. Approximately one-third of the medication is placed at this point. The needle is then redirected posteriorly and anteriorly, where the remainder of the agent is injected. A successful injection is often attended by almost immediate relief of pain and increased range of shoulder motion. Specific sites of inflammation may be difficult to localize and a general periarthritis may be present; local steroid injections into sites similar to those described for supraspinatus tendinitis frequently give relief. Injection into the sheath of the long head of the biceps is made immediately over the tendon at the anterior aspect of the shoulder as it passes through the bicipital groove of the humerus. Approximately one third of the medication is inserted at the site of maximal tenderness. The needle is then redirected in a superior and inferior direction to complete the injection. Small rotator cuff tears may be associated with pain and secondary inflammation. Local steroids injected into the site of pathology provide symptomatic relief.

Several areas of inflammation may be present in the same patient; injection should be made into all areas for maximal success. It is well to caution the patient to avoid overexerting the joint when injections have been made into areas of tendinitis, since steroid-induced atrophy may decrease the tensile strength of the tendon and predispose it to rupture. This complication is uncommon but does occur, especially in athletes.

Epicondylitis of the Elbow. Inflammation in the area of tendon origins at the lateral or medial epicondyle of the elbow secondary to chronic stress is common. Local injections are first made into the site of maximal tenderness of the involved epicondyle. The needle is then redirected into several areas peripheral to the site of maximal tenderness in order to achieve an effective result.

Tendinitis of the Fingers. Tenosynovitis of the flexor tendons of the hands is common and produces the so-called "trigger finger" (see Chapter 15). Although the patient often complains that the finger itself is the site of difficulty, the pathologic changes are usually located in the area of the distal palmar crease. Local steroids should be injected into this latter area at the site of maximal tenderness, crepitus or nodule formation.

Stenosing Tenosynovitis at the Wrist (DeQuervain's Disease). Inflammation of the abductor pollicis longus and extensor pollicis brevis tendons is usually secondary to chronic trauma. Symptoms include pain in the area of the radial styloid and weakness of grip. Local steroid injection is made directly into the tendon sheath at the site of maximal tenderness, followed by injection along the tendon sheath in a proximal and distal direction.

Olecranon Bursitis. Inflammation and swelling of the olecranon bursa occurs in various connective tissue diseases, in gout and following nonspecific trauma. Treatment includes direct aspiration of the bursa followed by the local introduction of steroids.

Greater Trochanteric Bursitis. Inflammation of the bursa over the greater trochanter of the hip is a common cause of pain in this area. The patient complains of tenderness in a localized region and symptoms are accentuated by pressure when the patient is lying on the involved side. Injection therapy is simple and effective. The needle is placed directly into the area of maximal tenderness and local steroid with lidocaine is introduced. Steroid should also be injected circumferentially to the site of maximal tenderness.

Anserine Bursitis and Medial Collateral Ligament Inflammation at the Knee. Bursitis of the anserine bursa at the medial aspect of the knee is common. Tenderness is noted at the edge of the medial tibial plateau; steroid injection is made directly into the area of tenderness just beneath the medial collateral ligament. Inflammation of the medial collateral ligament itself may produce similar symptoms; steroid injection is directed somewhat more superficially into the area of ligamentous inflammation.

Ischial Tuberosity Bursitis. Pain and tenderness at the base of the buttock are symptoms of ischial tuberosity bursitis. Pain is aggravated by sitting. Relief is usually obtained with local steroid injection over the bony prominence of the ischial tuberosity.

Bursitis at the Bunion Joint. Acute inflammation of the bursa at the medial aspect of the first metatarsophalangeal joint may simulate symptoms of acute gout or rheumatoid arthritis. Treatment involves aspiration of fluid followed by injection of local steroid into the bursal sac.

Trigger Areas of Spasm. Tender areas of muscle spasm frequently can be palpated in patients with localized or diffuse primary fibrositis. Relief of symptoms with local steroid injection is often good to excellent. Steroid with lidocaine is injected directly into the site of maximal tenderness. Further injections are made circumferentially to the site of maximal pain. Injections may be required in several trigger areas at the same time in order to obtain maximal relief.

Costochondritis and Tietze's Syndrome. Inflammation of the costal cartilages may cause severe, annoying chest pain. Tenderness is usually localized to specific areas of involvement. Localized swelling due to inflammation of one or more costal cartilages is seen in patients with Tietze's syndrome. Local injections of steroid with lidocaine provide effective relief. A 20- or 22-gauge needle is directed at a 45° angle down to the rib at the site of maximal tenderness or swelling. A perpendicular approach is hazardous because injection deep to the rib is more likely if the patient moves inappropriately. Although injection close to the rib surface is desirable, good results are usually obtained even with more superficial injections, since the steroid-lidocaine suspension diffuses sufficiently for an effective result. Repeat injections at intervals of days or weeks may be required for permanent relief. As noted, great care must be taken to avoid visceral structures deep to the rib cage.

Ganglia. A ganglion is a cystic swelling in the area of a tendon sheath or joint capsule, from which structures they appear to be derived. They occur most commonly on the dorsum of the wrist but may be seen elsewhere. Most ganglia are asymptomatic but tenderness may be bothersome. Spontaneous disappearance is common. Specific treatment may be required for relief of tenderness or for cosmetic reasons. Most cases respond to aspiration of the cyst contents through a large-bore needle followed by injection of local steroid.

Figure 21-9.   Injection for carpal tunnel syndrome. (Courtesy, Dr. A. Mackenzie)

Carpal Tunnel Syndrome. Compression of the median nerve may be secondary to inflammatory or infiltrative diseases at the wrist. Temporary relief usually can be obtained by local steroid injection. The landmarks for injection include the palmaris longus tendon medially and the flexor carpi radialis tendon laterally. The median nerve runs in the groove between these two tendons or lies just under the palmaris longus. Injection is made over the median nerve at the wrist, just proximal to the palm (Fig. 21-9). A 22-gauge needle is usually satisfactory and is less likely to cause inadvertent damage than larger needles. One and a half to 2 ml of steroid-lidocaine mixture is a satisfactory volume for injection. The initial injection is made at a 45° angle directed away from the palm, parallel and superficial to the nerve. The remainder of the material for injection is then placed distally under the transverse carpal ligament after appropriate redirection of the needle. The needle should be withdrawn immediately if radiation of nerve pain is noted, to avoid injection into the nerve itself. Proper injection is often, but not always, associated with a lidocaine-induced nerve block in the distribution of the median nerve.

Tarsal Tunnel Syndrome. This syndrome represents an entrapment neuropathy of the posterior tibial nerve as it passes through the tunnel beneath the flexor retinaculum on the medial side of the ankle. Injection is made inferior and posterior to the medial malleolus in a fan-like manner. The posterior tibial artery which courses through the same tunnel should be identified by palpation prior to injection, and intravascular injection avoided.

REFERENCES

1. Hollander, J. L., Jessar, R. A. and Brown, E. M. Jr.: Intra-synovial corticosteroid therapy: a decade of use. Bull Rheum Dis 11:329, 1961.

2. Fitzgerald, R. H.: Intrasynovial injection of steroids: uses and abuses. Mayo Clinic Proc 51:655, 1976.
3. Jessar, R. A., Ganzell, M. A. and Ragan, C.: The action of hydrocortisone in synovial inflammation. J Clin Invest 32:480, 1953.
4. Weissman, G. and Thomas, L.: Studies on lysosomes. II. The effect of cortisone on the release of acid hydrolases from a large granule fraction of rabbit liver induced by an excess of vitamin A. J Clin Invest 42:661, 1963.
5. Persellin, R. H. and Kee, L. C.: Effects of steroid hormones on human polymorphonuclear leukocyte lysosomes. J Clin Invest 54:919, 1974.
6. Zuckner, J., Machek, O. and Ahern, A. N.: Hydrocortisone tertiary-butylacetate for intra-articular therapy in rheumatic diseases. Ann Rheum Dis 15:258, 1956.
7. Wright, V., Chandler, G. N., Morison, R. A. H. et al.: Intra-articular therapy in osteo-arthritis. Ann Rheum Dis 19:257, 1960.
8. Hollander, J. A.: Intrasynovial corticosteroid therapy in arthritis. Maryland Med J 19(3):62, 1970.
9. Traut, E. F.: Procaine and procaine amide hydrochloride in skeletal pain. JAMA 150:785, 1952.
10. Miller, J. H., White, J. and Norton, T. H.: The value of intra-articular injections of osteoarthritis of the knee. J Bone Joint Surg 40B:636, 1958.
11. Gray, R. G., Tenenbaum, J. and Gottlieb, N. L.: Local corticosteroid injection treatment in rheumatic disorders. Semin Arthritis Rheum 4:231, 1981.
12. Gottlieb, N. L. and Risken, W. G.: Complications of local corticosteroid injections. JAMA 243:1547, 1980.
13. Moskowitz, R. W. et al.: Experimentally induced corticosteroid arthropathy. Arthritis Rheum 13:236, 1970.
14. Mankin, J. H. and Conger, K. A.: The acute effects of intra-articular hydrocortisone on articular cartilage in rabbits. J Bone Joint Surg 48A:1383, 1966.
15. Behrens, F., Shepard, N. and Mitchell, N.: Alteration of rabbit articular cartilage by intra-articular injections of glucocorticoids. J Bone Joint Surg 57A:70, 1975.
16. Steinberg, C. L., Duthie, R. B. and Piva, A. E.: Charcot-like arthropathy following intra-articular hydrocortisone. JAMA 181:851, 1962.
17. Alarcon-Segovia, D. and Ward, L. E.: Charcot-like arthropathy in rheumatoid arthritis. Consequence of overuse of a joint repeatedly injected with hydrocortisone. JAMA 193:1052, 1965.
18. Cassidy, J. T. and Bole, G. G.: Cutaneous atrophy secondary to intra-articular corticosteroid administration. Ann Int Med 65:1008, 1966.
19. McCarty, D. J.: Treatment of rheumatoid joint inflammation with triamcinolone hexacetonide. Arthritis Rheum 15:157, 1972.
20. Koehler, B. E., Urowitz, M. B. and Kellinger, D. W.: The systemic effects of intra-articular corticosteroid. J Rheumatol 1:117, 1974.
21. Ellison, R. W. and Flatt, A. E.: Intra-articular Thiotepa in rheumatoid disease. Arthritis Rheum 14:212, 1971.
22. Ansell, B. M. et al.: Evaluation of intra-articular colloidal gold [198]Au in the treatment of persistent knee effusions. Ann Rheum Dis 22:435, 1963.
23. Bridgman, J. F., Bruckner, F. and Bleehan, N. M.: Radioactive Yttrium in the treatment of rheumatoid knee effusions. Ann Rheum Dis 30:180, 1971.
24. Gumpel, J. N.: Clinical application and investigation of radioactive colloids in the treatment of arthritis. Review of published and personal results. Ann Rheum Dis 32(Suppl):29, 1973.
25. Gumpel, J. N., Farran, H. E. A. and Williams, E. D.: Use of Yttrium-90 in persistent synovitis of the knee. II. Direct comparison of Yttrium colloid resins and Yttrium citrate. Ann Rheum Dis 33:126, 1974.
26. Stevenson, A. C.: Biological effects of radiation. Ann Rheum Dis 32(Suppl):19, 1973.
27. Dolphin, G. W.: Biological hazards of radiation. Ann Rheum Dis 32(Suppl):23, 1973.
28. Goode, J. D. and Howey, E.: Effect of premedication with intra-articular hydro-

cortisone on the retention of [198]Au in the knee joint in rheumatoid arthritis. Ann Rheum Dis 32(Suppl):43, 1973.
29. Roberts, S. D. and Gillespie, P. J.: Effect of immobilization on retention of [90]Y. Ann Rheum Dis 32(Suppl):46, 1973.
30. Steinbrocker, O. and Neustadt, D. H.: Aspiration and Injection Therapy in Musculoskeletal Disorders. New York, Harper and Row, 1972.
31. Swezey, R. L.: Chapter 36, Rehabilitation aspects in arthritis. In McCarty, D. J. (editor): Arthritis and Allied Conditions, 9th Ed. Philadelphia, Lea & Febiger, 1979.
32. Wrenn, R. N., Goldner, J. L. and Markee, J. L.: An experimental study of the effect of cortisone on the healing process and tensile strength of tendons. J Bone Joint Surg 36A:588, 1964.
33. Ismail, A. N., Balakrishnan, R. and Rajakumar, M. K.: Rupture of patella ligament after steroid infiltration: report of a case. J Bone Joint Surg 51B:503, 1969.

CHAPTER 22

STEROID MANAGEMENT IN STRESS SITUATIONS

Clinical manifestations of adrenal insufficiency may develop during stress situations in patients who are receiving or who have received corticosteroid therapy. Among the more common situations in which this complication arises are surgical procedures, obstetric delivery and intercurrent infection. The availability of rapidly-acting steroid preparations allows effective management of this untoward reaction. On the other hand, prevention of this complication by appropriate prophylactic supplementation of steroids is desirable when possible.

Several different methods of steroid supplementation can be utilized. Effective use depends upon a working knowledge of the pharmacology of available agents. The rapidity and duration of clinical action varies not only with the chemical nature of the steroid used, but also with the route of administration.[1-6] Although efforts have been made to correlate half-life values of various corticosteroids in the circulation, the relationships between circulating half-life and potency and duration of action are imprecise. Evaluations of the extent and duration of hypothalamic-pituitary-adrenal (HPA) suppression following steroid therapy are based on clinical observations of adrenal crisis developing in response to stress, and on experimental studies utilizing measurements of adrenal and pituitary function.[7-14] The latter experimental investigations utilize measurements such as plasma cortisol and urinary 17-hydroxycorticoids with and without adrenal stimulation, response to insulin-induced hypoglycemia, and HPA response to metyrapone administration. Adrenal gland atrophy and suppression of adrenal response have been described as soon as days to several weeks following steroid administration.[7-9] Recovery of function may require as long as 9 to 12 months following cessation of therapy depending on dose and duration of steroid use.[11-13] Pituitary-adrenal suppression is less likely to occur in patients given steroid therapy on an alternate day basis as compared to drug administration in daily divided doses.[15] Similarly, daily single dose therapy appears to reduce the likelihood of developing

suppression if the agent is given in the morning to simulate the normal di-
urnal steroid rhythm.[16] Long-acting steroid preparations such as dexamethasone will, however, produce HPA suppression even if administered
on an alternate day or single daily dose regimen. There is no evidence from
available data that ACTH can prevent or reverse development of steroid-
induced HPA suppression.[13]

Despite clinical and experimental observations, data do not always per-
mit an accurate estimate of the duration of steroid treatment which will
dispose a patient to shock under the stress of surgery or severe illness. If
hypothalamic-pituitary-adrenal suppression is suspected, one may do
ACTH or metyrapone testing, or one may treat the patient as though adrenal cortical insufficiency is present. Although there is usually a steady
improvement in HPA responsiveness from the time steroid therapy is
stopped, a period of 9 to 12 months or longer may be required to achieve
normal responses, as noted.

The following programs represent general methods of management of
stress situations in patients with a history of steroid therapy; other procedures can be safely substituted if based on knowledgeable application of
the various steroid agents available for therapeutic use.

SURGICAL STRESS

Prophylactic steroid supplementation is indicated prior to surgery in patients who are presently receiving corticosteroids. Steroid supplementation
must also be considered in patients who have received corticosteroids in a
potentially suppressive dose prior to surgery. Exact guidelines are difficult
to specify since there are, as noted, differences of opinion as to the minimum time and dosage required for adrenal suppression, and the time period
required for recovery of the hypothalamic-pituitary-adrenal axis.[17] This is
further complicated by gaps between clinical and biochemical evidence of
HPA recovery. In general, prednisone 15 to 20 mg/day, or its equivalent,
given on a daily divided dose schedule for 10 to 14 days or more should
be considered suppressive. Routine steroid supplementation for such patients is usually recommended if steroids have been administered in the 3-
month interval prior to surgery. Routine supplementation may also be
utilized in patients who have received steroids at intervals of 3 to 12 months
prior to surgery if the dose and duration of administration suggest possible
continued suppression. Alternatively, in the latter group of patients, the
need for supplementation may be evaluated by rapid adrenal stimulation
studies.[18,19] As one such example, the patient is given 250 μg of synthetic
ACTH (cosyntropin) intramuscularly and a plasma cortisol level is obtained 30 to 60 minutes later. A cortisol level greater than 20 μg/100 ml
with a minimum increment of 6 μg/100 ml over baseline, or a two-fold
response is considered normal. On a practical basis, when steroids have

been administered many months prior to surgery, it is reasonable to withhold supplementation and observe the patient closely over the stress period.

Hypothalamic-pituitary-adrenal (HPA) axis suppression is more likely to occur for prolonged periods in patients administered steroids in high doses for an extended time. Accordingly, both dose and duration of steroid therapy should be taken into account in assessing whether or not a patient may have impaired adrenal response when seen. In patients who have received steroid therapy on an alternate day or single daily dose morning schedule, prophylactic therapy may not be required, but close observation of the patient for possible HPA suppression is prudent. Steroids administered intermittently by intramuscular or intra-articular routes should also be considered as potentially suppressive when given frequently or in high doses. Patients with residual evidence of hypercortisonism may be susceptible to adrenal insufficiency, regardless of the interval since prior steroid administration.

These are only general guidelines to which patients should be considered for steroid supplementation at the time of surgical stress. The final decision regarding use of such therapy also involves certain variables, such as the extent of the planned surgical procedure and contraindications to steroid use. Although relatively few patients receiving prior low-dose steroids for short intervals are likely to develop adrenal insufficiency under stress, it is generally safer to err in the direction of overuse of supplementation. Complications are minimal and the support against unanticipated stress is reassuring.

As noted, various techniques for steroid supplementation of patients in stress situations can be utilized, based on the pharmacodynamics of the steroid agents used. The following recommendations represent examples of steroid supplementation schedules.

Major Surgery

In patients for whom extensive, prolonged major surgery is planned, cortisone acetate, 100 mg IM, may be administered every 12 hours beginning 48 hours before surgery. Cortisone acetate administered intramuscularly achieves therapeutic effectiveness only after 18 to 24 hours; this program allows a reasonable period to attain an effective parenteral depot of the drug. An intravenous infusion of hydrocortisone sodium succinate, 100 mg per liter, may be added at the time of surgery, but it usually is not necessary. However, it should routinely be administered when the full 48-hour administration of intramuscular cortisone acetate has not been carried out. Postoperatively, cortisone acetate, 100 mg IM, is given the night of surgery. On the first postoperative day, 100 to 150 mg of cortisone acetate IM is administered; on day two, 75 mg; and on day three, 25 mg. The original preoperative oral dose of steroids is re-instituted when the patient is able to tolerate oral medications. When oral intake is delayed, parenteral administration of steroids in an equivalent daily dose is continued until the oral preparation can be substituted.

More rapid initiation of steroid supplementation may be accomplished by utilizing steroid preparations which have an accelerated onset of action, such as dexamethasone sodium phosphate, prednisolone sodium phosphate, or methylprednisolone sodium succinate. These agents have a rapid onset of action when given by either the intramuscular or intravenous route, with effective levels achieved in 30 to 60 minutes or less. In contrast to cortisone acetate, the use of these agents allows preparation of the patient for surgery without need for injections beginning two days prior, making their use advantageous for emergency surgery preparation as well as routine use. Dexamethasone sodium phosphate is recommended in a dose of 4 mg IM on call to the operating room, followed by IM administration every 12 hours on the day of surgery. Alternatively, prednisolone sodium phosphate may be administered in a dose of 40 mg IM on call to the operating room, and every eight hours on the day of surgery. The dose is reduced to 20 mg every eight hours on the second postoperative day. Both agents are tapered as appropriate over the subsequent postoperative course depending on the overall clinical status of the patient, and the ability to substitute oral medications. Rapid induction of steroid coverage may also be provided by intravenous "piggyback" infusion. Dexamethasone sodium phosphate is recommended in a dose of 4 mg IV every six hours. Alternative medications such as prednisolone sodium phosphate, 40 mg IV every six hours, or methylprednisolone sodium succinate, 40 mg IV every six hours may be used. Dosage reduction is carried out as indicated by patient need and operative circumstance.

Minor Surgery

Minor surgical procedures do not require extensive steroid supplementation. For short operative procedures, such as dilatation and curettage or cystoscopy, hydrocortisone sodium succinate, 100 mg IM is administered one to two hours before surgery. This dose is followed by 50 mg IM at four-hour intervals for several doses. A satisfactory alternative program is to administer the same agent intravenously, in a dose of 100 mg per liter of saline or glucose, just prior to and during surgery. The intravenous infusion is discontinued when the patient is stable and back on oral intake. Alternative preparations for use include dexamethasone sodium phosphate, prednisolone sodium phosphate or methylprednisolone sodium succinate administered by either the IM or IV route as described under major surgery. The dose may be more rapidly tapered and discontinued over the subsequent 24 hours postoperatively, depending upon the clinical status of the patient and the ability to resume oral steroid intake.

Patients undergoing dental extractions under short analgesia can be satisfactorily managed by administration of two to three times the usual oral dose of steroid several hours before extraction.

OBSTETRIC DELIVERY

Similar precautions and procedures for steroid supplementation should be considered at termination of pregnancy in patients receiving steroids for various illnesses. Although experimental studies in animals have shown some association between corticosteroid therapy and congenital abnormalities, clinical studies have demonstrated no definite hazard with respect to fetal development.[20,21] Increased doses of steroids should be utilized when indicated during the stress of normal or surgical delivery.

INTERCURRENT INFECTION

Steroid supplementation should also be considered at times of nonsurgical or obstetric stress, such as might occur in the presence of severe infection. Steroid supplementation to levels equivalent to twice the prior daily intake is adequate if the infection is mild. In the presence of severe infection, more intensive steroid supplementation may be required. Appropriate antibiotics should be utilized to treat the infectious process.

As noted earlier, the availability of steroid preparations with rapid onset of action has diminished the threat imposed by unexpected adrenal insufficiency. However, prevention of clinical adrenal insufficiency when possible is preferable to treatment of this complication. In patients in whom acute adrenal insufficiency intervenes, high doses of rapidly-acting steroid agents should be administered intravenously in whatever dosage is required to maintain corticosteroid support.

REFERENCES

1. Melby, J. C. and Silber, R. H.: Clinical pharmacology of water-soluble corticosteroid esters. Am Pract Digest Treat 12:156, 1961.
2. Melby, J. C. and St. Cyr, M.: Comparative studies on absorption and metabolic disposal of water-soluble corticosteroid esters in healthy subjects. Metabolism 10:75, 1961.
3. Buhler, D. R., Thomas, R. C., Jr. and Schlagel, C. A.: Absorption, metabolism and excretion of 6-methylprednisolone-³H, 21-acetate following oral and intramuscular administrations in the dog. Endocrinology 76:852, 1965.
4. Melby, J. C. and Dale, S. L.: Comparison of absorption, disposal and activity of soluble and repository corticosteroid esters. Clin Pharmacol Therapy 10:344, 1969.
5. Christy, N. P.: The Human Adrenal Cortex. New York, Harper & Row, 1971.
6. Cope, C. L.: Adrenal Steroids and Disease. 2nd Ed. Philadelphia, J. B. Lippincott Co., 1972.
7. Salassa, R. M., Bennett, W. A., Keating, F. R. et al.: Postoperative adrenocortical insufficiency. JAMA 152:1509, 1953.
8. Christy, N. P., Wallace, E. Z. and Jailer, J. W.: Comparative effects of predni-

sone and of cortisone in suppressing the response of the adrenal cortex to exogenous adrenal cortico-adrenocorticotropin. J Clin Endo Metab 16:1059, 1956.

9. Slaney, G. and Brooke, B. N.: Postoperative collapse due to adrenal insufficiency following cortisone therapy. Lancet 1:1167, 1957.
10. Plager, J. E. and Cushman, P., Jr.: Suppression of the pituitary-ACTH response in man by administration of ACTH or cortisol. J Clin Endo Metab 22:147, 1962.
11. Graber, A. L., Ney, R. L., Nicholson, W. E. et al.: Natural history of pituitary-adrenal recovery following long-term suppression with corticosteroids. J Clin Endo Metab 25:11, 1965.
12. Livanou, T., Ferriman, D. and James, V. H. T.: Recovery of hypothalamo-pituitary-adrenal function after corticosteroid therapy. Lancet 2:856, 1967.
13. Axelrod, L.: Glucocorticoid therapy. Medicine 55:39, 1976.
14. Nelson, A. M. and Conn, D. L.: Series on pharmacology practice: 9. Glucocorticoids in rheumatic disease. Mayo Clinic Proc 55:758, 1980.
15. Harter, J. G., Reddy, W. J. and Thorn, G. W.: Studies on an intermittent corticosteroid dosage regimen. N Eng J Med 269:591, 1963.
16. Myles, A. B., Bacon, P. A. and Daily, J. R.: Single daily dose corticosteroid treatment: effect on adrenal function and therapeutic efficacy in various diseases. Ann Rheum Dis 30:149, 1971.
17. Garber, E. K., Fan, P. T. and Bluestone, R.: Realistic guidelines of corticosteroid therapy in rheumatic disease. Sem Arth Rheum 11:231, 1981.
18. Wood, J. B., James, V. H. T., Franckland, A. W. et al: A rapid test of adrenocortical function. Lancet 1:243, 1965.
19. Kehlet, H. and Binder, C.: Value of an ACTH test in assessing hypothalamic-pituitary-adrenocortical function in glucocorticoid-treated patients. Br Med J 2:147, 1973.
20. Bongiovanni, A. M. and McPadden, A. J.: Steroids during pregnancy and possible fetal consequences. Fertil Steril 2:181, 1960.
21. Popert, A. J.: Pregnancy and adrenocortical hormones. Br Med J 1:967, 1962.

PART IV

APPENDIX

HISTORY AND PHYSICAL EXAMINATION FORMS

NAME: _____   Occupation: _____

ADDRESS: Age___ Sex___ Race___ Birthdate___

    Home: _____

    Business: _____   Referred by: _____

PHONE:

    Home: _____   Hospital #: _____

    Business: _____   Insurance: _____

    Family physician: _____

Date:

Chief Complaint:

_____

History of Present Illness:

_____

_____

_____

_____

_____

Systems Review:

General

Weight loss

Appetite

Fever, chills

Head

Eyes, ears, nose, throat

Cardiorespiratory

Gastrointestinal

Genitourinary

Menses

Bruising, bleeding

Connective tissue

Pleurisy

Hair loss

Psoriasis

Sun sensitivity

Skin rash

Dry mouth (eyes)

Canker sores

Iritis

Urethritis

Colitis

Heel pain

Back pain

Sciatica

Raynaud's

Drug allergy: _____

_____

_____

Contraceptive pills:

Past Medications (arthritis)	Response	Present medications and dose
Aspirin		
Indomethacin		
Sulindac		
Ibuprofen		
Fenoprofen		
Naproxen		
Tolmetin		
Meclofenamate		
Phenylbutazone (Oxyphenbutazone)		
Antimalarials		
Gold (I.M.)		
Auranofin		
P.O. Steroids		
I.M./I.V. Steroids		
I.A. Steroids		
Immunosuppressives		
Plasmapheresis		
Analgesics		
Other		

Past Medical History—Illness: Diabetes _____ Hypertension _____

Other _____

Surgery (where, surgeon)

Fx (Fracture):

Past roentgenograms and where done:

Rheumatic fever:

Pregnancies:

Family History:

M_____   Age_____   Illnesses_____

F _____   Age_____   Illnesses_____

Siblings: _____

Arthritis history: _____

Social History:

Home_____   Apartment_____

Lives with _____

Occupational activity _____Disability (date)_____

Tobacco _____

Alcohol _____

Physical therapy/occupational therapy _____

_____

ADL (Activities of daily living): _____

_____

Physical Examination:

Temp. _____ Pulse _____ BP_____

Ht. _____ Wt. _____ Chest expansion_____

General:

   Skin:

   Lymph:

   Head:

   EENT:

   Neck:

   Heart:

   Lungs:

   Abd:

   Pelvic:

   Rectal:

   Neurologic:

   Muscles:

   Pulses:

   Nodules:

   Tophi:

Musculoskeletal: (S=swelling, T=tenderness, L=limitation)

Cervical spine: LS spine:

	Rt.				Lt.	
S	T	L		S	T	L

Hands:

Wrists:

Elbows:

Shoulders:

TMJ (Temporomandibular):

AC (Acromioclavicular):

SC (Sternoclavicular):

Hips:

Knees:

Ankles:

Subtalar:

Feet:

Miscellaneous:

Diagnostic
    Impressions:

Proposed study and management:

Roland W. Moskowitz, M.D.

INDEX

Page numbers in *italics* indicate figures; page numbers followed by "t" indicate tables.